Monitoring for Health Hazards at Work

Fourth Edition

John W. Cherrie, BSc, PhD, FFOH
Institute of Occupational Medicine, Edinburgh, UK

Robin M. Howie, Grad Inst P, Dip Occ Hyg
Independent Consultant, Ednburgh, UK

Sean Semple, BSc, MSc, PhD
University of Aberdeen, UK

With contributions from **Adrian Watson**

D1082058

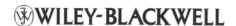

WILEY-BLACKWELL

A John Wiley & Sons, Ltd., Publication

This edition first published 2010
Previous editions published 1982, 1992, 2000 by Blackwell Publishing Ltd
© 2010 Blackwell Publishing Ltd

Blackwell Publishing was acquired by John Wiley & Sons in February 2007. Blackwell's publishing programme has been merged with Wiley's global Scientific, Technical, and Medical business to form Wiley-Blackwell.

Registered office
John Wiley & Sons Ltd, The Atrium, Southern Gate, Chichester, West Sussex, PO19 8SQ, United Kingdom

Editorial offices
9600 Garsington Road, Oxford, OX4 2DQ, United Kingdom
2121 State Avenue, Ames, Iowa 50014-8300, USA

For details of our global editorial offices, for customer services and for information about how to apply for permission to reuse the copyright material in this book please see our website at www.wiley.com/wiley-blackwell.

The right of the author to be identified as the author of this work has been asserted in accordance with the UK Copyright, Designs and Patents Act 1988.

Wiley also publishes its books in a variety of electronic formats. Some content that appears in print may not be available in electronic books.

Designations used by companies to distinguish their products are often claimed as trademarks. All brand names and product names used in this book are trade names, service marks, trademarks or registered trademarks of their respective owners. The publisher is not associated with any product or vendor mentioned in this book. This publication is designed to provide accurate and authoritative information in regard to the subject matter covered. It is sold on the understanding that the publisher is not engaged in rendering professional services. If professional advice or other expert assistance is required, the services of a competent professional should be sought.

Library of Congress Cataloging-in-Publication Data

Cherrie, J. W. (John W.)
    Monitoring for health hazards at work. – 4th ed. / John W. Cherrie, Robin M. Howie, Sean Semple ; with contributions from Adrian Watson.
        p. ; cm.
    Rev. ed. of: Monitoring for health hazards at work / Indira Ashton, Frank S. Gill. 3rd ed. 2000.
    Includes bibliographical references and index.
    ISBN 978-1-4051-5962-3 (pbk. : alk. paper)   1. Industrial toxicology.   2. Environmental monitoring.
I. Howie, Robin.   II. Semple, Sean.   III. Ashton, Indira. Monitoring for health hazards at work.
IV. Title.
    [DNLM: 1. Occupational Diseases–prevention & control.   2. Air Pollutants, Occupational–adverse effects.   3. Environmental Exposure–prevention & control.   4. Hazardous Substances–adverse effects.
5. Noise, Occupational–adverse effects.   6. Risk Assessment–methods. WA 440 C522m 2010]
    RA1229.A84 2010
    615.9′02–dc22

                                                                                                    2009048111

A catalogue record for this book is available from the British Library.

Set in 9.5/12pt Palatino by Aptara® Inc., New Delhi, India
Printed in Singapore by Ho Printing Singapore Pte Ltd

1   2010

Contents

List of Illustrations, ix

List of Instruction Sheets, xiv

Preface, xvi

Acknowledgements, xviii

Units and Abbreviations, xix

Part 1 Introduction

Chapter 1 Occupational Hygiene and Risk Assessment, 3
        1.1 Introduction, 3
        1.2 Hazard and risk, 7
        1.3 Risk assessment, 7
        1.4 The stages of a risk assessment, 8
        1.5 Who should carry out risk assessment, 12

Chapter 2 Identifying Hazards, 13
        2.1 Introduction, 13
        2.2 Identifying hazards, 13
        2.3 Example of hazard identification, 15
        2.4 Conclusions arising from a hazard assessment, 16

Chapter 3 Exposure, Exposure Routes and Biological Monitoring, 18
        3.1 Introduction, 18
        3.2 Measuring exposure, 21
        3.3 Biological monitoring, 22
        3.4 Exposure assessment: what the legislation requires, 22
        3.5 Conclusions, 23

Chapter 4 The Exposure Context, 25
        4.1 Context for measurement, 25
        4.2 Sources of hazardous substances, 25

4.3 Dispersion through the workroom, 27
4.4 Receptor, 29
4.5 Jobs and tasks, 29

Chapter 5 Why Measure?, 31
5.1 Introduction, 31
5.2 Reasons for undertaking monitoring, 31

Chapter 6 How to Carry Out a Survey, 34
6.1 Introduction, 34
6.2 Planning the survey, 34
6.3 Workplace monitoring, 35
6.4 Monitoring strategies, 37
6.5 Quality assurance and quality control, 39
6.6 Survey checklists, 41

Chapter 7 Analysis of Measurement Results, 48
7.1 Introduction, 48
7.2 Dealing with variability in measurement results, 48
7.3 Summary statistics and data presentation, 50

Chapter 8 Hygiene Reports and Records, 53
8.1 Measurement records, 53
8.2 Survey reports, 55

Part 2 Inhalation Exposure

Chapter 9 Dust and Fibrous Aerosols, 63
9.1 Introduction, 63
9.2 Airborne dust, 63
9.3 Fibres, 65
9.4 Measurement of airborne dust levels, 66
9.5 Measurement of flow rate, 73
9.6 Pumps, 74
9.7 Direct-reading aerosol monitors, 75
9.8 Calibration of a rotameter or electronic flow calibrator by using the soap-bubble method, 76
9.9 The measurement of inhalable airborne dust, 80
9.10 The measurement of airborne respirable dust by using a cyclone sampler, 83
9.11 The sampling and counting of airborne asbestos fibres, 84
9.12 The choice of filter and filter holder to suit a specific dust, fume or mist, 88
9.13 To trace the behaviour of a dust cloud by using a Tyndall beam, 89

Chapter 10 Gases and Vapours, 92
  10.1 Introduction, 92
  10.2 Collection devices, 94
  10.3 Containers, 100
  10.4 Direct-reading instruments, 101
  10.5 To measure personal exposure to solvent vapours using an adsorbent tube, 102
  10.6 Sampling for gases by using a bubbler, 104
  10.7 To measure the short-term airborne concentration of a gas by using a colorimetric detector tube, 106
  10.8 To measure a vapour concentration using a diffusive sampler, 108

Chapter 11 Bioaerosols, 111
  11.1 Introduction, 111
  11.2 Classification of microorganisms, 112
  11.3 Viruses, 112
  11.4 Bacteria, 113
  11.5 Moulds and yeasts, 114
  11.6 Allergens, 115
  11.7 Principles of containment, 115
  11.8 Handling microorganisms, 116
  11.9 Monitoring bioaerosols, 117
  11.10 Measurement of endotoxins and allergens, 120
  11.11 Interpretation of sample results, 121

Part 3 Dermal and Ingestion Exposure

Chapter 12 Dermal and Ingestion Exposure Measurement, 125
  12.1 Introduction, 125
  12.2 Occupations where dermal exposure is important, 125
  12.3 Local and systemic effects, 126
  12.4 How do we know if dermal exposure is an issue?, 127
  12.5 What do we measure?, 128
  12.6 Methods for dermal exposure measurement, 129
  12.7 Sampling strategy, 132
  12.8 Liquids and solids, 132
  12.9 Biomonitoring and modelling of dermal exposure, 134
  12.10 From exposure to uptake, 135
  12.11 Controlling dermal exposure, 136
  12.12 Inadvertent ingestion exposure, 136

Part 4 Physical Agents

Chapter 13 Noise, 143
  13.1 Introduction, 143

13.2 Pressure and magnitude of pressure variation, 143
13.3 Frequency, 144
13.4 Duration, 147
13.5 Occupational exposure limits, 147
13.6 Equipment available, 148
13.7 Sound level meters and personal noise dosimeters, 148
13.8 Personal noise dosimeters, 151
13.9 Calibration, 152
13.10 To measure workplace noise using a SLM, 153
13.11 To measure workplace noise using a PND, 155
13.12 To measure the spectrum of a continuous noise by octave band analysis, 157
13.13 To determine the degree of noise exposure and the actions to take, 159

Chapter 14 Vibration, 161
14.1 Introduction, 161
14.2 Vibration, 163
14.3 Occupational exposure limits, 165
14.4 Risk assessment, 165
14.5 Measurements and measurement equipment, 166
14.6 To measure hand–arm vibration, 167
14.7 Control of vibration, 171

Chapter 15 Heat and Cold, 173
15.1 Introduction, 173
15.2 Heat stress, 175
15.3 Measurement equipment, 176
15.4 Personal monitoring, 181
15.5 Measurement of the thermal environment, 182
15.6 Predicted Heat Strain Index, 185
15.7 Risk assessment strategy, 186
15.8 Cold, 188
15.9 To calculate the wind chill factor, 189

Chapter 16 Lighting, 191
16.1 Introduction, 191
16.2 Lighting Standards, 192
16.3 Equipment available, 193
16.4 Calibration, 193
16.5 To measure lighting, 194
16.6 Control, 197

Chapter 17 Ionising Radiation, 199
17.1 Introduction, 199
17.2 Ionising radiation, 200

17.3 Background radiation, 201
17.4 Basic concepts and quantities, 201
17.5 Types of radiation, 202
17.6 Energy, 204
17.7 Activity, 204
17.8 Radiation dose units, 205
17.9 Dose limits, 206
17.10 Derived limits, 207
17.11 Procedures to minimise occupational dose, 207
17.12 Personal dosimetry and medical surveillance, 209

Chapter 18 Non-Ionising Radiation, 216
18.1 Introduction, 216
18.2 Ultraviolet radiation, 218
18.3 Infrared radiation, 220
18.4 Microwaves and radiowaves, 220
18.5 Lasers, 222

Part 5 Assessing the Effectiveness of Control

Chapter 19 Introduction to Control, 227
19.1 Introduction, 227
19.2 Specific control measures, 228
19.3 The effectiveness of control measures, 231

Chapter 20 Ventilation, 233
20.1 Introduction, 233
20.2 Air pressure, 234
20.3 Measurement equipment, 235
20.4 Ventilation measurement records, 242
20.5 Measurement of air flow in ducts, 246
20.6 Measurement of pressure in ventilation systems, 252
20.7 To measure the face velocity on a booth or hood, 254
20.8 To measure the face velocity on a fume cupboard, 255
20.9 To measure the performance of a suction inlet, 257

Chapter 21 Personal Protective Equipment, 260
21.1 Introduction, 260
21.2 Components of an effective PPE programme, 260
21.3 Face-fit testing using a particle counter, 269

Part 6 Risk Assessment and Risk Communication

Chapter 22 Risk Assessment, 275
22.1 Introduction, 275
22.2 Identify all hazardous substances or agents, 276

22.3 Identify the likely levels of exposure, 276

22.4 Identify all persons likely to be exposed, 278

22.5 Assess whether the exposures are likely to cause harm, 279

22.6 Consider elimination or substitution, 279

22.7 Define additional control measures necessary to reduce the harm to acceptable levels, 280

Chapter 23 Risk Communication, 282

23.1 Introduction, 282

23.2 Risk perception, 282

23.3 Trust, 283

23.4 Communication, 284

23.5 An example of quantitative risk assessment to aid risk communication, 285

Equipment Suppliers, 288

Chemical Analytical Services, 290

Index, 291

List of Illustrations

1.1   An idealized exposure–response relationship.
3.1   A simple conceptual model of exposure to hazardous substances: (a) inhalation; (b) dermal; (c) ingestion; (d) injection.
4.1   The ratio of near- (NF) to far-field (FF) exposure levels in different conditions.
4.2   Exposure over a working shift.
7.1   Results from ten measurements of inhalable dust in a packing plant.
7.2   Results from 100 measurements of inhalable dust in a packing plant.
7.3   A log–probability plot showing data from ten measurements of exposure during bag filling.
9.1   The ISO/CEN/ACGIH sampling conventions for health-related aerosol fractions. (Reproduced with permission from *Occupational Hygiene*, 3rd edition, edited by Kerry Gardiner and J. Malcolm Harrington, Blackwell Publishing Ltd., 2005, p. 187.)
9.2   Dust sampling equipment worn by operator, with IOM inhalable sampler in blown-up inset. (Reproduced with permission from SKC Ltd.)
9.3   (a) Multi-orifice sampler (HSE). (b) IOM inhalable sampler (HSE). (c) Conical inhalable sampler (HSE). (Reproduced with permission *Monitoring for Health Hazards at Work*, 3rd edition, by Indira Ashton and Frank S. Gill, Blackwell Publishers Ltd., 2000. pp. 6–7.)
9.4   Cyclone respirable sampler (HSE). (Reproduced with permission *Monitoring for Health Hazards at Work*, 3rd edition, by Indira Ashton and Frank S. Gill, Blackwell Publishers Ltd., 2000, p. 9.)
9.5   The CIP10-R respirable dust sampler. (Reproduced with permission from *Occupational Hygiene*, 3rd edition, edited by Kerry Gardiner and J. Malcolm Harrington, Blackwell Publishing Ltd., 2005, p. 194.)
9.6   The MRE 113 respirable dust sampler (Reproduced with permission *Monitoring for Health Hazards at Work*, 3rd edition, by Indira Ashton and Frank S. Gill, Blackwell Publishers Ltd., 2000, p. 9.)
9.7   The cowl sampler used for asbestos and other fibrous dusts. (Reproduced with permission from *Occupational Hygiene*, 3rd edition, edited by Kerry

Gardiner and J. Malcolm Harrington, Blackwell Publishing Ltd., 2005, p. 203.)

9.8   (a) A TSI Sidepak direct-reading dust monitor (Reproduced with permission from *Occupational Hygiene*, 3rd edition, edited by Kerry Gardiner and J. Malcolm Harrington, Blackwell Publishing Ltd., 2005, p. 197.) (b) SKC Split 2 sampler (Reproduced with permission from *Occupational Hygiene*, 3rd edition, edited by Kerry Gardiner and J. Malcolm Harrington, Blackwell Publishing Ltd., 2005, p. 197.) (c) Casella Microdust sampler. (Reproduced with permission from Casella Measurement Ltd.) (d) Output from a Sidepak sampler showing variation in aerosol concentration during work task.

9.9   An electronic flow calibrator. (Reproduced with permission from Casella Measurement Ltd.)

9.10 Apparatus used to calibrate a rotameter. (Reproduced with permission *Monitoring for Health Hazards at Work*, 3rd edition, by Indira Ashton and Frank S. Gill, Blackwell Publishers Ltd., 2000, p. 16.)

9.11 Typical rotameter calibration chart.

9.12 The Walton–Beckett eyepiece graticule. (Reproduced with permission *Monitoring for Health Hazards at Work*, 3rd edition, by Indira Ashton and Frank S. Gill, Blackwell Publishers Ltd., 2000, p. 28.)

9.13 Acetone vapouriser used to prepare samples for microscopic analysis. (Reproduced with permission from JS Holdings.)

9.14 Layout of Tyndall beam apparatus (A&G Marketing). (Reproduced with permission *Monitoring for Health Hazards at Work*, 3rd edition, by Indira Ashton and Frank S. Gill, Blackwell Publishers Ltd., 2000, p. 33.)

10.1 A single-gas detector with optional datalogger. (Reproduced with permission from Draeger Safety UK Ltd.)

10.2 Typical impinger samplers (SKC Ltd). (Reproduced with permission *Monitoring for Health Hazards at Work*, 3rd edition, by Indira Ashton and Frank S. Gill, Blackwell Publishers Ltd., 2000, p. 54.)

10.3 Adsorbent tubes. (Reproduced with permission from SKC Ltd.)

10.4 Badge type diffusive sampler. (Reproduced with permission from 3M United Kingdom PLC.)

10.5 Tube-type diffusive sampler. (Reproduced with permission from Draeger Safety UK Ltd.)

10.6 Colorimetric detector tube sampler and a range of tubes. (Reproduced with permission from Draeger Safety UK Ltd.)

10.7 Gas-tight sampling bags. (Reproduced with permission from SKC Ltd.)

10.8 A portable Fourier-transform infrared analyser. (Reproduced with permission from Quantitech Ltd.)

10.9 A MultiRAE photo-ionisation monitor. (Reproduced with permission from RAE Systems UK)

11.1 A multi-stage liquid impinger. (Reproduced with permission from Burkard Manufacturing Co. Limited)

11.2 Cascade impactor for bioaerosols. (Reproduced with permission from Casella Measurement Ltd.)

12.1 Typical arrangement of patches used in patch-sampling methods. (Reproduced with permission *Occupational Hygiene*, 3rd edition, edited by Kerry Gardiner and J. Malcolm Harrington, Blackwell Publishers Ltd., 2005, p. 395.)

13.1 Change in acoustic pressure with time for a pure tone. (Reproduced with permission from *Occupational Hygiene*, 3rd edition, edited by Kerry Gardiner and J. Malcolm Harrington, Blackwell Publishing Ltd., 2005, Figure 17.1).

13.2 Change in acoustic pressure with distance for a pure tone. (Reproduced with permission from *Occupational Hygiene*, 3rd edition, edited by Kerry Gardiner and J. Malcolm Harrington, Blackwell Publishing Ltd., 2005, Figure 17.2).

13.3 The weighting curves used in noise measurement. (Reproduced with permission from *Occupational Hygiene*, 3rd edition, edited by Kerry Gardiner and J. Malcolm Harrington, Blackwell Publishing Ltd., 2005, Figure 17.8).

13.4 Simple sound level meters. (Reproduced with permission from Casella Measurement Ltd.)

13.5 Octave band monitoring with a sound level meter. (Reproduced with permission from Casella Measurement Ltd.)

13.6 A noise dosemeter. (Reproduced with permission from Casella Measurement Ltd.)

13.7 A selection of hearing protection devices (muffs, reusable inserts and disposable inserts). (Reproduced with permission from Moldex-Metric AG & Co. KG)

14.1 x, y, z coordinates. (Reproduced with permission from *Occupational Hygiene*, 3rd edition, edited by Kerry Gardiner and J. Malcolm Harrington, Blackwell Publishing Ltd., 2005, p. 252.)

14.2 The relationship between displacement, velocity and acceleration for a simple mass and spring system.

14.3 Vibration measurements in practice. (Reproduced with permission from Bruel & Kjaer UK Ltd.)

15.1 Kata thermometer. (Reproduced with permission from Ashton and Gill)

15.2 Globe thermometer with glass thermometer. (Reproduced with permission from Ashton and Gill)

15.3 Integrating heat stress monitor. (Reproduced with permission from Quest Technologies)

15.4 Portable heat strain monitor. (a) monitor on belt (b) schematic arrangement of sensors (Reproduced with permission from Quest Technologies)

15.5 Arrangement of thermometers on a stand. (Reproduced with permission from Ashton and Gill)

16.1 The light meter. (Reproduced with permission from Castle Group)

17.1   The electromagnetic spectrum.

17.2   Decay of an unstable nuclide to a stable one. (Reproduced with permission *Monitoring for Health Hazards at Work,* 3rd edition, by Indira Ashton and Frank S. Gill, Blackwell Publishers Ltd., 2000. pp. 165.)

17.3   Decay of carbon 14. (Reproduced with permission *Monitoring for Health Hazards at Work,* 3rd edition, by Indira Ashton and Frank S. Gill, Blackwell Publishers Ltd., 2000. pp. 165.)

17.4   An example of decay in stages: lead to bismuth to polonium to lead. (Reproduced with permission *Monitoring for Health Hazards at Work,* 3rd edition, by Indira Ashton and Frank S. Gill, Blackwell Publishers Ltd., 2000. pp. 166.)

17.5   A Geiger–Muller counter. (Reproduced with permission from Thermo Fisher Scientific.)

17.6   A scintillation detector. (Reproduced with permission from Berthold Technologies (UK) Ltd.)

17.7   Two thermoluminescent detectors (TLDs). (Reproduced with permission from Mirion Technologies, Inc.)

17.8   Two film badges. (Reproduced with permission from Loxford Equipment Company Ltd.)

18.1   A broad-spectrum UV monitor along with the weighting. (Reproduced with permission from LOT-Oriel Ltd (for International Light))

18.2   A hand-held monitor for IRA and part of IRB. (Reproduced with permission from LOT-Oriel Ltd (for International Light))

18.3   A leak monitor for microwave ovens. (Reproduced with permission from ETS-Lindgren)

19.1   Diagram showing the incorrect placement of a hood while welding, i.e. too far from the source.

19.2   Operators placing their head between the emission source and the extraction hood.

20.1   Portable inclined manometer.

20.2   Magnehelic diaphragm pressure gauge. (Reproduced with permission *Monitoring for Health Hazards at Work,* 3rd edition, by Indira Ashton and Frank S. Gill, Blackwell Publishers Ltd., 2000. p. 89.)

20.3   Digital micromanometer. (Reproduced with permission from TSI Instruments Ltd.)

20.4   Electronic vane anemometer.

20.5   Heated sensor anemometer. (Reproduced with permission from TSI Instruments Ltd.)

20.6   Pitot-static tube. (Reproduced with permission from JS Holdings.)

20.7   Principle of operation of pitot-static tube. (Reproduced with permission from *Occupational Hygiene,* 3rd edition, edited by Kerry Gardiner and J. Malcolm Harrington, Blackwell Publishing Ltd., 2005, p. 443.)

20.8   Measuring positions for placing pitot-static tubes in circular ducting. (Reproduced with permission from Gardiner and Harrington.)

20.9   Log-Tchebycheff rule for traverse points in a rectangular duct. (Reproduced with permission from Gardiner and Harrington.)

20.10   Face of booth showing measurement positions. (Reproduced with permission *Monitoring for Health Hazards at Work*, 3rd edition, by Indira
Ashton and Frank S. Gill, Blackwell Publishers Ltd., 2000. p. 106.)

20.11   Extract slot showing measured air speed results and plotted contours.
(Reproduced with permission *Monitoring for Health Hazards at Work*,
3rd edition, by Indira Ashton and Frank S. Gill, Blackwell Publishers
Ltd., 2000. p. 110.)

21.1   A selection of respiratory protection: (a) disposable respirator FFP1; (b)
half-mask respirator; (c) powered hood TH2; (d) full facepiece respirator; (e) full masks breathing apparatus. (Reproduced with permission
from Draeger Safety UK Ltd.)

21.2   Face-fit testing kit – PortaCount. (Reproduced with permission from
TSI Instruments Ltd.)

List of Instruction Sheets

Chapter 9

9.8 Calibration of a rotameter or electronic flow calibrator by using the soap-bubble method, 76

9.9 The measurement of inhalable airborne dust, 80

9.10 The measurement of airborne respirable dust by using a cyclone sampler, 83

9.11 The sampling and counting of airborne asbestos fibres, 84

9.13 To trace the behaviour of a dust cloud by using a Tyndall beam, 89

Chapter 10

10.5 To measure personal exposure to solvent vapours using an adsorbent tube, 102

10.6 Sampling for gases by using a bubbler, 104

10.7 To measure the short-term airborne concentration of a gas by using a colorimetric detector tube, 106

10.8 To measure a vapour concentration using a diffusive sampler, 108

Chapter 13

13.10 To measure workplace noise using a SLM, 153

13.11 To measure workplace noise using a PND, 155

13.12 To measure the spectrum of a continuous noise by octave band analysis, 157

Chapter 14

14.6 To measure hand–arm vibration, 167

Chapter 15

15.5 Measurement of the thermal environment, 182

15.9 To calculate the wind chill factor, 189

Chapter 16

16.5 To measure lighting, 194

Chapter 20

20.5 Measurement of air flow in ducts, 246
20.6 Measurement of pressure in ventilation systems, 252
20.7 To measure the face velocity on a booth or hood, 254
20.8 To measure the face velocity on a fume cupboard, 255
20.9 To measure the performance of a suction inlet, 257

Chapter 21

21.3 Face-fit testing using a particle counter, 269

Preface

The methods for measuring exposure to hazards in the workplace have progressively developed over the last 50 or more years. A major impetus for improving ways of assessing workers' exposure to chemical, biological and physical hazards in the UK was the introduction of the Health and Safety at Work (etc.) Act in 1974, which required employers to ensure that tasks and work environments were 'safe and without risks to health...'. Subsequent regulations made under the Act have strengthened the role for measurement as part of a modern approach to health and safety at work. Recent developments have seen greater standardisation of approaches to measurement and an increasing understanding of the role of exposure measurement in the context of assessing risks to health. Over the last 10 years there has been increasing interest in how best to quantify dermal exposure to chemicals and in the future we expect to see more interest in measurement of chemicals inadvertently ingested from contaminated hands or objects. Today, methods for measuring hazards at work are being applied throughout the world, and in the future the process of globalisation and standardisation will ensure greater uniformity in approaches to measurement.

The earlier editions of this book provided a very practical introduction to the topic, with helpful practical advice about how to undertake specific measurements of everything from hazardous airborne dusts to hot stressful environments. We had used the book in teaching occupational hygiene students and to help support other health and safety professionals develop their skills and had found it invaluable. When we were asked to take on the job of revising and updating the text for the fourth edition, we took the opportunity to think carefully about the changes in practice that had taken place and to reflect these in the text while retaining the practical 'how to do it' approach that had made the book unique.

The text of this fourth edition has been completely reorganised into 6 separate sections and 25 chapters. The sections cover background material necessary to understand the context within which measurements are made, and then we deal with measurement of exposure to inhalation hazards, dermal and ingestion hazards and physical agents such as noise, heat and radiation. The final sections deal with measurements to assess the effectiveness of risk management measures such as local ventilation or personal protection, and risk assessment/risk communication. We believe that these provide a comprehensive introduction to the topic that will help the reader understand how measurements should be made and their results communicated to the workforce.

We hope that the book will be a useful source for students interested in learning about the practical aspects of occupational hygiene measurements. However, we have also included information on many new techniques and emerging areas of occupational hygiene practice and hope that there is also much that will be useful to established professionals who perhaps relied on previous editions of the book in the earlier part of their career. As with the earlier editions we have tried to ensure that the text is accessible to a wide range of health and safety professionals, including safety advisors, occupational health nurses, ergonomists, occupational physicians and occupational hygienists.

It is important to realise that the measurement methods we describe in this book are tools that can be used to assess the degree of risk and guide further preventative actions where necessary. In doing this the readers will need to use a wider knowledge base encompassing the underpinning legislation, toxicology, other sciences, engineering and management techniques. These topics are beyond the scope of the present work. In addition, there is a need to apply sound professional judgment in deciding what type of measurements will be helpful and in interpreting the results that are obtained. There is no substitute for good academic or professional education or training. In the UK, the British Occupational Hygiene Society (www.BOHS.org) regulates a system of qualifications that covers most of the techniques described in this book. Internationally, the Occupational Hygiene Training Association (OHTA) provides a similar role. There are also relevant postgraduate courses available in universities in the UK and throughout the world.

We are interested to receive feedback from readers about the book and to continue to support those interested in measurement of health hazards and other aspects of occupational hygiene. Visit www.OH-world.org for more information.

John W. Cherrie
Robin M. Howie
Sean Semple
January 2010

Acknowledgements

We owe a great deal to the authors of the earlier edition of this book – Frank Gill and Indira Ashton. They recognised the need for a simple practical introduction to monitoring for health hazards at work, and their text provided a wealth of material that we have reused and recycled in this edition. We are also grateful to the many colleagues and friends who have offered advice and provided comments on earlier drafts of the text. In particular, we wish to thank Finlay Dick, Alastair Robertson, Adrian Watson, Adrian Hirst, Richard Graveling, Andy Gillies, Bob Rajan and Brian Crook. Adrian Watson also provided initial draft material for the chapters on lighting and vibration, which was invaluable in revising these sections of the book.

The authors would also like to thank the many companies who have provided information and photographs of measurement equipment to illustrate the book.

Of course, the book would have never been finished without the support of our wives and families, for which we are most grateful.

Units and Abbreviations*

The more common units used in workplace environmental measurement

Unit	Dimension	SI	Imperial	Conversion
Length	L	m	ft	ft $\times$ 0.3048 = m
		mm	in	in $\times$ 25.4 = mm
Area	L^2	m^2	ft^2	ft^2 $\times$ 9.29 $\times$ 10^{-2} = m^2
		mm^2	in^2	in^2 $\times$ 645.2 = mm^2
Volume	L^3	m^3 (1000 litre)	ft^3	ft^3 $\times$ 2.832 $\times$10^{-2} = m^3
		1 (litre)	gallon	gallon $\times$ 4.546 = litre
Mass	M	kg	lb	lb $\times$ 0.4536 = kg
		g (gram)	oz	oz $\times$ 28.35 = g
		mg	grain	gr $\times$ 64.79 = mg
Airborne concentration of substance				
(Mass)	$\dfrac{M}{L^3}$	mg m^{-3}	grain ft	gr ft^{-3} $\times$ 2288 = mg m^{-3}
(Volume)	—	—	parts per million (ppm)	
(Particle)	—	mp cm^{-3}	mp ft^{-3}	(millions of particles per cm^3 (ft^3))
Acceleration	$\dfrac{L}{T^2}$	m s^{-2}	ft sec^{-2}	ft s^{-2} $\times$ 0.305 = m s^{-2}
		gravity = 9.81 m s^{-2}		
Density	$\dfrac{M}{L^3}$	kg m^{-3}(g l^{-1})	lb ft^{-3}	lb ft^{-3} $\times$ 16.02 = kg m^{-3}
Flow rate				
(Mass)	$\dfrac{M}{T}$	kg s^{-1}	lb hr^{-1}	lb hr^{-1} $\times$ 1.26 $\times$ 10^{-4} = kg s^{-1}
(Volume)	$\dfrac{L^3}{T}$	m^3 s^{-1}	ft^{-3} min^{-1}	ft^3 min^{-1} $\times$ 4.719 $\times$ 10^{-4} = m^3 s^{-1}
			gall hr^{-1}	gall hr^{-1} $\times$ 1.263 $\times$ 10^{-6} = m^3 s^{-1}
Force	$\dfrac{ML}{T^2}$	N (Newton) (N = kg m s^{-2})	lb$_f$	lb$_f$ $\times$ 4.448 = N

*In this book SI units are used throughout; however, conversions from Imperial to SI are given in the list of common units. Also, we use the form mg m^{-3} when presenting units rather than mg/m^3, although both are acceptable in practice.

Unit	Dimension	SI	Imperial	Conversion
Temperature	–	K (Kelvin) °C (degree Celsius)	°F	(°F-32) × 0.5555 = °C °C + 273.15 = K
Energy/ Heat quantity	$\frac{ML^2}{T^2}$	J (Joule) Ws = Nm kW hour	Btu	Btu × 1055 = J kW hour × 3.6 × 10^6 = J kilocalorie × 4187 = J
Heat flow/ Power	$\frac{ML^2}{T^3}$	W	HP Btu hr^{-1}	HP × 745.7 = W Btu hr^{-1} × 0.291 = W
Latent heat	$\frac{L^2}{T^2}$	kJ kg^{-1}	Btu lb^{-1}	Btu lb^{-1} × 2.326 = kJ kg^{-1}
Specific heat	$\frac{L}{T^2\,temp}$	kJ kg^{-1} °C	Btu lb^{-1} °F	Btu lb^{-1} °F × 4.187 = kJ kg^{-1} °C
Pressure	$\frac{M}{T^2L}$	Pa (Pascal) = N m^{-2} bar (×10^5 = Pa)	lb$_f$ ft^{-2} lb$_f$ in^{-2} in water (4°C) in mercury (0°C)	lb ft^{-2} × 47.88 = Pa lb in^{-2} × 6895 = Pa in H$_2$O × 249.1 = Pa in Hg × 3386 = Pa
Torque	$\frac{ML^2}{T^2}$	Nm	lb$_f$ ft	lb$_f$ ft × 1.356 = Nm
Velocity	$\frac{L}{T}$	m s^{-1}	ft min^{-1} ft s^{-1}	ft m^{-1} × 5.08 × 10^{-3} = m s^{-1} ft s^{-1} × 0.305 = m s^{-1}
Viscosity				
(Dynamic)	$\frac{M}{TL}$	Pa s (Ns m^{-2}) Poise (dyne s cm^{-2})	lb.s ft^{-1}	lb.s ft^{-1} × 47.88 = Pa s Poise × 0.1 = Pa s
(Kinematic)	$\frac{L^2}{T}$	m^2 s^{-1} Stokes (cm^2 s^{-1})	ft^2 s^{-1} in^2 s^{-1}	ft^2 s^{-1} × 9.29 × 10^{-2} = m^2 s^{-1} in^2 s^{-1} × 6.452 × 10^{-4} = m^2 s^{-1} Stokes × 10^{-4} = m^2 s^{-1}
Luminous intensity		candela (Cd)	candle (int)	candle × 0.981 = Cd
Luminous flux		lumen (1m) (lm = 1Cd sr)		
Illuminance		lux (lx = 1m m^{-2})	foot candle lumen ft^{-2}	ft candle × 0.1076 = lx lm ft^{-2} × 0.1076 = lx
Luminance		Cd m^{-2}	foot lambert candela in^{-2}	ft lambert × 3.426 = Cd m^{-2} Cd in^{-2} × 1550 = Cd m^2
Radiation activity	dis s^{-1}	Bq	Ci	1Ci = 3.7 × 10^{10}Bq = 3.7 × 10^4 MBq = 0.037 TBq 1 mCi = 37 × 10^6 Bq = 37 MBq = 3.7 × 10^{-5} TBq 1 μCi = 37 000 Bq = 0.037 MBq = 3.7 × 10^{-8} TBq 1 Bq = 2.7 × 10^{-5} μCi = 2.7 × 10^{-8} mCi = 2.7 × 10^{11} Ci 1 MBq = 27 μCi = 0.027 mCi = 2.7 × 10^{-5} Ci 1 TBq = 2.7 × $10^7$11Ci = 2.7 × 10^4 mCi = 27 Ci

Radiation absorbed dose	$\dfrac{J}{kg}$	Gy	rad	$1Gy = 1J\,kg^{-1} = 100\ rad$
	kg			$1mGy = 100\ mrad$
				$1\mu Gy = 0.01\ mrad$
Dose equivalent	$rad \times Q \times N$	Sv	rem	$1Sv = 100\ rem$
				$1mSv = 100\ mrem$
				$1\mu Sv = 0.1\ mrem$

Temperature	°Celsius	°Fahrenheit	$°F = (°C \times 1.8) + 32$
	−40	−40	
	−30	−22	
	−20	−4	
	−10	14	
	0	32	
	10	50	
	20	68	
	30	86	
	40	104	
	50	122	
	60	140	
	70	158	
	80	176	
	90	194	
	100	212	

Useful abbreviations

ACoP	Approved Code of Practice – from the HSE
ACTS	The UK Advisory Committee on Toxic Substances (www.hse.gov.uk/aboutus/meetings/iacs/acts/)
ALARP	As low a reasonably practicable
ANSI	American National Standards Institute (www.ansi.org/)
BOHS	British Occupational Hygiene Society (www.BOHS.org)
CAD	Chemical Agents Directive (details at http://europa.eu/)
CAS Number	A unique identifying number assigned to a hazardous substance by the Chemical Abstracts Service (www.cas.org/)
CIBSE	Chartered Institute of Building Services Engineers (www.cibse.org/)
COMAH	Control of Major Accident Hazards Regulations (www.hse.gov.uk/comah/)
ECHA	European Chemicals Agency (http://echa.europa.eu/)
EU	European Union (http://europa.eu/)
HPA	Health Protection Agency (www.hpa.org.uk/)
IARC	International Agency for Research on Cancer (www.iarc.fr)
IDLH	Immediately Dangerous to Life or Health (www.cdc.gov/niosh/idlh/idlh-1.html)
ILO	International Labour Organization (www.ilo.org)
IOELV	Indicative Occupational Exposure Limit Values from the EU (http://ec.europa.eu/social/main.jsp?catId=153&langId=en&intPageId=684)
IUPAC	The International Union of Pure and Applied Chemistry (www.iupac.org/)
NOEL	No observed effect level

SI	Système international d'unités (www.bipm.org/en/si/)
STEL	Short-term Exposure Limits (See EH40)
TLV	Threshold Limit Value is a type of OEL used in the USA and elsewhere. TLV's are published by the American Conference of Governmental Industrial Hygienists (www.ACGIH.org/tlv/)
WASP	Workplace Analysis Scheme for Proficiency. A quality assurance scheme for occupational hygiene analysis managed for HSE by the Health and Safety Laboratory (www.hsl.gov.uk/centres-of-excellence/proficiency-testing/wasp.aspx)
WATCH	The Working Group on the Assessment of Toxic Chemicals, which is a subcommittee of ACTS (www.hse.gov.uk/aboutus/meetings/iacs/acts/index.htm)

Abbreviations in the text

ACDP	Advisory Committee on Dangerous Pathogens (www.dh.gov.uk/ab/ACDP/)
ACGIH	American Conference of Governmental Industrial Hygienists (www.acgih.org/)
ACH	Air Changes per Hour (ventilation)
ALARA	As Low As Reasonably Achievable
ALI	Annual Limits of Intake (radiation)
APF	Assigned Protection Factor (respirator)
ART	Advance REACH Tool (www.advancedreachtool.com/)
BMGV	Biological Monitoring Guidance Values (details in HSE publication EH40, www.hse.gov.uk/COSHH/)
BS EN	British Standard – European Norm (www.standardsuk.com/)
CA	Control of Asbestos regulations (www.hse.gov.uk/asbestos/regulations.htm)
CE	Conformity marking system for products (www.bsigroup.com/en/ProductServices/About-CE-Marking/)
CEN	European Committee for Standardisation (www.cen.eu/)
CFU	Colony Forming Units
CHIP	Chemical (Hazards Information and Packaging for Supply) Regulations (www.hse.gov.uk/chip/)
CLW	Control of Lead at Work regulations
CNW	Control of Noise at Work regulations (www.hse.gov.uk/noise/regulations.htm)
COSHH	Control of Substances Hazardous to Health Regulations (www.hse.gov.uk/coshh/)
COSHH-Essentials	An initiative from the HSE designed to help small and medium size companies manage supplied chemicals at work (www.coshh-essentials.org.uk/)
CVW	Control of Vibration at Work regulations (www.hse.gov.uk/vibration/)
DAC	Derived Air Concentrations (radiation)
DL	Derived Limits (radiation)
DNA	Deoxyribonucleic acid
EH40	The guidance document published annually by HSE Books, which contains the complete list of UK OEL's. EH40 (www.hse.gov.uk/COSHH/)
ELF	Extremely Low Frequency (radiation)
EMF	Electro-Magnetic Field

FFP	Filtering Facepiece (respirator)
FTIR	Fourier Transform Infrared spectroscopy (chemical analysis)
GHS	Globally Harmonised System for the classification and labelling of hazardous substances (www.hse.gov.uk/ghs/)
GMP	Good Manufacturing Practice
HPLC	High-performance liquid chromatography (chemical analysis)
HSE	Health and Safety Executive (www.hse.gov.uk)
HSG	Health and Safety Guidance publications (from HSE)
HVL	Half-Value Layer (radiation)
ICNIRP	International Commission on Non-Ionizing Radiation Protection (www.icnirp.de/)
ICRP	International Commission on Radiological Protection (www.icrp.org/)
IOM	The Institute of Occupational Medicine. An independent research and consulting organisation in Scotland (www.IOM-world.org)
IR	Infrared (also IRA, IRB and IRC to signify parts of the infrared spectrum)
IREQ	Required clothing insulation (thermal)
ISLM	Integrating Sound Level Meter
ISO	International Standards Organisation (www.iso.org)
LAA	aboratory Animal Allergy
LEL	ower Explosive Limit
$L_{EP,d}$	Daily noise exposure level
$L_{EP,w}$	Weekly noise exposure level
LEV	ocal Exhaust Ventilation
LPS	ipopolysaccharide
MDHS	Methods for the Determination of Hazardous Substances (www.hse.gov.uk/pubns/mdhs/)
MMMF	Man-Made Mineral Fibres. Also known as synthetic mineral fibres or man-made vitreous fibres (those MMMF with a glassy structure)
MMVF	Man-Made Vitreous Fibres (see MMMF)
MRE	Mining Research Establishment
MSDS	Material Safety Data Sheet (see also SDS, which is the preferred terminology)
MDHS	Methods of Determination of Hazardous Substances (www.hse.gov.uk/pubns/mdhs/index.htm)
NIOSH	National Institute for Occupational Safety and Health (www.cdc.gov/niosh)
OECD	Organisation for Economic Co-operation and Development (www.oecd.org/)
OEL	Occupational Exposure Limit (http://osha.europa.eu/en/topics/ds/oel)
OVA	Organic Vapour Analyser
PAH	Polycyclic Aromatic Hydrocarbons
PF	Protection Factor (respirator)
PND	Persona Noise Dosimeter
PNIHL	Personal Noise Induced Hearing Loss
PPE	Personal Protective Equipment (www.hse.gov.uk/pubns/indg174.pdf)
PPE	Personal Protective Equipment
P_{peak}	Peak sound pressure level
PTFE	Polytetrafluoroethylene
PUF	Polyurethane Foam
PVC	Polyvinylchloride
Q	Quality factor (radiation)
REACH	Registration, Evaluation, Authorisation and restriction of Chemicals regulations (http://ec.europa.eu/environment/chemicals/reach/reach_intro.htm)

RNA	Ribonucleic Acid
RPE	Respiratory Protective Equipment (www.hse.gov.uk/pubns/guidance/rseries.htm)
SCOEL	Scientific Committee on Occupational Exposure Limits. An independent committee set up by the EU (http://ec.europa.eu/social/main.jsp?catId=153&langId=en&intPageId=684)
SDS	Safety Data Sheet
SEG	Similarly Exposed Group of workers
SIMPEDS	Safety in Mines Personal Dust Sampler
SPL	Sound Pressure Level
TLD	Thermoluminescent Dosimeters
TWA	Time-Weighted Average concentration (See EH40)
UKAS	UK Accreditation Service (www.ukas.com/)
UV	Ultraviolet (also UVA, UVB and UVC to signify different parts of the UV spectrum)
VBNC	Viable But Non Culturable
VOC	Volatile Organic Compound
WBGT	Wet-Bulb Globe Temperature
WEL	Workplace Exposure Limits (www.hse.gov.uk/COSHH/table1.pdf)
WHO	World Health Organization (www.who.int/topics/occupational_health/en/)

Multiples of SI units

Name	Symbol	Factor
tera	T	10^{12}
giga	G	10^{9}
mega	M	10^{6}
kilo	k	10^{3}
hecto	h	10^{2}
deca	da	10^{1}
deci	d	10^{-1}
centi	c	10^{-2}
milli	m	10^{-3}
micro	μ	10^{-6}
nano	n	10^{-9}
pico	P	10^{-12}
femto	f	10^{-15}
atto	a	10^{-18}

1 Introduction

1 Occupational Hygiene and Risk Assessment

1.1 Introduction

"When you can measure what you are speaking about, and express it in numbers, you know something about it; but when you cannot measure it, when you cannot express it in numbers, your knowledge is of a meager and unsatisfactory kind..."

Lord Kelvin, *Popular Lectures and Addresses*

Scientists have always known that measurement is fundamental to making accurate statements about the world around us. The pioneers of occupational health were also enthusiastic about measuring exposure, even when this involved considerable effort to get reliable data. In recent years, it has become less fashionable to rely on measurement data and we have seen the development of sophisticated computer-based systems to estimate exposures, or health and safety professionals rely on their judgment to come to a conclusion about the risks in a particular situation. We support these approaches but we also recognise that which was clear to Lord Kelvin more than 100 years ago: measurements can provide a precise, reliable and objective description of a situation that is generally superior to the alternatives.

The science of human exposure encompasses assessment and control of exposure to hazardous agents that arise from work, in the home or elsewhere in the environment. It does not really matter whether you want to measure the exposure to diesel engine exhaust particulate of someone working as a truck driver or the exposure of someone else in the street where the truck is unloading: the underlying science is the same. Where differences do arise, they are in relation to who has responsibility to manage the exposures and what legislative regime applies. Occupational health professionals are concerned with establishing and maintaining a safe and healthy working environment. Occupational hygienists are the occupational health professionals who are focused on the prevention of ill health by intervening in the workplace to eliminate or reduce exposures to hazardous agents. There are other occupational health and safety specialists who may deal with different aspects of health and work, for example occupational physicians and nurses, safety advisors and ergonomists. However, no matter what the specific expertise of the individuals they should all be aware of the principles of occupational hygiene to help them in their job.

Hazardous agents may be chemicals, loud noise, unseen radiations or many other things. The discipline of occupational hygiene groups hazardous agents into three categories: *physical, chemical* or *biological* agents. Psychological stressors are generally seen as being outside the remit of occupational hygiene. Physical agents include noise, vibration, electromagnetic radiation, ionizing and non-ionizing radiation, excessively hot or cold environments and abnormal atmospheric pressures. Chemical agents include harmful dusts, liquids, gases and vapours. Biological agents include bacteria, viruses and other materials of biological origin that are harmful to health. For convenience chemical and biological agents are often grouped together as substances hazardous to health.

The basis for occupational hygiene is the link between exposure to a hazard and the risk of illness arising from that exposure, where the 'hazard' is the potential for harm and the 'risk' is the chance that that harm may arise in a particular situation. In general, it is assumed that the higher the exposure someone experiences, the greater the risk to their health. Figure 1.1 shows an

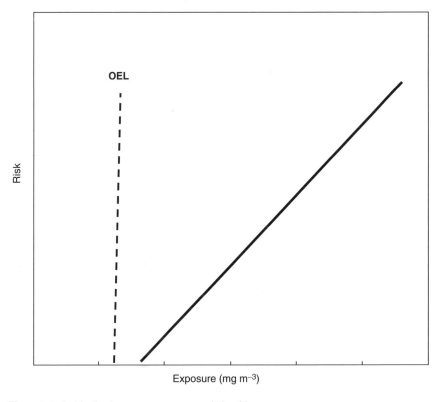

Figure 1.1 An idealized exposure–response relationship.

idealized exposure–response relationship for a hazardous agent, which epitomizes the causal link between these two measures. The point at which the line cuts the horizontal axis is the threshold for this particular agent and exposure less than this value will not cause any adverse effects. It is clear that limiting the exposure below the threshold will prevent anyone becoming ill and in these circumstances an occupational exposure limit (OEL) should ideally be defined at this point; i.e. it is a health-based OEL. Note that in this book we use the term OEL to refer in a general way to limit values for exposure.

In practice, the setting of occupational exposure limits is more complex than the identification of a simple unambiguous threshold, but the general principle of restricting exposure below some value, to ensure risk is minimised, is still valid. In some cases we cannot identify whether the exposure–response relationship contains a threshold below which the hazardous agent has no effect; i.e. the exposure–response line passes through the origin on the graph. The main types of hazardous agents that may be in this category are carcinogens that act on the structure of DNA – so-called genotoxic carcinogens. Also, people express a range of different susceptibilities to hazardous agents and although in theory, there may be a threshold for a given agent it may be that some individuals will still be affected at lower exposures. For example, someone with asthma may react to quite low concentrations of an irritant gas when others do not experience any ill effects. Finally, there may be factors that make it impracticable to set a limit at a threshold, for example it may not be technically or economically feasible to restrict exposure to the level of a low threshold and society deems that the benefits from production or use of this material outweigh the health risks from the exposure.

There are many systems that are in place to derive OELs: some are based on national legislation and are used to enforce the law in the workplace; some are national or international advisory limits without any direct link to legislation and some are international limits with the intention of harmonizing practice. In Great Britain, there is a system for workplace exposure limits (WELs) for substances hazardous to health, which are linked to the legal provisions of the Control of Substances Hazardous to Health (COSHH) regulations. Each country in Europe has its own limits, but the European Union has set uniform minimum standards for OELs for some hazardous substances through the efforts of the Scientific Committee for Occupational Exposure Limits (SCOEL), which aims to identify health-based OELs. The European Commission then uses the scientific advice from SCOEL to make proposals for indicative occupational exposure limits based only on the scientific advice given or binding limits where socioeconomic or technical feasibility factors are taken into account in the decision. International bodies provide advisory limits for radiation and other physical agents, and these may then be incorporated into national legislation or guidance.

Harm may be caused by exposure to a hazardous agent. The degree of harm depends on the hazardous properties of the agent, the intensity and duration of exposure and the person's response to the exposure. Exposure is conventionally characterised by two independent factors: the intensity of the exposure and the duration of the individual's exposure. For chemicals, where the person inhales the substance, the intensity is usually the average concentration of that substance in the air breathed into the nose or mouth. In the workplace, concentration is generally measured in terms of the mass of the hazardous substance per cubic metre of air, for example mg m^{-3}, or in parts of the substance by volume per million parts of air, i.e. ppm. However, the units of exposure should really be something like mg m^{-3} h, i.e. the product of intensity and duration, but it is conventional to express exposures in units of concentration only and to make the duration a standard period, normally either 8 h or 15 min. So for example, a painter exposed to 10 mg m^{-3} of toluene for 4 h out of an 8-h shift would have an exposure of 40 mg m^{-3} h but we would normally say that the painter's 8-h average exposure was 5 mg m^{-3}, i.e. $40/8 = 5$. If the exposure is to be assessed over a 15-min period then the sample is normally collected for this duration. In the case of our painter, the 15-min exposure might be measured on a number of occasions partway through the shift when it was judged the exposure level was highest.

If exposure is measured by collecting a number of samples over an 8-h period then it is conventional to take the average of these, allowing for the different duration of each sample – this is called a time-weighted average (TWA). For example, we could have measured the painter's exposure during the first hour when she was preparing the job, for the next 3 h when she was painting and then for the final 4 h when she was doing paperwork in the office. The results from this monitoring are shown in Table 1.1.

The 8-h TWA exposure level ($E_{8\text{-h TWA}}$) is calculated by multiplying each exposure level in the table by the corresponding duration, summing them all and then dividing by the total duration (i.e. 8 h). Mathematically this is written as

$$E_{8-h\,\mathrm{TWA}} = \frac{\sum_{i=1}^{n} E_i t_i}{8}$$

where E_i are the exposure levels, t_i the durations and n the number of samples collected over the 8 h. If you calculate the 8-h TWA for the results in the table you will see that it is also 5 mg m^{-3}, i.e. $(4 \times 1 + 12 \times 3 + 0 \times 4)/8 = 40/8 = 5$.

For hazardous substances, exposure may occur by several different routes; i.e. the substance may enter the body by inhalation, by ingestion, by injection or by passing through the skin. For most chemicals the science was

Table 1.1 Toluene exposure measurements for a painter.

Activity	Duration of sample (h)	Exposure level (mg m^{-3})
Preparation	1	4
Painting	3	12
Paperwork	4	0

originally developed to address problems from inhalation, principally because this was considered the most important route for the majority of substances. This means that for the other routes of exposure the measurement methodologies and the concept of an OEL are less coherently developed. Also, for physical agents there are differences in the units of measurement and in the approaches used to obtain a measure of exposure, but again these issues are dealt with in the later sections of this book.

1.2   Hazard and risk

We saw earlier that a hazard is a situation that has the potential to cause harm to a person, e.g. exposure to toxic chemicals, absorption of energy transmitted as microwaves or exposure to loud noise. Risk is the possibility of that hazard causing harm to a particular individual or group of individuals in a given time period. Hazard and risk can be expressed in words, numbers or any other way, as long the information is meaningful. However, it should be clear that if you cannot come into contact with a hazard, i.e. you are not exposed, then the risk is zero.

The type of harm that may occur is an important aspect of a hazard. As each hazard may cause a range of harm, from minor injury to death, the type of harm must be specified. For example, exposure to a substance may carry a risk of causing respiratory tract irritation or cancer, and it is obvious that the latter consequence would be the more serious outcome. This is partly because cancer is a life-threatening illness and irritation is generally a nuisance, and partly because once the cancer has been initiated it tends to be irreversible whereas the irritation will mostly cease soon after exposure has ended.

In assessing risk, care should be taken to ensure that possible accidental exposures are properly considered and there is not just a focus on routine conditions. Accidental exposures may include spillages, activities such as cleaning and maintenance, which can disturb deposited material making a hazardous substance airborne again, entry into confined spaces that contain hazardous substances without proper protective equipment, and wearing contaminated personal protective clothing. Rules that prohibit eating, drinking, smoking, applying cosmetics, nail biting and so on can help prevent substances hazardous to health entering the body by inadvertent ingestion. Advice about washing and showering can reduce the risk from dermal exposure.

1.3   Risk assessment

Risk assessment is the process of making decisions about the acceptability of the risk and the need to take precautionary or protective measures. Risk assessments are part of the wider systems designed to ensure effective management of health and safety in the workplace, but they are a key component that is necessary for the protection of health.

The outcome of a workplace risk assessment is usually expressed in terms such as the *risks are acceptable,* the *risks are unacceptable* or the outcome of the *risk assessment is uncertain* and further information is required to arrive at an appropriate conclusion. One would generally start by making a qualitative assessment of the risks by using all of the relevant available information. For example, if a laboratory technician is using a very small quantity of a low-toxicity liquid in a fume cupboard while wearing appropriate protective gloves then it will almost certainly be the case that the risks from handling the chemical are acceptable, and any further investigation would be unnecessary. In contrast, people working in a factory where the noise levels were so loud that you cannot hear someone next to you talking are probably exposed to unacceptable risks to their hearing and the most important thing to do is ensure that a suitable noise control strategy is implemented as soon as possible. However, it may be necessary to obtain some simple quantitative data to arrive at a satisfactory conclusion or it may be that measurements of exposure are needed to convince management that the risks are unacceptable and that they need to take action. This type of data may be obtained by measuring exposure.

Any measurements need to be interpreted in terms of risk and for most situations the OEL provides the best way of doing this; exposures above the limit being unacceptable. Where there are no published OELs then a more considered approach is needed to evaluate the risks and in these circumstances it will be necessary to seek the advice of an occupational hygienist or other relevant scientific or medical expert.

1.4 The stages of a risk assessment

1.4.1 Identify the hazard

Workplace risk assessments are best carried out with the cooperation of the relevant managers and workers. They will have access to the sort of information that is needed to come up with an appropriate conclusion and they will also be able to help identify possible solutions where the risks are considered unacceptable.

The first stage in risk assessment is to define the scope and state which area, task or activity is to be assessed. You may choose to start by drawing a hazard map of the area, or a flow diagram of the tasks or activities to be assessed. Check that you have covered all relevant activities including cleaning, breakdowns and maintenance. Then list the physical, chemical or biological hazards associated with each activity, taking care to consider process-generated agents and remembering to identify accidental exposures. Examine the workplace layout and the process to identify where different hazardous agents may interact and make a note of the environmental conditions such as air temperature, humidity and general ventilation. It is often useful to seek out published information from trade associations, regulators, e.g. the Health and Safety Executive (HSE) or other reputable information sources.

Risks that are reasonably foreseeable should be noted and some preliminary decisions taken on their significance. The risks judged to be insignificant should be noted to indicate that they have been considered but the significant ones will require more attention.

1.4.2 Decide who might be affected and how

List all types of personnel who may be exposed to the hazards, including how many people are in each group, the split by gender and any other relevant demographic information. Some workers such as new and young workers, new or expectant mothers and people with disabilities may be at particular risk and there may be specific legal obligations in respect of them.

It is usual to identify work groups or types of employees such as process workers, maintenance workers, welders, office workers and so on, and non-employees such as contractors, customers or neighbours. If appropriate, you should also record more specific job titles represented in each group.

1.4.3 Evaluate the risks

Identify the possible types of harm that could be realised, for example whether there is a chance of acute or chronic effects. Then make an estimate of the exposure that the identified groups of workers and non-workers may experience. The sorts of things that need to be considered here are the following:

- Who is carrying out the work;
- What work processes and equipment are used;
- What methods of work and materials are used;
- What are the frequency and duration of operations;
- What conditions are there in the work environment, including the presence of general ventilation, lighting and other factors; and
- Are there any legal or good practice requirements specific to the activity?

In deciding whether there is adequate control, you should also consider the principles of good practice for the control of exposure to substances hazardous to health as laid down in the COSHH regulations. These principles, which can be extended to physical agents, are the following:

- Design and operate processes and activities to minimise emission, release and spread of substances hazardous to health.
- Take into account all relevant routes of exposure: inhalation, skin absorption, injection and ingestion, when developing control measures.
- Control exposure by measures that are proportionate to the health risk.
- Choose the most effective and reliable control options to minimise the escape and spread of substances hazardous to health through the workplace.
- Provide suitable personal protective equipment, in combination with other control measures, where adequate control of exposure cannot be achieved by other means.

- Check and regularly review all control measures for their continuing effectiveness.
- Inform and train all employees about the hazards and risks from the substances with which they work, and the use of control measures developed to minimise the risks.

There is no easy way to estimate the exposure once you have assembled the information about the work task. In some cases, it is possible to argue that the risks are acceptable because of observations made during the information gathering process. For example, if the noise levels are sufficiently low as to not interfere with communication, if there are no signs of dust being emitted from a powder transfer workstation, if the hand tool does not appear to vibrate during use then we may eliminate possible unacceptable risks from noise, chemicals and vibration, respectively. In some situations it may be possible to draw upon your previous experience with similar processes in other workplaces.

Hazards with risks judged to be insignificant should be noted to indicate that they have been considered. For example, in a workroom where the temperature is 25–30°C, there is little chance of any serious risk from heat strain, but the conditions may contribute to the discomfort of workers, particularly if they are engaged in manual work or need to wear protective clothing that limits their ability to lose heat. However, if the risk is judged to be unacceptable, then protective measures are required. The best approach is to identify what control measures are needed and then compare these against the measures that are being taken. Where there is uncertainty some exposure monitoring may be necessary and these data can then be compared with an appropriate limit value.

1.4.4 Take preventative and protective measures

If the risk is unacceptable then measures are required to either prevent or control the risk. Where control measures are being taken then you must check that they are reducing the risk to an acceptable level. It may be helpful to check the controls are functioning as originally installed and are regularly maintained. If they were initially judged adequate then regular maintenance and testing will help ensure continued control.

It is often appropriate to think about whether it is possible to modify the process to eliminate some or all of the hazardous agents. For example, by replacing a welding process where hazardous gases and fumes are emitted to a system involving bolts to join the metal pieces. However, one must always be alert to changes that just alter the hazard without really reducing the risk. In the example mentioned earlier, there may be no real advantage if the bolts were fixed using power tools with associated exposure to noise and vibration. For hazardous substance there is also the possibility of moving to a less hazardous material or to a material that gives rise to a lower emission into the work environment.

Special consideration should be given to personal protective equipment (PPE) worn by operators, particularly where the equipment is heavy or difficult to wear, as this may not be worn correctly. It is often asserted that PPE should be 'the last resort', i.e. that PPE should only used if it is not possible to achieve adequate control by other forms of intervention, and it is a requirement of the British health and safety regulations that PPE should be used in this way.

Whenever a control measure is introduced, its effectiveness should only be checked by objective measurements or observations. These checks could include using methods such as dust lamps, smoke tubes, direct reading dust monitors, photoionization detectors or sound level meters.

There is an increasing base of information available about good control practice and the types of control measures that should be implemented on specific work processes. A number of guidance sheets have been published by the British HSE for hazardous substances as part of the COSHH Essentials initiative (www.COSHH-Essentials.org.uk). This type of information provides a guide as to the level of control that is needed to ensure the risks are properly controlled.

1.4.5 Record the significant findings

At the end of the risk assessment process, you must be in a position to demonstrate that the assessment was suitable and sufficient. In particular, that:

- A thorough investigation was made;
- You asked those who might be affected by the hazards for their input;
- You considered all the significant hazards;
- The precautions that were put in place were reasonable and the resultant risk was low.

If the current controls are insufficient to properly control the risk then further measures must be introduced. Any recommendations for further control measures should be identified in the written record of the assessment.

In our view, it is good practice to always record a risk assessment, although if there is a small number of people exposed and the hazard is relatively slight then it may not be necessary to make an extensive written record of the assessment.

1.4.6 Review the assessment regularly and revise it if necessary

Risk assessments must be reviewed at suitable intervals or if there has been an important change to the work process or work environment. If any cases of injury and ill health are identified amongst workers on a process then the risk assessment should be immediately reviewed to ensure that it is still valid.

1.5 Who should carry out risk assessment

To undertake a risk assessment you need to have an appropriate level of training, knowledge and experience. Some regulations or official guidance specify that the risk assessment should be undertaken by a competent person, but you should assume that competence is required by everyone undertaking this type of work. However, the level of competence may vary from one situation to another, and for example someone assessing the risk in a large petrochemical site will need to have a greater level of competence than another individual assessing the risk for an office environment. A competent person must be able to recognise their own limitations and when they need further assistance from someone more experienced. This may involve assistance from within the company or external advisors, experts or consultants. Usually, larger companies have specialists such as safety professionals, occupational hygienists and engineers to assist; smaller organisations will need to outsource such advice.

References and further reading

Sadhra SS. (2005). Principles of risk assessment. In: *Occupational Hygiene*, 3rd edition (Gardiner K, Harrington, JM, eds). Oxford, UK: Blackwell Publishing.

HSE (1999). *Five Steps to Risk Assessment*. INDG163. Sudbury, UK: HSE Books. Available at www.hse.gov.uk/pubns/indg163.pdf.

HSE (2004). *A Step by Step Guide to COSHH Assessment*. HSG 97. Sudbury, UK: HSE Books.

HSE (2003). *COSHH Essentials Easy Steps to Control Chemicals*. HSG 193. Sudbury, UK: HSE Books.

The *Scientific Committee on Occupational Exposure Limits* (SCOEL) provides scientific advice to the European Commission to underpin regulatory proposals on exposure limits for chemicals in the workplace. Available at http://ec.europa.eu/social/main.jsp?catId=153&langId=en&intPageId=684.

More information on good control practice techniques is available at HSE's *COSHH Essentials* website. www.coshh-essentials.org.uk/.

HSE's COSHH website provides information about the regulations and how to comply with them, plus a list of WELs. www.hse.gov.uk/coshh/.

HSE information about the calculation of exposure with regard to the specified reference periods, with examples. Available at http://www.hse.gov.uk/coshh/calcmethods.pdf.

2

Identifying Hazards

2.1 Introduction

There is sometimes the perception that our workplaces are relatively hazard-free and that workplace risks to health are now well controlled. However, there are on an average two people killed and 6000 injured from work activities every working day in Britain. If hazards were well identified and the risks they posed managed and understood, then we would not see over 750,000 workers taking time off from work because of work-related ill health resulting in 31 million working days being lost each year. There are also still thousands of people dying from occupational cancers or chronic respiratory disease each year. Unfortunately, there are still more people dying from occupational diseases in Great Britain than those die in road traffic accidents. Improving hazard identification and the subsequent evaluation, control and communication of risks is necessary if we are to see workers' health protected with the resulting advantages that would bring to society.

The costs of failing to identify hazards and controlling their risks in monetary terms can also be high. The following list provides some examples of the potential hidden costs from occupational exposures:

- Compensation for injury/death;
- Medical treatment;
- Replacement labour and training;
- Increased insurance premiums;
- Poorer business image and lost custom;
- Lost time;
- Plant and equipment damage;
- Environmental damage;
- Poor workforce morale.

This chapter provides a framework and guidance for hazard identification.

2.2 Identifying hazards

The ability to identify materials, physical agents, and procedures that have the ability to cause harm to health is central to risk assessment. As we have seen hazardous agents can broadly be categorised into three groups:

- Chemical agents: gases, vapours, liquids and solids of any element or compound;
- Physical agents: noise, heat, cold, ionising and non-ionising radiation, including visible light;
- Biological agents: any living organism or part or product of an organism.

Those responsible for workplace health have traditionally focussed on the first two of these hazard groups primarily found in the extraction and manufacturing industries. However, with the increasing shift to a service-based economy in the developed world, there is greater awareness of the emergence of new hazardous agents. Hazards have also to be re-examined as we begin to use materials in new ways. For example, nano-materials, which are particles smaller than 100 nm (one ten thousandth of a millimetre), may pose entirely different health risks due to their very small size and structure.

So what makes a material hazardous? If we consider chemical substances then the British Control of Substances Hazardous to Health (COSHH) regulations provide us with some guidance. COSHH defines hazardous substances as the following:

- Substances that are very toxic, toxic, harmful, irritant or corrosive;
- Substances with an workplace exposure limit;
- A biological agent;
- Dust of any kind in high concentrations;
- Any other substance that has comparable hazardous properties.

The Chemical (Hazard Information and Packaging for Supply) Regulations (often referred to as CHIP regulations) create a duty on the supplier to classify substances and to provide labels identifying if a material is very toxic, toxic, harmful, irritant or corrosive. These labels are used as a primary source of information for compiling a list of chemical hazards in the workplace. The CHIP regulations were amended in 2009 to introduce a new Globally Harmonised System (GHS) for the classification, labelling and packaging of substances and mixtures.

Suppliers must also provide users with a safety data sheet (SDS – sometimes referred to as a material safety data sheet or MSDS), which provides information relating to the chemical hazards and advice on how to use the agent safely. Of course, process-generated emissions of hazardous substances will not have a SDS or be labelled and you will need to gather the necessary information about these hazards from published sources.

Other sources of information are lists of workplace exposure limits. In Great Britain, the HSE guidance document 'EH40' outlines airborne exposure limits and details risk information for many chemical substances considered to be hazardous. Similar systems exist in many other countries.

Physical agents are sometimes less obvious than chemicals: for example unless you are aware that there is a microwave source inside a particular piece of process equipment you may not realise that there is the potential for exposure to this type of radiation. In most cases, it is difficult or impossible to detect radiation emissions without some sort of measurement device and so to identify the hazard you must thoroughly understand the process. Loud noise is more easily understood and detected. In general, if it is difficult to conduct a conversation with someone close to you without raising your voice then the noise level may be hazardous. Hot work conditions may be hazardous if the air temperature is consistently above 30°C, particularly if the person has to do strenuous physical work and/or they are wearing impervious protective clothing. However, in general with physical agents it is necessary to obtain some further information about the magnitude of exposure before one can be certain whether the conditions are hazardous.

The basic framework for hazard identification in any workplace would utilise all or most of the following steps:

- A walk-through survey of the workplace noting the main processes, tasks, areas, materials used and products (with by-products) produced.
- Compilation of a list of chemicals used and produced in the workplace. This may be obtained from SDSs, existing COSHH assessment records, ordering/purchasing data or directly from labels on bulk containers used on the site. If SDSs are unavailable then labels on containers will provide a supplier telephone number. Suppliers are required by law to provide an SDS for their product on request.
- Identification of any dust, vapour, mist or process fume that is generated throughout the workplace by using information provided by the process management and/or using other information sources about the process.
- Consideration of the use of any biological materials or the possibility of processes that may allow the growth of micro-organisms such as cooling systems, water storage tanks or metalworking fluid sumps in engineering workshops.
- The existence of physical hazards should also be examined. Is there noisy plant or machinery? Is vibrating equipment used? Do workers have to work in hot or cold conditions? Is the lighting of the work area suitable and sufficient for the task being performed? Are there sources of ionising or non-ionising radiation used or produced by the process?
- Discussions with management, union representatives and shop-floor workers are invaluable ways of identifying hazards. Human resource data on staff turnover within sections, sickness and accident rates can also help pinpoint problems within a workplace.

2.3 Example of hazard identification

It is useful to consider an example of hazard identification in a work setting. We examine the hazards involved for a team of workers laying telecommunications cabling. The procedure involves digging up road surfaces, digging trenches, laying cabling, refilling the trench and re-laying the road surface. What are the hazardous agents involved in this task?

The list of hazards to health could include the following:

- Exposure to ultraviolet radiation from the sun while working outdoors;
- Exposure to noise, hand–arm vibration, dust and diesel fumes from the use of pneumatic jack-hammers;
- Exposure to noise and whole-body vibration from driving tracked plant and equipment;
- Exposure to dust generated during the road breaking, digging and filling processes;
- Exposure to vapours and aerosols from hot asphalt used to re-lay the road surface;
- Exposure to biological agents in sewage and standing waters.

There are other possible hazards depending on the exact nature of the task but this list provides an example of the mixture of physical, chemical and biological agents that should be considered in any hazard identification process.

2.4 Conclusions arising from a hazard assessment

An important initial output of the hazard identification process is being able to prioritise actions for those hazards that pose immediate and clearly unacceptable risks. For example, the identification of the use of a material that is now banned due to adverse health effects does not require further risk assessment or measurement but simply removal of that agent from the workplace. Similarly, if there are hazards that can be removed by housekeeping or basic maintenance then these changes can also be carried out at this stage. However, for many hazards there is the need to assess the risks they pose, to measure the workers' exposure and to control exposure to reduce risks to acceptable levels.

References and further reading

HSE (2002). *CHIP for Everyone*. HSG 228. Sudbury, UK: HSE Books.
HSE (2005) *COSHH: A Brief Guide to the Regulations*. INDG 136. Sudbury, UK: HSE Books. Available at http://www.hse.gov.uk/pubns/indg136.pdf.

A list of symbols, abbreviations, risk and safety phrases used on labels and safety data sheets. Available at http://www.hse.gov.uk/chip/phrases.htm.
International Programme for Chemical Safety (IPCS). INCHEM: Authoritative information on the health hazards of chemicals. Available at http://www.inchem.org/.
The US National Toxicity Program Report on Carcinogens. Available at http://ntp.niehs.nih.gov/go/19914.
The NIOSH Pocket Guide to Chemical Hazards provides a source of general industrial hygiene information on several hundred chemicals. Available at http://www.cdc.gov/niosh/npg/.

CCOHS – Canada's national occupational safety and health resource center. www.ccohs.ca/.

Information on physical agents. Available at http://www.ccohs.ca/oshanswers/phys_agents/.

Information on biological agents. Available at http://www.ccohs.ca/oshanswers/biol_hazards/.

Information about chemicals. Available at http://www.ccohs.ca/oshanswers/chemicals/.

3   Exposure, Exposure Routes and Biological Monitoring

3.1   Introduction

Occupational hygiene is built on recognition, evaluation and control of physical, chemical and biological agents within the workplace. It relies on the identification of a hazard, then the ability to quantify the risk to health from that hazard and finally, having the experience and skill to recommend appropriate measures to control that risk. Exposure assessment is key to the evaluation phase of occupational hygiene.

Exposure assessment is the process of quantifying how much of a material comes into contact with a person in a given environment. In occupational hygiene, the judgement can range from simple measures, such as 'exposed' or 'unexposed', through to quantitative indices of level (e.g. mg m^{-3} of air) or cumulative exposure (e.g. mg m^{-3} h).

Figure 3.1 shows a simple 'conceptual' model of the exposure process for hazardous substances. Exposure to hazardous substances can occur in a variety of ways. Chemicals or biological agents may enter the body by inhalation, ingestion, injection or by transfer through the unbroken skin. Inhalation of dusts, fibres, gases and vapours can cause adverse health effects either directly on the respiratory tract or indirectly when the material is inhaled and transferred through the blood to produce effects in the brain, liver, kidneys or other organs. Similarly, dermal exposure may also result in local effects such as skin irritation, or can produce effects elsewhere in the body if the substance is able to pass through the skin and into the blood system. Solvents and other substances that easily dissolve in fats and oils have been found to be particularly able to cross the unbroken skin. Many national OEL systems now have a skin (sk) notation that alerts occupational health and safety professionals and others to the ability of the material to pass through the unbroken skin.

Chemicals can also enter the body by ingestion – either inadvertently or intentionally. For this to occur there must be transfer of the hazardous substance to the mouth, usually by hand contamination, and then the material must be absorbed across the gastrointestinal wall and into the blood. Coarse aerosols that deposit in the upper airways will be trapped in the mucous lining of the airway and eventually be swallowed into the gut. Ingestion in workplace settings is particularly important for pharmaceutical materials, some metals and pesticides.

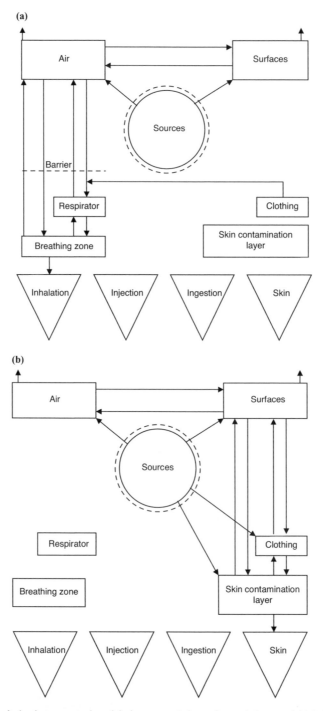

Figure 3.1 A simple conceptual model of exposure to hazardous substances: (a) inhalation; (b) dermal; (c) ingestion; (d) injection.

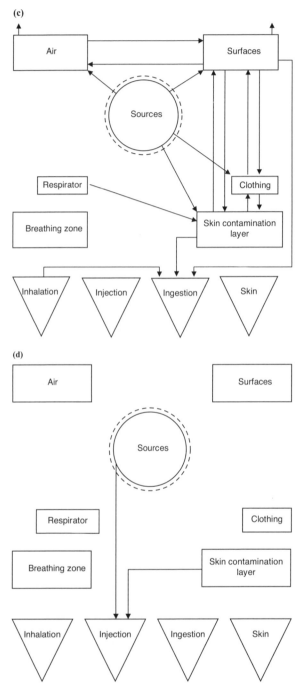

Figure 3.1 A simple conceptual model of exposure to hazardous substances: (a) inhalation; (b) dermal; (c) ingestion; (d) injection. (*Continued*)

Finally, injection – the direct entry of material into the blood or other body tissue – is rare in most occupational scenarios. However, needle-stick injuries in hospitals, which are fairly common, or accidents with high-pressure systems can produce exposure by this route.

In Figure 3.1, the dotted lines are intended to represent some form of barrier, for example around the source represents local control measures such as exhaust ventilation systems applied to the source. Contaminant passes out from the source to one or more compartments, for example the air in the workroom or the walls, benches, floors or tools used by the worker, which are all grouped in the surfaces compartment. The triangular boxes represent the uptake of chemical contaminant into the body by one of the four routes we have identified.

3.2 Measuring exposure

Inhalation exposure can be measured by a monitoring device worn by the worker; this is known as personal monitoring. Alternatively, the concentration of a hazardous substance may be measured in a workspace or at a fixed location, which is known as static or area monitoring. Exposures will vary throughout the workroom and in time, and so personal monitoring is necessary to determine an individual worker's exposure and hence demonstrate compliance with regulations and occupational exposure limits (OELs). This technique involves positioning a sampling device in the 'breathing zone' of workers, the air volume within about 30 cm of their nose and mouth. Static sampling will generally tend to underestimate personal exposures but may be useful when examining the effectiveness of control measures or to identify sources.

The methods that may be employed to measure exposure to a wide range of hazardous substances are detailed in the Health and Safety Executive (HSE) *Methods for Determination of Hazardous Substances* (MDHS) series available in full at the HSE website. These documents provide detailed procedures for both sampling and laboratory analyses of the resultant materials. Where there is no MDHS for a material, an extensive list of methods is also available from the US National Institute of Occupational Safety and Health (NIOSH) in their *Manual of Analytical Methods* – and can be accessed via the NIOSH Pocket Guide for Chemicals online.

The process of measuring dermal exposure in workplaces is much less developed and is not standardized in the same way as inhalation exposure measurements. Measurements can be made by three different approaches: interception methods using patches or whole-body suits to collect the contaminant; removal techniques such as wiping or washing the skin; or visualisation methods using fluorescent tracer techniques. Each type of sampling has advantages and disadvantages and each measures a different aspect of exposure. For example, patches, normally 10 cm^2, measure the amount of material deposited over a part of the body and, by a process of multiplication, can be used to provide an estimate of the total dermal exposure. Differences in the type of material used for patch samplers, the body locations sampled and the patch–substance interaction will all increase the variability of any measurement made. Ingestion exposure is even more difficult to quantify and techniques for measurement are currently being developed.

3.3 Biological monitoring

Biological monitoring is the process of examining how much of a substance has entered the worker's body by measuring the level of contaminant, or a breakdown product specific to that contaminant, in human tissue or body fluids such as saliva, urine, hair, blood or exhaled breath. Biological monitoring has the advantage of integrating the exposures received from all exposure routes and can also provide information on the effectiveness of personal protective equipment (PPE) used to reduce uptake from either airborne exposure or potential dermal exposure. The usefulness of biological monitoring is often limited by the availability of a suitable method to measure the material in body fluids, the half-life of the material in the body and variability in how the body metabolises the substance. The HSE publish Biological Monitoring Guidance Values (BMGVs) for certain substances such as isocyanates, chromium VI and mercury. These are available, together with advice on the timing of collection of samples in relation to the exposure or work-shift, from the HSE publication EH40. Biological monitoring for lead in blood is also required under the Control of Lead at Work (CLW) regulations where exposure is deemed to be significant.

3.4 Exposure assessment: what the legislation requires

Exposure assessment is central to the legislative framework designed to protect workers' health in the Britain. For hazardous substances, which include biological and chemical agents, the Control of Substances Hazardous to Health (COSHH), the Control of Asbestos (CA), or the CLW regulations require the employer to make an assessment of the risk to health of workers and anyone else who might be exposed due to their work activity.

Regulation six of the COSHH regulations outlines the need for this risk assessment to consider the hazardous properties of the substance, 'the level, type and duration of exposure', the circumstances of the work, including the amount of the substance involved; activities, such as maintenance, where there is the potential for a high level of exposure; in circumstances where the work will involve exposure to more than one substance hazardous to health, the risk presented by exposure to such substances in combination; and any relevant OEL. Workplace exposure limits (WELs) are used to define adequate control of a hazardous substance within the COSHH regulations and similar control levels or standards are employed for the CLW and CA regulations.

While the assessment of risk requires judgement of the 'level' or 'degree' of exposure, if the assessment indicates that an exposure limit could be exceeded then, according to regulation 10 of COSHH, exposure monitoring is required. Monitoring is also mandatory when failure of control measures could result in serious health effects. In general, monitoring for hazardous substances where it is required should be carried out at least once every 12 months. In addition to the legal requirements of legislation, exposure data can be used to observe trends. Assessing exposure levels can often provide a measure of improvements in effectiveness of controls or new working methods.

Records of exposure monitoring carried out to comply with regulations should include the results together with details of when, where and the duration of the monitoring, the monitoring procedures employed, processes in progress at the time and the names of those employees who were sampled. In most cases, records of personal exposure monitoring must be kept for at least 40 years.

The Control of Noise at Work (CNW) regulations require employers, whose workers may be exposed to loud noise, to make a suitable and sufficient assessment of the risks to health, which should identify the measures required to comply with the regulations. The assessment could be based on:

- Observation of working practices;
- Reference to data on the probable levels of noise from any equipment used in the workplace; and
- If necessary, measurement of the level of noise to which employees may be exposed.

The CNW regulations contain action levels and exposure limit values expressed as daily or weekly personal noise exposure and peak sound pressure.

The Control of Vibration at Work (CVW) regulations came into force in 2005. These regulations provide daily exposure action and limit values for hand–arm and whole body vibration. The wording of the regulations in relation to assessment is very similar to those for noise. There are no other specific legal obligations concerning monitoring of other physical agents, although there are plans to introduce further legislation in Europe for artificial optical radiation and electromagnetic fields.

3.5 Conclusions

Exposure assessment and biological monitoring are important elements in ensuring control of risks from hazardous substances. In workplaces, there is a range of legislation requiring employers to assess the nature and degree of workers' exposure. While there are many tools available to help in the process of exposure assessment it is important to remember that exposure is often a complex, multi-route process. Simple solutions to complex problems often lead to inadequate control and an increased risk to health, or conversely, expensive and unnecessary measures making industry uncompetitive.

References and further reading

Aw TC. (2005). Biological monitoring. In: *Occupational Hygiene*, 3rd edition (Gardiner K, Harrington JM, eds). Oxford, UK: Blackwell Publishing.

HSE (1997). *Biological Monitoring in the Workplace: A Guide to its Practical Application to Chemical Exposure*. HSG 167. Sudbury, UK: HSE Books.

UK Legislation is available to download from the Office of Public Sector Information. Available at www.opsi.gov.uk/.

HSE Methods for Monitoring Hazardous Substances – MDHS. Available at http://www.hse.gov.uk/pubns/mdhs/.

NIOSH Methods for Monitoring Hazardous Substances. Available at http://www.cdc.gov/niosh/nmam/.

CHAPTER 4

The Exposure Context

4.1 Context for measurement

Exposure varies, from day to day, from one worker to another doing the same job, from one job to another within a plant, from one plant to another with the same process and so on. Measuring the exposure on one occasion will tell you what the exposure was for that individual on that day but this is not really what we want to achieve, we want to be sure that we know something about all of the workers on a process or a plant or in several plants. Ideally, if we are trying to control exposure below the OEL then we want to know that only a small proportion of exposures exceed the limit at our work site. To do this we should make sufficient measurements of exposure to be sure that we have a reliable picture of the actual exposures experienced, but we are almost always constrained by the amount of resource available and we have to do the best possible jobs with what is available to us.

To be able to reach a valid conclusion about exposure from a limited number of measurements we need to understand those factors in the workplace that can influence the variability in exposure. For example, it is clear that if the process is running at half of its maximum capacity then exposure to noise and hazardous substances will be lower than when the process is running full out. In this section we explain how the process, the worker and the workplace environment can influence the level of inhalation exposure so that we can better understand how to interpret our exposure measurement data. We will focus on inhalation of hazardous substances, although the principles apply to all areas of occupational hygiene practice.

The approach we have taken is to use a simple model of how all of these factors interact so that their relative importance can be better understood. The model is technically known as a "source-receptor" model and it can help trace the pathway that the hazardous substance follows as it is emitted from a source and travels through the workplace to the breathing zone of the worker, i.e. the receptor. In fact this is the model shown in Figure 3.1a.

4.2 Sources of hazardous substances

The source or sources may be an open container of solvent sitting on a work-bench or a wallboard that is being cut with a saw; it could be paint that is to be applied to a vehicle or a powder about to be compressed into a tablet in a pharmaceutical plant. The key thing about a source is that it has the potential to release the hazard into the area where people are working. Although as we have said it is possible to have multiple sources for the sake of simplicity, we will continue the model description for the simplified case where there is just one source.

For chemicals, the source can be characterized in terms of three factors:

- The intrinsic ability of the material to release aerosols, gases or vapours – referred to as the *substance emission potential;*
- The amount of energy being input to the source as part of the process, or the *activity emission potential* and
- The effectiveness of any local control measures, such a local ventilation – the *localized control* factor.

The substance emission potential is dependent on the dustiness of solid materials, the ease with which aerosols can be generated from liquids or the ability of liquids to evaporate into the air. Dustiness has been measured for a range of powders by using a variety of test apparatus involving dropping the materials from a fixed height or agitating the material in a rotating drum or a vibrating container. Some investigators have used simulations of the process to assess differences in dustiness of solids, e.g. drilling into rock. There is no defined mathematical relationship between the material properties and the dustiness, but the powder size distribution, the surface properties of powders, the cohesiveness of aggregates and the moisture content of the material are all important. The intrinsic properties of liquids that determine evaporation are predominantly the vapour pressure of the liquid and the composition of the mixture. Some products containing solids and liquids, e.g. paints, can form a solid film across the liquid surface reducing the amount of evaporation of the liquid components.

Second, the handling of the material can influence the emission from a source – more energy input equates to higher emissions. See the following for example:

- Dropping a powder from a greater height will increase the airborne dust generated;
- Heating a liquid will increase the emissions from evaporation;
- Vigorously bubbling air through a liquid will increase evaporation and aerosol formation compared to an undisturbed liquid;
- Using a pneumatic chipping hammer will produce more airborne dust from a rock surface than a hammer and chisel.

The amount of materials being handled in a process will also dictate the emissions and so a laboratory scale pharmaceutical process will emit less dust than the same process scaled up to handle ten times the mass of product – all other things being equal.

The third factor that determines the strength of emissions from a source is the effectiveness of any local controls such as local ventilation or some form of enclosure around the source. If we took the pharmaceutical process that we are scaling up from the laboratory prototype and designed a number of additional local controls, for example by placing the powder handling stages inside a ventilated cabinet then it might be that rather than exposures being higher in the full-scale process they could be lower.

There is one type of source that is worth some further description, these are passive or fugitive emission sources. These sources are often due to uncontrolled factors, for example equipment leaks, evaporation from spills or draughts blowing settled dust around. The key difference with these sources is that it is almost impossible to apply local controls to them because by their very nature they tend to be unpredictable in terms of where and when they will happen. Fortunately, passive sources are generally much less important in terms of worker exposure than active emission sources.

4.3   Dispersion through the workroom

Once the hazard has escaped from the local region around the source it is free to disperse throughout the workroom air because of airflow, either from the many different 'random' airflows present in any room – a phenomenon referred to as turbulent diffusion – or because of some directed airflow coming, for example, from an air-supply vent, or from an open door or window. The dispersion process can be quite complex, but it is possible to simplify the way we think about these processes by dividing the work area into two 'virtual' regions: the 'near-field' and the 'far-field'. The near-field is essentially everything that is within touching distance of the worker; i.e. this is a region centred on the worker and it moves with her as she moves around the workroom. The far-field is everything else in the workroom. Then all we need to do is think whether a source is in the near- or far-field to decide how important it is. In most situations near-field sources are between about two and ten times more important than far-field sources. In the model shown in Figure 3.1, this would correspond to splitting the air compartment into two regions.

An example of a near-field source would be a worker weighing powder from a drum by using a scoop, where the source is the process of emptying the scoop onto the weigh scales. This would be a far-field source for this woman's supervisor who works in the general vicinity of the process but is not directly involved.

The relationship between near- and far-field exposure levels depend on three factors: the volume of the workroom, the quantity of general ventilation air flowing in and out of the workroom and the duration of the task. Figure 4.1 shows how the ratio between the near- and far-field changes with the size of the workroom and the general ventilation rate, described in 'air-changes per hour' (ACH). For example, for a large room (3000 m^3) with a low level of general ventilation (0.3 ACH) the near-field exposure level is likely to be about eight times higher than the far-field level; and so in this case if the supervisor was working alongside an operator who was exposed to 10 mg m^{-3}

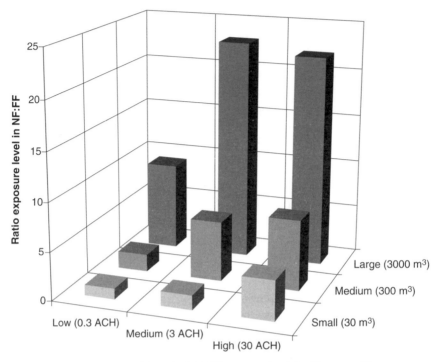

Figure 4.1 The ratio of near- (NF) to far-field (FF) exposure levels in different conditions.

of airborne dust then they would probably have exposure at around 1.25 mg m^{-3}, i.e. an eighth of the operator's level.

Figure 4.1 also shows that for small rooms with low ventilation rates the concentration is fairly uniform throughout; i.e. the ratio of near- and far-field levels is close to one. This kind of environment is described as a 'confined space' and they present particular problems in terms of control because of the possibility of high levels of exposure arising from relatively small sources. For a task involving a volatile liquid carried out for 8-h in a confined space the exposure could be more than 10 or 20 times higher than the level that would occur if the same operation had been undertaken in a large well-ventilated space.

The third factor is the duration of the task and here the difference between near- and far-field will be greater if the task is only carried out for a relatively short time, i.e. less than about an hour, compared to longer durations. The task duration is less important for larger and better ventilated rooms.

One factor that can reduce exposure during transmission is the presence of barriers away from the source such as plastic curtains dividing a workroom into smaller areas (i.e. segregation) or the presence of an enclosure around the worker separating him from the sources (i.e. separation).

4.4 Receptor

The exposure level in the breathing zone of an individual is the summation of all of the exposures coming from sources in the far-field and near-field, modified by the effect of the room size, general ventilation and task duration as already described. The final inhaled exposure that the person receives may be modified if they are wearing a respirator, which will remove part of the contaminant before it is inhaled. Respirator effectiveness depends on a number of different factors, but most important are the design of the respirator and the personal factors involved with the wearing of the device. For example, a full-face respirator will give a higher level of protection than a half-mask device, unless of course the person wearing it does not fit it correctly to the face or the respirator does not fit their face. Respirators can provide a very high level of protection when compared with the effectiveness of other control measures, such as local ventilation. However, they can come with a 'high cost' in terms of discomfort to the wearer and if the respirator is not worn then it provides no protection. Respirators are therefore often considered as the 'last resort' for exposure control.

4.5 Jobs and tasks

A workday generally encompasses several tasks and the exposure can differ from one to the next. If a process operator spends 2 h in preparatory work, 4 h running the process and 2 h finishing and cleaning their work equipment then their exposure profile may be something like that shown in Figure 4.2.

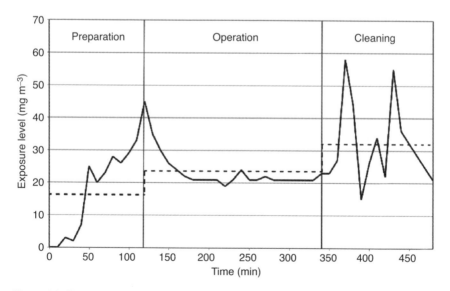

Figure 4.2 Exposure over a working shift.

In Figure 4.2, the solid line shows the level of exposure measured every 10 min throughout the shift and the dotted line is the average exposure over each of the three tasks.

It is important to understand which tasks are undertaken and particularly the duration of each task as this is a major determinant of exposure. For example, if on the day that monitoring was undertaken there was a problem with the production run and the processing took 6 h; and as a consequence there was no time to finish up and this was done by the following shift then the measured exposure might be expected to be lower because the cleaning work is the part of the job that has the potential to give high exposure, up to almost 60 mg m^{-3} on occasions.

References and further reading

Tielemans E, Schneider T, Goede H, Tischer M, Warren N, Kromhout H, van Tongeren M, van Hemmen J, Cherrie JW. (2008). Conceptual model for assessment of inhalation exposure: Defining modifying factors. Annals of Occupational Hygiene 52(7): 577–586.

5 Why Measure?

5.1 Introduction

There are many different reasons for monitoring. It may be that measurements are needed to be sure that the conclusion that has been arrived at as part of a risk assessment is valid, it is possible that we wish to monitor exposure to evaluate whether we are in compliance with an occupational exposure limit (OEL), perhaps we need to evaluate the effectiveness of a particular control measure in reducing the exposure of workers. The following sections briefly discuss a number of different reasons for undertaking a monitoring survey and how the purpose behind the investigation will determine the strategy that should be adopted for monitoring. These are not the only reasons for undertaking monitoring but they will also illustrate the key approaches to monitoring.

5.2 Reasons for undertaking monitoring

5.2.1 To support a risk assessment

Most risk assessments are made without having extensive monitoring data available. However, there are some circumstances where it can be useful to have objective or quantitative data to support the conclusions of the assessment. For example, it may be that you are uncertain whether a specific toxic chemical is emitted as a process-generated emission; i.e. it is not one of the raw materials or final products. In this case, it may be appropriate to collect an air sample at a fixed location close to the process and ask that the sample be analysed for the presence of the chemical of interest.

In some cases, it may be that you are uncertain about the conclusion from a risk assessment made by one of your colleagues, or your boss wants to see something more than your judgement that the risks in a process are unacceptable before they sanction an investment in new control technology. In this case, it might be appropriate to identify those workers who are most likely to be exposed to the highest exposure levels in the process and to make measurements of their exposure. Because you expect the exposures to be above the OEL, the results should provide the confirmatory evidence you are looking for. In any case it is probably not necessary to have a large number of measurements in this type of situation.

5.2.2 To assess compliance with an OEL

The majority of exposure measurements are made to assess compliance with an OEL. In this case, a standard sampling methodology should be used and the duration of the measurements should be sufficient to make reliable estimates of either the long-term or short-term exposure, for whichever the compliance is being assessed. There are no formal procedures specified by the Health and Safety Executive (HSE) to decide when a situation is in compliance or not. We consider that it is sufficient for compliance with a long-term OEL that there should be 90% of measurements below the limit value (i.e. on average 1 in 10 measurements could be above the OEL).

5.2.3 To make a comparison with existing data

In some circumstances you may be interested to repeat some measurements that were made on a previous occasion, for example you may have convinced the company management to install some new local ventilation and want to gather information about the effectiveness of the control measures. In this case, you will need to make measurements of exposure before and after the installation of the ventilation so that you can see how much the average exposure has been reduced. It is important to make a careful record of the process and environmental conditions that prevailed on each occasion and to make sure that they match as far as possible. For example, if the original measurements were made when the process was running at full capacity it would not be appropriate to repeat the measurements during a quiet period when the machines were running only at half capacity; in this case, the exposures might be expected to be lower just because of the process conditions. It is also a good idea in this type of investigation to collect some fixed location samples at strategic points, some close to the process and some further away. If there are other emissions in the vicinity of the machine then these may interfere with the assessment of the change in exposure and the more distant samples will help your interpretation in these circumstances.

5.2.4 To provide baseline information on the exposure distributions within a plant

This is a much more extensive type of monitoring exercise where the purpose is to collect detailed information about the distribution of exposures for all groups of workers in a plant. It implies a collection of a large number of measurements over an extended time period. In many cases with repeated measurements made on the same workers so that you can understand how much exposures vary between people and over time. This type of investigation is rare and is probably only merited when there is some serious concern about the risks in a plant.

5.2.5 To underpin a research study

Some occupational hygienists become involved in research studies to quantify exposures for use in epidemiological studies, to validate measurement methods, compare different methods of measurement or for some other purpose. This type of investigation is very specialized, and in most cases needs specialist expertise to design the measurement strategy.

References and further reading

HSE (2006). *Monitoring Strategies for Hazardous Substances*. HSG 173. Sudbury, UK: HSE Books.

BSI (1996). *Workplace Atmospheres — Guidance for the Assessment of Exposure by Inhalation to Chemical Agents for Comparison with Limit Values and Measurement Strategy*. BS EN 689. London: BSI. (Note: This standard has come in for some criticism, e.g. from Prof Hans Kromhout from the University of Utrecht.)

Kromhout H. (2002). Design of measurement strategies for workplace exposures. *Occupational and Environmental Medicine* 59(5): 349–354.

6 How to Carry Out a Survey

6.1 Introduction

We have previously looked at the main reasons for undertaking measurement of exposure to health hazards in the workplace and the basis of sampling strategies. Ensuring compliance with an exposure limit is one of the most common aims of the survey, as are assessing the effectiveness of control measures and providing re-assurance to the workforce or neighbouring population. It is therefore important to make sure that the design of a survey will address the primary aim and will allow conclusions to be drawn that answer the underlying question being asked. In this chapter we discuss the planning of a measurement survey and the design of an appropriate monitoring strategy.

6.2 Planning the survey

Preparation and planning are the key elements of successful surveys. Contact with the management of the factory or production line where the survey will take place should be initiated at an early stage. This will help to determine the equipment that can be used, the most appropriate time to carry out the visit and any limiting features of the work process, site or workforce that could have a bearing on the measurements. One of the commonest problems that can arise during a survey stems from the failure of the management to understand that the measurements should be carried out at a time that is representative of 'normal' work conditions. You should avoid completing a survey at a quiet time or when machinery is down for maintenance because the results gained will not tell you much about typical exposures. A visit to the site should be made wherever possible before any monitoring is carried out. If the site is too distant to make a visit then a plan and photographs of the areas to be surveyed should be obtained. A telephone conversation with the line manager or health and safety manager to gather details of the number of workers in each area, tasks, processes and materials used are invaluable. Copies of any relevant risk assessment reports should also be obtained.

We have provided some examples of basic checklists for survey items as a guide (see Section 6.6). These checklists should be supplemented if additional items are required and in the light of experience of a particular worksite or industrial sector. The checklists also contain items of protective clothing as you may be uncertain about whether the level of risk is acceptable. Health and safety professionals need to protect themselves and set a good example to others. Always follow the company policy on wearing respirators, hearing defenders or other items of personal protective equipment. It is also important to make sure that all measurement equipment to be used during the survey is calibrated by a competent individual or organisation and maintained according to the manufacturers' instructions.

Photographs of the workplace and particular processes can be a useful aid to memory or to illustrate some point in the report, although permission must always be sought to take them. Similarly, a video camera can also serve to show process control failures or visible emissions from sources.

We strongly recommend that you take some time and write down the purpose that you wish to achieve from the survey. For example, this might be the following:

• Does the styrene inhalation exposure for workers in the widget department, averaged over both 8 h and 15 min, exceed the WEL?

  or

• Is long-term exposure to respirable mica dust for workers on the packing machine lower than before the local ventilation system was upgraded?

6.3 Workplace monitoring

Workplace monitoring can be divided into either routine or operational monitoring. Routine monitoring allows you to keep a check on whether exposures are satisfactory for continuing operations. It is a confirmatory activity but may include provision for the detection of the onset of abnormal or emergency conditions. Operational monitoring provides information about a particular operation, procedure or workplace. It is useful where routine monitoring is not feasible or when specific procedures are carried out.

Special monitoring is carried out for various reasons such as to check the adequacy of control equipment; to examine an operation that is carried out under abnormal conditions; to confirm design specifications; to settle disputes; or to investigate certain features of exposure. Special monitoring is therefore of limited duration with clear objectives and is terminated once the problems are identified or decisions are taken about appropriate routine or operational monitoring.

Ideally, a comprehensive monitoring programme should include the measurement, evaluation and recording of all exposures incurred by all employees involved in a particular work activity. The methods used for monitoring that should be considered are the following: (1) personal monitoring; (2) workplace or area monitoring; (3) the measurement of surface contamination where necessary and (4) biological monitoring.

A system of monitoring should aim to:

- Specify the type and extent of monitoring that must be carried out;
- Select suitable instruments, dosimeters and analytical techniques;
- Test, calibrate and maintain equipment;
- Identify the descriptive information about the work and workplace that should be recorded at the time of the measurements;
- Carry out monitoring and sample collection;
- Analyse, process and interpret monitoring data;
- Maintain monitoring records;
- Produce a system for reporting the monitoring results in an appropriate form to management, supervisors, employees, safety representatives and other interested parties;
- Check on reproducibility and quality assurance of monitoring techniques;
- Correlate monitoring data with medical and other observations made, particularly exposure determinants;
- Check the implementation of recommendations resulting from monitoring data.

In terms of planning a larger survey it is usually an advantage to involve at least two people, one of whom need not be involved in the technical aspects, but is available to record results and note the workplace operations that are taking place. The amount of work that can be done in a shift will depend upon the layout of the work area to be surveyed. For example, in the case of an airborne dust survey, no investigator should be expected to have more than ten sampling pumps running simultaneously without the help of an assistant, and if the area to be covered involves several workrooms or large distances between workers then even fewer samples per investigator should be collected.

The location where sampling is being carried out should be supervised throughout the measurements, not only to make a note of the type of activities that are being carried out, but also to watch the equipment to minimise the risk of accidental or deliberate interference with the measurements. Noise dosimeters often show characteristic peaks a few minutes after the surveyor has left the workplace as workers and their colleagues shout into or tap the microphone. Other deliberate actions may have a more long-term effect on the results; these include removing the sampling device and leaving it in the staff room or locker leading to an underestimation of exposure. Alternatively, workers who have an interest in exaggerating their exposures may place the sampling device near to an emission source or can introduce handfuls of the material directly on to the sampling head. Careful explanation of the nature of the survey to the workers, together with encouraging their involvement and interest in the results can help prevent these actions and can be time well spent in the planning or initial stage of any survey. In most cases deliberate tampering produces extreme results. In these situations you should 'do a reality check' and discount the results if they are implausible.

6.4 Monitoring strategies

Decisions must be made about the appropriate monitoring strategy to meet the need of the survey. When and how the monitoring will be carried out should be specified and the measuring or sampling methods to be used must be determined. The locations and sampling frequency must be decided and consideration must be given to how the results are to be interpreted and presented. For example, sampling may be carried out on a representative group of workers only or may be carried out among individuals doing selected tasks when exposures are likely to be high. Where the aim of the survey is to compare exposures at two time points, it is important to ensure as far as possible that the basic conditions are similar, e.g. production rate, materials handled, and weather. It is good practice to write down the sampling strategy before undertaking the work and to think carefully whether it will achieve the overall aim of the survey. Writing it down will help you be sure you have a good plan.

Sampling strategies such as that described earlier are not suitable if excursions above the occupational exposure limit (OEL) could cause serious, irreversible health effects because even if an excursion is identified it is too late as the individual's health is already damaged.

Selecting individuals for sampling from a group of workers can be an efficient way of organising the monitoring effort. However, you must try as far as possible to choose workers who are similarly exposed, for example because they do the same or a similar job. This is because we are trying to protect all of the workers and therefore any results that we obtain from the subset of people sampled should also be relevant to the rest of the group. Groupings have the practical advantage that resources can be concentrated on those workers with the highest exposure as the variability in exposure levels should be smaller for well-defined groups than for the exposed workforce as a whole. However, it is necessary to verify that groups have been properly selected by critical study of the work patterns and examination of the preliminary sampling data. If you have chosen your groups well, you will have what is called a 'similarly exposed group' (SEG), sometimes, perhaps a little optimistically, also known as a 'homogeneous exposure group'.

When it is possible to clearly identify times where higher exposures occur, e.g. because of high emissions from certain working activities or based on screening measurements, then the sampling periods can be selected to contain these episodes. This approach is called 'worst case sampling'.

To obtain the best estimate of exposure a structured approach is necessary. This should be based on knowledge and experience of the site. It may be helpful to carry out an initial appraisal of the area to be monitored; followed by a basic survey and then finally a more detailed survey. The results of these may indicate if some form of regular monitoring is required.

The initial appraisal can serve the following purposes:

- Indicate, identify or define the problem;
- Show the range and pattern of exposure, highlighting the likely variability of results;
- Provide the order of magnitude of the exposures to compare with published national, international or company standards;
- Identify what protective equipment is required for the assessor to safely carry out the survey.

From this information a more detailed survey can be planned with confidence. Alternatively, it could show that further measurement is unnecessary.

A preliminary risk assessment should suggest whether full-shift sampling is necessary or whether sampling over a shorter period could be more appropriate. It is often better to carry out a number of part-shift samples than one sample for the full-shift. For example, an operative may work in an area for part of the shift where exposure is high but for the remaining time they may be in an area where exposure is low. A full shift sample will indicate the worker's average exposure on that day, but would not indicate how much of that exposure was obtained from the high-exposure source. At times, spot samples or samples taken during the shift to coincide with natural gaps for meal breaks or rest periods may be more useful. In general, it is advisable to ensure that at least 6 h out of an 8-h shift are sampled, and it is preferable to sample for the whole of the working time. Samples of less than 6 h duration may provide higher or lower results than should be the case with 8 h sampling; i.e. the data are more variable.

Whenever possible personal monitoring should be carried out which, for airborne pollution, should be in the breathing zone of the worker. However, this is not always possible and static monitoring may be the only recourse available. For example, it is unwise to ask a worker to carry a glass bubbler containing a liquid reagent as it may break or spilt, sometimes the noise monitor available may be too bulky to be worn as a personal sampler. In these cases, a static sampler placed as close to the worker as possible has to suffice but it must be realised that it may underestimate the true exposure. As described earlier, the difference between static and personal samples will be greatest where the static samples are collected in the background of larger rooms; in these circumstances static sample measurement results can be about a tenth of personal sample results.

There are two basic approaches for the selection of employees to be sampled if representative exposure data are required for a group of people who undertake substantially the same work and are exposed to the same substance(s). The best approach is to select individuals at random from the group, which, if sufficient measurements are made, avoids any selection bias. In most situations we believe it is better to select those to be sampled randomly. Various authorities give advice on how to choose, recommending minimum numbers based upon the total size of the workforce employed on that process. For small workplaces it is best to sample everyone that is available and willing to participate. The HSE provide advice on monitoring strategies in their guidance note HSG 173. They recommend monitoring one in five persons of each group for worst case monitoring and five in ten persons of each group for representative monitoring. The US NIOSH sampling strategy manual suggests that out of a group of eight employees seven should be selected; out of a group of 15, 12 should be selected; and out of a group of 50, 18. This pre-supposes that all the chosen employees will agree to be sampled and that sufficient sampling equipment and personnel are available.

Careful notes of the positioning, timing and type of monitoring employed should be taken during the survey. Pre-prepared standard record sheets should be drawn up, which should at least contain the following information:

- The location of the sample to include reference to a sketch plan or photograph of the workplace;
- Whether the sample was personal, that is taken in the breathing zone of a worker, or static, i.e. at a fixed position;
- If static, how close it is to the source of pollution, noise or radiation;
- If personal, the employees' names and job being undertaken;
- The results of the measurement: airborne concentration, noise level or dose, radiation level or dose;
- The date, time and duration of the sampling period;
- Details of any special conditions prevailing at the time that may make the results untypical;
- Whether personal protective equipment (PPE) was being worn during the sampling period and, if so, the type.

The next chapter outlines how the results of the measurement survey should be used and how exposure data should be interpreted but it is important to maintain focus on the reason for the survey throughout the measurement–analysis–reporting chain. This will ensure that the company and workforce receive a report that provides solutions to their problems.

6.5 Quality assurance and quality control

There are a number of simple quality assurance or quality control procedures that should be applied to monitoring to help ensure the reliability of the final results. In Britain, there is also a system to accredit organisations that undertake sampling and analysis, which is run by the organisation UKAS (www.UKAS.com).

The key first step for reliable measurement is to use a consistent system for numbering samples so that every sample that you collect or every measurement that you make is uniquely identified. The sample-identifying number should be on the sample holder and all of the relevant records sheets. Ideally, you should also keep a log of numbers that have been used and in which work sites and departments so that you can easily cross-check your data.

Any measurement equipment that is used should be calibrated as recommended by the manufacturer. So for noise measurements, the sound level meter or dosimeter should generally be calibrated on each occasion it is used and sometimes it is prudent to calibrate the instrument more frequently. For air sampling using pump systems, the flow measurement system should be calibrated at least once each year and this should be done in a way that verifies the accuracy of the reading of flow rate. Sometimes it is recommended that it should be calibrated against a 'primary standard', although more frequent comparison of a working flowmeter should be made with a secondary calibration device. Calibration of flowmeters against a primary standard is not difficult, but there are also organisations that can provide this service for you.

Where several air samples are taken during a single measurement exercise it is good practice to also obtain a proportion of 'field blanks', which are samples that have been taken to the worksite and handled in exactly the same way as the other samples with the exception that no air is drawn through the sampling media. We suggest that one in ten samples you send for analysis should be field blanks. In most cases, these samples will return a zero or very low result. However, if you obtain a significant amount of chemical on a blank then it is an indication of some contamination of all of the samples and some further investigation is needed to identify the problem.

A further step that can be used to check the reliability of the analytical procedures is to prepare a sample 'spiked' with a known amount of the chemical and submit it to the laboratory for analysis along with the batch of samples from the workplace. Spiked samples can be prepared for vapours by using a micropipette to dose the sampling media with an appropriate quantity of the substance of interest in the analysis. If the result returned by the laboratory is markedly different from the amount spiked onto the sample then it is again a trigger for some further investigation. Of course this procedure must be carefully carried out to ensure that the sample is accurately loaded with the chemical.

Where samples are analysed by a laboratory there should be additional quality assurance applied during the analytical work and this should be a normal part of their service. The best way to guarantee a consistent level of quality in any analysis is to choose a laboratory that has been accredited under the UKAS scheme.

6.6 Survey checklists

Table 6.1 Dust survey equipment check list

Item as required	Amount	Packed	Returned
Adhesive tape			
Camera			
Carrying case			
Clip board			
Cyclone filter holder			
Dust lamp			
Electronic calculator			
Filters (weighed)			
Filter holders and covers			
Forceps or tweezers			
Harnesses			
Knife			
Labels			
Membrane filters			
Paper			
Pens and pencils			
Petri dishes or storage tins			
Plastic bags			
Pumps – high flow			
Pumps – medium flow			
Results sheets			
Rotameter and calibration chart			
Safety pins			
Scissors			
Screwdrivers (small)			
Smoke tube kit			
String			
Tape measure			
Tripods			
Tubing			
Timer or stop watch			
Safety clothing:			
Shoes			
Goggles			
Helmet			
Respirator			
Gloves			
Overalls			
Ear defenders			

Table 6.2 Gases and vapours survey equipment check list

Item as required	Amount	Packed	Returned
Adhesive tape			
Adsorbent tubes			
Bubblers (empty)			
Bubblers (full)			
Bubbler reagent			
Camera			
Carrying case			
Clip board			
Colorimetric detector tubes and pump			
Direct reading instrument			
Electronic calculator			
Filters			
Filter holders			
Forceps or tweezers			
Harnesses			
Knife			
Labels			
Passive samplers			
Paper			
Pens and pencils			
Plastic bags			
Pumps – low flow			
Pumps – medium flow			
Result sheets			
Rotameter and calibration chart			
Safety pins			
Sampling bags: mylar or tedlar			
Scissors			
Screwdriver (small)			
Smoke tube kit			
String			
Tape measure			
Tripods			
Tubing (check bore)			
Vacuum tubes			
Timer or stop watch			
Safety clothing:			
Shoes			
Goggles			
Helmet			
Respirator			
Gloves			
Overalls			
Ear defenders			

Table 6.3 Thermal survey equipment list

Item as required	Amount	Packed	Returned
Adhesive tape			
Camera			
Carrying case			
Clip board			
Distilled water			
Dry bulb thermometers			
Electronic calculator			
Globe thermometer (large) and charts			
Globe thermometer (small) and charts			
Heat index charts			
Kata thermometer and charts			
Natural wet bulb thermometer: wicks and beakers			
Paper			
Pens and pencils			
Reflective foil and corks			
Results sheets			
Swing psychrometer (whirling hygrometer)			
Smoke tube kit			
Spare thermometers			
Spare wicks			
Tape measure			
Thermos flask and hot water			
Timer or stop watch			
Tripod:			
Stand			
Boss heads			
Clamps			
WBGT meter or other direct reading monitor			
Safety clothing:			
Shoes			
Goggles			
Helmet			
Respirator			
Gloves			
Overalls			
Ear defenders			

Table 6.4 Ventilation survey equipment check list

Item as required	Amount	Packed	Returned
Anemometer, heated head type			
Anemometer, digital or vane type			
Aneroid barometer			
Camera			
Calibration charts			
Carrying case			
Clip board			
Diaphragm pressure gauge			
Drill and bit for hole boring in ducts			
Electronic calculator			
Manometers			
Manometer liquid			
Marker pen			
Paper			
Pen and pencils			
Pitot-static tubes			
Plasticine or 'Blu-tack'			
Plugs for holes in ducts			
Results sheets			
Smoke tube kit			
Tape measure			
Thermometer			
Timer or stop-watch			
Tracer gas			
Tracer gas detector			
Tubing for gauges and manometers, blue and red			
Safety clothing:			
Shoes			
Goggles			
Helmet			
Respirator			
Gloves			
Overalls			
Ear defenders			

Table 6.5   Noise survey equipment check lists

Item as required	Amount	Packed	Returned
Batteries, spare for meters			
Calibrator			
Camera			
Carrying case			
Clip board			
Dosimeters			
Electronic calculator			
Microphones for meters			
Microphone extensions for meters			
Octave band analyser			
Paper			
Pens and pencils			
Pistonphone calibrator			
Results sheets			
Screwdriver (small)			
Sound level meters			
Tape measure			
Tape recorder, connections and tapes			
Tripods			
Timer or watch			
Safety clothing			
Shoes			
Goggles			
Helmet			
Respirator			
Gloves			
Overalls			
Ear defenders			

Table 6.6 Lighting survey equipment check list

Item as required	Amount	Packed	Returned
Calibration charts			
Camera			
Carrying case			
Clip board			
Daylight factor meter			
Electronic calculator			
Photometer			
CIBSE Code			
Measuring tape (10 m)			
Paper			
Pens and pencils			
Photometer			
Results tables and plans			
Screwdriver (small)			
Tape measure			
Safety clothing:			
Shoes			
Goggles			
Helmet			
Respirator			
Gloves			
Overalls			
Ear defenders			

References and further reading

HSE (2006). *Monitoring Strategies for Hazardous Substances.* HSG 173. Sudbury, UK: HSE Books.

NIOSH (1977). *Occupational Exposure Sampling Strategy Manual.* NIOSH Publication No. 77-173. Cincinnati, OH: NIOSH. Available at www.cdc.gov/niosh/docs/77-173/. (Note: The NIOSH publication is rather old and is in the process of being updated. Search the internet to check whether the updated version has been published. There is an excellent commentary on proposed guidance on sampling strategies: Ogden T. (2009). Proposed British–Dutch guidance on measuring compliance with occupational exposure limits. *Annals of Occupational Hygiene* 53: 775–777.)

7 Analysis of Measurement Results

7.1 Introduction

Understanding measurement results is an important step in coming to a reliable conclusion. This is particularly the case because exposure is variable between people doing the same job and for the same person from one day to the next. In addition, we are often faced with a limited number of measurement results. Using simple statistics can assist you in your evaluation. In this chapter we discuss simple methods that can be used to summarise exposure measurements to bring out the key information.

7.2 Dealing with variability in measurement results

In a bagging plant, a safety advisor made a single measurement of 8 h average exposure to inhalable dust and then sent the sample for analysis. The result that came back showed that the exposure was 100 mg m^{-3}. As one might imagine, she was shocked but she also realized that exposures could vary for many different reasons. After making several enquiries, she was unable to identify any particular reason for the high result. She decided to make a further nine measurements over the next 2 weeks and the results from these are shown in Figure 7.1. These results ranged from <0.5 to 40 mg m^{-3}. It would be easy to conclude that the situation is either completely unpredictable or there is something wrong with the measurement or analysis method. In reality, this is fairly typical of an exposure scenario and in fact, the more data obtained the more the overall picture becomes clearer. Figure 7.2 summarises the results from 100 measurements made in this scenario and it can be seen that the data are starting to form a coherent picture or 'distribution'.

This type of distribution is close to what is often found in occupational hygiene measurements. It is asymmetrical with the majority of measurements towards the lower values and a long 'tail' to the right with a decreasing number of data points. This is often said to be approximated by the statistical distribution known as a log-normal distribution.

It is important to understand that if you only make one measurement in this type of situation it is possible to get a very low measurement, a very high measurement or something in between, and coming to a valid conclusion from this limited information is not possible. The more measurements that are made the greater the confidence that can be placed on any interpretation. After making

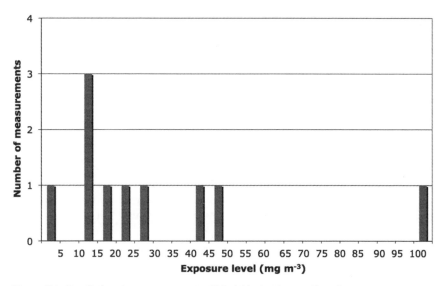

Figure 7.1 Results from ten measurements of inhalable dust in a packing plant.

100 measurements in the scenario outlined here we can be fairly sure that the measurements are typically less than about 25 mg m^{-3} and only about 4% of the results are likely to be above about 100 mg m^{-3}.

These data were for bagging titanium dioxide in an old plant that had no local ventilation on the bagging workstation – the operator was wearing respiratory protection. It is straightforward with this large set of information to

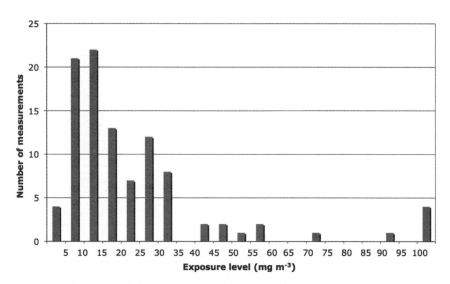

Figure 7.2 Results from 100 measurements of inhalable dust in a packing plant.

conclude that the results show that exposure was above the WEL for this material, which is 10 mg m^{-3} for inhalable dust. When more than about 5% of measurements are above the limit then it is probably sensible to conclude that the limit is exceeded; in this example about half of the results are above 10 mg m^{-3}.

7.3 Summary statistics and data presentation

A set of monitoring data from a single scenario can be summarised by calculating the arithmetic average (mean), geometric mean and geometric standard deviation, although you should only do this if the measurements are all made on the same basis, e.g. 8-h average samples. These summary statistics should only be calculated if the measurements are representative of long-term (i.e. 8-h), short-term (i.e. 15-min) average exposure or some other standardized time period over a workday, and are from the same situation. Samples collected for different durations or from different scenarios should not be considered together when calculating simple summary statistics. In general, you can use the geometric mean to indicate the median of the distribution; i.e. about half of the measurement results should be above and below the geometric mean. The arithmetic mean is more useful in comparing the risk between groups of workers.

The arithmetic mean is calculated by adding all of the measurements together and dividing by the total number of measurements. If E_1, E_2 etc. up to E_n are the exposure measurements, where n is the number of measurements, then the mean exposure E_{ave} is

$$E_{ave} = \frac{\sum_{i=1}^{n} E_i}{n}$$

It is possible to use a computer spreadsheet to calculate the mean and other summary statistics. Further information about the calculation of summary statistics can be found in any elementary statistics textbook. If you use Excel spreadsheets then you can use the functions 'Average' and 'Geomean' to calculate the arithmetic and geometric means for a set of measurements.

In addition to calculating summary statistics, it is often useful to graph your data on what is know as a log–probability plot, which shows the same information that we saw in the histograms but in a more informative way. For example, Figure 7.3 shows a log–probability plot for ten measurements of 8-h inhalable dust exposure level collected for a worker filling sacks with titanium dioxide powder at a workstation where local ventilation had been installed. The horizontal axis is exposure level in mg m^{-3} and the vertical axis is probability (between 0.01 and 0.99). Note the scales on both axes have irregular intervals, the horizontal is the logarithmic scale and the vertical follows a probability scale. The dots represent the measurements. In this type of plot if the data are approximated by a log-normal distribution then they should fall

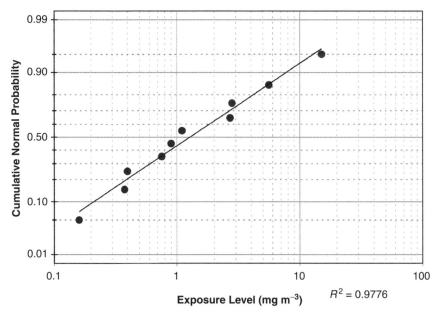

Figure 7.3 A log–probability plot showing data from ten measurements of exposure during bag filling.

on a straight line. It is clear that in this example the data are approximately log-normal.

We can use this type of plot to estimate percentile points of the distribution, e.g. the 90th percentile. On the graph find the 0.90 (90%) on the vertical axis and look across to the point where it crosses the trend line through the data points; in this example it is about 8 mg m^{-3}. This shows that we would expect that on about 90% of occasions the exposure during this bagging task would be less than 8 mg m^{-3}. In this case, we can conclude that the exposures are below the WEL even though there is one measurement above the limit.

In interpreting any set of measurements it is important to take account of contextual information collected at the same time as the samples were obtained. For example, in the two bagging plants described in this section it is important to know that the one that was associated with the higher results had no local ventilation while the lower results came from a situation with effective ventilation. Remember, where the context for a set of measurements differs then it is appropriate to summarise the measurement data separately for each context.

There are many new statistical analysis techniques for monitoring data based on what are known as Bayesian methods. These allow the investigator to use both their judgement about what they expect the exposure level to be and the available measurement data to come to a decision about whether the exposure exceeds the limit value. Some of these developments are described by Professor Gurumurthy Ramachandran (2008) in a recent scientific paper. While these are interesting developments we believe they are beyond the scope of this book.

References and further reading

Kromhout H, van Tongeren M, Burstyn I. (2005). Design of exposure measurement surveys and their statistical analyses. In: *Occupational Hygiene*, 3rd edition (Gardiner K, Harrington JM, eds). Oxford, UK: Blackwell Publishing.

Ramachandran G. (2008). Toward better exposure assessment strategies—The new NIOSH initiative. Annals of Occupational Hygiene 52(5): 297–301. Available at http:// annhyg.oxfordjournals.org/cgi/reprint/52/5/297.

8   Hygiene Reports and Records

8.1   Measurement records

The information that is written in notebooks or sample record sheets from any monitoring survey is the most important record from the investigation. In most cases it is still easiest to use paper to record the details of a survey, and making notes during the investigation should be second nature to anyone undertaking a monitoring survey.

The records from a survey will allow a full interpretation of the results at the time a report is prepared and provide a long-term source of information about any measurement data, which may be useful should any further questions arise about the work at a later date. It is sometimes surprising how useful monitoring records can be after their immediate use, for example to demonstrate to a regulatory inspector that the company has been in compliance with the law or to help defend accusations of negligence in a civil court case. However, just as important is the possibility of using the records to show that the efforts the organisation is making to control exposures are actually working or to help in interpreting the results from health surveillance such as lung function testing on workers exposed to airborne dust.

The basic information that should be collected and recorded during a survey includes the following:

- Details of the premises where the monitoring was carried out, including the workplace and department.
- Details of the process being carried out and the tasks that the worker undertook, including how long each task approximately took to complete. In particular, it is of interest to know whether the processes operated continuously or almost continually or whether they were episodic or irregular, e.g. as in a batch process.
- Where the work was carried out, including a sketch plan of the work area.
- The names and other relevant information to identify the employees' samples, including their job title and whether they were male or female. The exact location where fixed position measurements were made.
- Details of any products or materials being handled or processed, including details of any chemicals – perhaps by obtaining copies of the relevant safety data sheets.

- The substances for which samples are being collected and the methods that will be/were used to analyse them. It is important to specify the reference to the written methodology being followed, e.g. HSE MDHS 14.
- Details of the sampling strategy used, e.g. the way that workers were selected for sampling, the reason for collecting samples and why they were collected at specific times during the day. Sampling strategies are often broadly categorised as 'worst case' – where the workers judged to be most likely to be exposed to higher levels are selected for monitoring, or 'representative'.
- Relevant details of the sampling such as the duration and flowrate through the sampling media, and the results of the monitoring.
- Details of who collected the samples and the organisation or individual who carried out any analysis.

In addition, it is important to make a record of the main items of contextual information that describe the determinants of the exposure level. These may most easily be described by work process or task; i.e. the information generally does not need to be recorded for each sample collected. The main items that should be recorded are the way that the materials were handled in the task or process, the presence and likely effectiveness of any local control measures, and the intrinsic properties of the materials, for example how dusty the materials appeared to be if you are monitoring airborne dust. In addition, records should be kept of whether the work was done outside or inside a building, and if so the size of the building (approximately in cubic metres) and the level of general ventilation (categorised as good or poor – natural or mechanical).

The main items of contextual information that should be recorded at a personal level are the wearing of a respirator and other forms of personal protective equipment (PPE). It is important to record the manufacturer of the PPE and the type or model number. Some information about how long the equipment is worn and an assessment of the likely effectiveness in protecting the individual will be helpful when interpreting the monitoring data. Details of any training in the use of PPE may be held separately in the company files, but if not the investigator should make a note of this also.

More general comments about what happened during a monitoring exercise can also be useful, for example noting periods when the process did not operate because of maintenance problems.

These records may be kept on paper or can be transferred to electronic media, but it is important that you try to retain as much of the original detail as possible. For this reason we recommend archiving any original paper records to a scanned electronic format. Information about measurement quality assurance and/or quality control, e.g. calibration data, should be kept alongside the monitoring records.

There have been attempts to standardise the main records from monitoring by using computer databases. A group of European occupational hygienists proposed a 'standard' for monitoring chemical hazards, and in the United States a separate but similar standard was proposed for chemicals and noise measurements (Lippmann et al., 1996; Rajan et al., 1997). These provide what is known as the core information for storage and provides the minimum set of database elements for workplace exposure databases for chemical agents.

With the introduction of regulations controlling the use of chemicals in Europe and particularly the REACH (*R*egistration, *E*valuation, *A*uthorization and restriction of *CH*emicals) regulations, there have been moves to improve the quality of information in monitoring records. The guidance published with these regulations specifies the information that should be available to justify the use of monitoring data in connection with this legislation. Also, there are moves to develop an Advanced REACH Tool (ART) for exposure assessment, which will contain a database for exposure measurements containing all of the key data elements.

8.2 Survey reports

Measurement of exposure to hazardous substances is almost always carried out to answer a question: for example, is legislation being complied with? or is there a danger to health? or are controls operating properly? The measurements made should provide the data that can be interpreted to answer that question. The art of interpreting and presenting the data is the key to good communication of the results and the delivery of a high-quality report is central to this process.

The final written report tends to be the primary output of the measurement process. It is the means by which information is transferred in a clear and concise manner and is often the tool used by management to reach decisions about the acceptability or otherwise of the measured levels, the need for change and the need to invest in that change. It is important to remember that decisions about health, safety and the environment are rarely made in isolation within an organisation and solutions to exposure problems often have to compete for limited resources within tight budgets. A persuasive and good quality report can help ensure that appropriate decisions can be made. Also, the report is the main long-term record of the results of the survey.

8.2.1 General principles of writing a good report

The ABC of report writing is alacrity, brevity and clarity.

Alacrity – A report finally delivered some 6 months after the measurements were made is likely to be out of date, have limited persuasive capacity ('things have changed since then') and at worst may have allowed workers to continue to be exposed to dangerous levels during the delays. A report should be timely and be provided to the person commissioning the survey as soon as possible on completion of the data collection and interpretation.

Brevity – Keep it brief and to the point. Answer the question posed by the individual or organisation that asked for the measurements to be done.

Extra data, observations or points of interest can be provided at any verbal debrief or in an annex, but the report itself should provide the results and associated solutions in as short a format as possible. A brief executive summary at the beginning of the report should also be provided – this should give the interested reader the key findings, priorities and solutions within a page of text.

Clarity – Consider the audience. Who is the report aimed at? The language and level of technical data should be matched to the experience and understanding of those who will read the report. In most cases, it is always a good idea to keep technical jargon to a minimum, or where it is necessary to include jargon then put it in a technical annex to the report.

More generally, reports should be written in the third person unless it is an expert witness report for a court where there is a need to indicate the observations or opinions relate directly to the author. Where abbreviations are used it is important to make sure that they are fully defined in the text and perhaps also within a glossary at the end or beginning of the report. Sentences should be short, and paragraphs should be used to introduce each new idea or concept. Numbering of sections and paragraphs can be useful in referring to results and in discussions relating to the report at a later stage. Units of measurement should be given and should be consistent throughout the report, for example changing between mg m^{-3} and ppm for vapour exposure measurement data in a report will lead to confusion. Choose one and stick to it. Ideally, you should use the units that are used in the relevant regulations or official guidance.

8.2.2 Report structure

A typical report should contain most of the following elements:

- A title page, including the name and address of the organisation that carried out the measurements;
- A unique report number;
- Name and address of the person who commissioned the survey;
- The name of the person who carried out the survey;
- A contents page;
- A short summary;
- An introduction and statement of the problem, i.e. the purpose of the survey;
- Outline of the relevant legislation;
- A description of the work process, including the conditions prevailing during the measurements;
- Methods used to collect the samples, including the sampling strategy;
- Details of quality assurance procedures;
- Results and discussion;
- Conclusion and recommendations, which should make reference to relevant OELs or other authoritative guidance;

- Name and signature of the investigator;
- References;
- Appendices.

The *title page* should summarise the nature of the report and make it clear what was measured, where and when. The title page should also provide a reference number (this may also be present on the footer of each page, together with a page number, date and total number of pages). In addition, the title page should provide the date of the report; the name and address of the commissioning company; the address of the work site where the measurements were made; contact details of the organisation carrying out the survey; the name, qualifications and signature of the person who prepared the report; and the name, qualifications and signature of the person who has reviewed and checked the report.

A *table of contents* is not always essential but for longer more detailed reports it can provide a useful and quick method of locating material.

The *summary* is essential and should provide the report 'in miniature'. It should cover the purpose of the survey, the main findings and any recommendations. It is often useful to consider that this may be the only page of your report that may be read by busy managers and non-technical staff. Spending time crafting a good executive summary is time well spent.

The *introduction* will state the background to the problem and clearly explain why the report was needed. It will also detail who commissioned the work, identify the sites visited, the dates the survey was carried out and any problems in completing the work as originally planned. This introduction may then lead on to a brief summary of the legislation relevant to the material or process being surveyed. A report of a survey of workers' exposure to lead sulphate would, for example, benefit from a short overview of the requirements of the Control of Lead at Work regulations.

A detailed *process description* is essential. This section will give a description of the area, plant and processes that were surveyed and will also detail the conditions prevailing at the time of the survey. It is useful to indicate how representative of the normal working practices the survey period was and to note unusual occurrences. If, for example, one of two production lines were down because of reduced output at the time of the survey, then this should be identified in this section and highlighted in the report discussion given that it may have had an affect on measured chemical concentrations, noise levels or other occupational exposures.

The *methods and measurement* section will outline the methods used. Referring to the use of previously published or standard methods such as the British HSEs methods for the determination of hazardous substances (MDHS) series is often sufficient. Details of the location, times, durations and names of any workers sampled should be set out in this section. Tables can be useful in summarising this data. Information relating to any quality assurance procedures including laboratory and field blanks and controls will also appear in this section.

The *results and discussion* section should provide a clear and simple presentation of results or observations with direct comparison to occupational exposure limits (OELs), where appropriate. A good discussion will also compare the results with any previous reports or pre-existing data held by the organisation or available within the wider scientific literature. The discussion will finally make an assessment of the risk to the workers' health and consider the need for control options utilising good control practice.

The *conclusions and recommendations* section is likely to be the most frequently read part of the report after the executive summary, and it should also present the key information. The conclusions of the report should answer the questions or concerns identified in the introduction and should clearly state if legislation is being complied with or if there is a breach of regulations, which has to be addressed. Recommendations should be clearly listed in the order of priority and the report should distinguish between measures that are essential and those that would represent good practice.

References supporting any methods used or comparison with standards or other data can be listed in their own section at the end of report or, if there are few of them, as footnotes within the body of the report. *Appendices* can also be used to provide additional data including equipment charts, graphs or raw data. Photographs, diagrams and maps of the area sampled may also be included in this section.

8.2.3   Common pitfalls and administrative points

Tables and graphs are excellent methods of communicating large amounts of measurement data. It is important to make sure that each table and figure has a title and a number and that they are presented at a sufficient size that makes them easy to read and understand. Check that the axes of graphs are labelled and that units are consistent with the text of the report.

It is essential to have the report reviewed before submission. Ideally, the report should be reviewed by someone for grammar, spelling, consistency and typographical errors, and for technical content, if necessary, by another person. While the spell-check facility of many software programmes can be a useful aid it should not be relied on completely. Have a final check of the report in hard copy format, if it is to be provided in this way, paying particular attention to printing errors with figures and graphics. If colour was used in the report make sure that the hard copy of the report is in a similar format and consider what information will be lost if the receiving organisation makes non-colour photocopies.

Finally, make sure your covering letter or accompanying email communication is of a high standard similar to the report you have just completed. This letter is likely to be the first impression of your work and it is important that it is well received. The covering letter should introduce the report and set the ground for any follow-up that may be required. Keep a copy of your report for your own records and always follow-up the delivery of the report to make sure it has been received, has been understood properly and to determine if there is a need for further explanation of your conclusions and/or recommendations.

References and further reading

Lippmann M, Gomez MR, Rawle GM. (1996). Data elements for occupational exposure databases: guidelines and recommendations for airborne hazards and noise. *Applied Occupational and Environmental Hygiene.* 11: 1294–1311.

Rajan B, Alesbury R, Carton B, Gerin M, Litske H, Marquart H, Olsen E, Scheffers T, Stamm R, Woldbaek T. (1997). European proposal for core information for storage and exchange of workplace exposure measurements on chemical agents. *Applied Occupational and Environmental Hygiene* 12: 31–39.

Tielemans E, Marquart H, de Cock J, Groenewold M, van Hemmen J. (2002). A proposal for evaluation of exposure data. *Annals of Occupational Hygiene* 46(3): 287–297. Available at http://annhyg.oxfordjournals.org/cgi/reprint/46/3/287.

Guidance on occupational hygiene reports from the Australian Institute of Occupational Hygienists. Available at www.aioh.org.au/downloads/documents/AIOH_OHReport Guideline.pdf.

2 | Inhalation Exposure

9   Dust and Fibrous Aerosols

9.1   Introduction

The inhalation of dust and fibres can lead to a variety of acute and chronic illnesses and disease. It is important to have reliable measurement methods available to assess the amount of material that workers inhale. Quantification of the exposure can then allow comparison with the requirements of regulations and occupational exposure limits (OELs) to ensure that the risk to health from breathing in such materials is acceptable. This chapter provides practical details of how to carry out measurements of airborne dust and fibres and some background to help interpret the data that the monitoring process generates.

9.2   Airborne dust

Airborne dust is ubiquitous; every operation and action at work releases a certain amount of dust into the air. Movement of people can release dust from clothing and skin. Even dust that has settled on floors and other horizontal surfaces can be made airborne by air currents as people move about their work. Windborne dust enters buildings particularly in dry weather and more so in densely populated areas. Add to that particles released by the operations within a workplace – handling and transfer of materials, machining, cutting, drilling, grinding, milling, sanding and planing of items being manufactured – and a dusty working atmosphere can be produced. Any dust in sufficient concentrations can cause discomfort and over a prolonged period may damage the lung. On the other hand, some dusts are distinctly harmful, giving rise to cancer, asthma, or other serious respiratory disorders.

How dust affects the health of those exposed is determined by the chemical or mineralogical composition of the material, its airborne concentration and by its particle size. The particle size influences the part of the lungs where the material is deposited, the fate of these particles once deposited and, in turn the effect on health. Large particles are deposited in the nose and upper airways of the lung whilst smaller ones are deposited further into the lung. Particles that penetrate the nose or mouth can deposit in the upper airways, i.e. the bronchi and bronchioles, where they may be caught up in the mucous layer lining the lung airways and be cleared to the gut via the ciliary movement of the cells on the airway walls. Very small particles can reach the deepest parts of the lung, the alveoli, where the oxygen transfer with the blood takes place.

Some very small particles are breathed out again and some are removed by body cells but others remain and may cause physical and chemical reactions that can be harmful in both the short and long term, sometimes leading to permanent lung damage.

Particles suspended in air are referred to as an "aerosol". Particle size is measured in micrometres (μm), or a 1000th part of a millimetre; for comparison a human hair is about 30 μm in diameter. Unfortunately, most particles of dust are irregular in shape and rarely spherical or circular, therefore it is difficult to accurately assess their geometric size. However, the important feature related to size is how dust behaves when it is airborne, particularly how rapidly it settles in still air. In the field of occupational health, the term 'aerodynamic diameter' is used to describe particle size. The aerodynamic diameter is the diameter of a spherical particle with a density of 1000 kg m^{-3} that settles at the same speed as the particle in question; thus in this way any irregularly shaped particle can be assigned an aerodynamic diameter.

Inhaled dust reaches different parts of the lung, depending upon its aerodynamic diameter. When measuring aerosols we wish to select a particular size of airborne dust because of the importance of size in determining heath effects. Collaboration between the main international organisations involved with measurement of aerosols[1] has produced agreement on the definition of health-related aerosol fractions. These are termed the *inhalable* fraction, *thoracic* fraction and *respirable* fraction, and are best described by means of the graph shown in Figure 9.1 and briefly below:

- The inhalable fraction, which includes the thoracic and respirable fractions, is defined as the mass fraction of total airborne particles that are inhaled through the nose and/or mouth;
- The thoracic fraction, which includes respirable fraction, is defined as the mass fraction that penetrates the respiratory system beyond the larynx;
- The respirable fraction is defined as the mass fraction that penetrates to the unciliated airways of the lung, known as the alveolar region, where the gas exchange takes place.

The respirable aerosol fraction is represented by a cumulative log-normal curve having a median aerodynamic diameter of 4.25 μm and a standard deviation of 1.5. From the curve in Figure 9.1 it can be seen that dust particles with an aerodynamic diameter larger than about 10 μm cannot reach this region of the lung.

Dust from coal, sand and most hard rocks is particularly harmful if within the respirable size because of its potential to damage the lung where oxygen is taken up; whereas coarser dust, pollens, spores and mists are larger but inhalable and can cause problems in the upper respiratory passages. Fumes from

---

[1] The International Standards Organisation (ISO), the European Committee for Standardisation (CEN) and the American Conference of Governmental Industrial Hygienists (ACGIH).

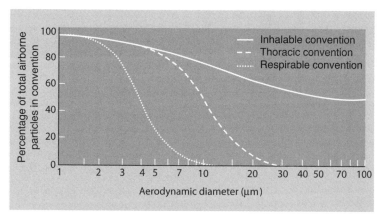

Figure 9.1 The ISO/CEN/ACGIH sampling conventions for health-related aerosol fractions. (Reproduced with permission from *Occupational Hygiene*, 3rd edition, edited by Kerry Gardiner and J. Malcolm Harrington, Blackwell Publishing Ltd., 2005, p. 187.)

vaporised metal contain particles that are very small, below 1 μm, and these can give rise to metal fume fever and more serious acute or chronic effects on the lung or elsewhere in the body. When determining the concentration of airborne dust it is important to understand what size of dust is required to be measured as this influences the method of sampling.

Very small particles, known as nanoparticles, present particular problems for the lung. These particles are smaller than 0.1 μm in diameter or 100 nm (a nanometre is 1000th part of a micrometre). There is good scientific evidence to show that particles a few tens of nanometres in diameter may be considerably more harmful than particles of the same material with diameters in the micrometre size range. Nanoparticles are found in association with a number of industrial processes, particularly combustion-related, but there is increasing use of manufactured nanoparticles in new products and processes.

9.3 Fibres

Fibres are a special type of particles that are longer than they are wide by a ratio of 3:1 or more (the ratio of particle length to diameter is known as its aspect ratio). Their aerodynamic diameter is more closely related to their width rather than their length. Fibres form an important group of particles as they include highly toxic materials, such as asbestos, which can cause respiratory cancer or other respiratory disease. The harmfulness of fibres is in part due to their size and shape, and in part to their biopersistence; i.e. how long they will remain in the lung once they are deposited there. Some types of asbestos may remain in the lung for several decades while many synthetic fibres will dissolve in the fluids in the lung within months or a few years.

Fibres can be classified into four groups: natural organic, natural mineral, synthetic organic and synthetic mineral.

Natural organic fibres include material from plants, such as cotton, hemp, jute, sisal, i.e. the natural constituents of textiles, plus wood fibres and other similar materials. Animal hairs are not normally included here because their aerodynamic diameter is generally not respirable.

Natural mineral fibres are obtained from the earth's crust, consisting of various types of asbestos, wollastonite, sepiolite and other minerals. They can have great strength, excellent fire resistance and good thermal insulation properties. These fibres have been used for thermal insulation on boilers and steam pipes, in acoustic ceiling tiles, in wall panels, roof panels and many other building and industrial applications. Asbestos is subdivided into two mineral groups: serpentines (hydrated magnesium silicates) and amphiboles (calcium, magnesium, sodium and iron silicates). The only serpentine mineral to have a fibrous form is known as chrysotile (white asbestos): when an airborne sample of chrysotile is viewed under a microscope most fibres appear to have a curly shape similar to some organic fibres. The amphiboles have several fibrous forms, for example: crocidolite (blue asbestos), amosite (brown asbestos), tremolite, actinolite and anthophyllite. The last three varieties were used much less commercially and are only occasionally encountered in construction materials. When airborne samples of amphiboles are viewed under a microscope they appear to be straight, needle-like fibres. Morphology is only one indication of fibre type and more elaborate techniques are required to positively identify the fibre. Asbestos fibres less than 3 μm in diameter are considered respirable – that is, they may reach the gas-exchange parts of the lungs (alveoli) where they may cause damage to the body tissue. Methods of sampling for airborne asbestos fibres are described later in this chapter.

Synthetic organic fibres include a wide range of textile and other materials. As far as hazards to health are concerned the main synthetic fibre is para-aramid, although other very fine durable fibres are increasingly being produced. Other synthetic organic fibres mainly used in the textile industry are nylon, orlon, crimplene and rayon. They typically have a physical diameter larger than 3 μm and generally don't produce many respirable-size fibres.

Synthetic mineral fibres are mainly used as a replacement for asbestos and in lower temperature thermal insulation, and are made of a variety of substances such as glass, rock, carbon/graphite and refractory ceramic fibres. These fibres can have a significant fraction with diameter less than 3 μm, i.e. in the respirable range. The methods for measuring synthetic mineral fibres are similar to those used for asbestos. Synthetic mineral fibres are sometimes known as man-made mineral fibres or machine-made mineral fibres (MMMF) and for glassy fibres man-made vitreous fibres (MMVF).

9.4 Measurement of airborne dust levels

There are two basic methods of measuring airborne dust: (a) collection of the aerosol onto a filter and (b) use of direct-reading instruments that directly detect the aerosol.

The first, and most common, method is to draw a known volume of air through a pre-weighed filter by means of an air pump. Weighing the filter before and after sampling determines the mass of dust collected. By dividing that mass by the total volume of air drawn through the filter, an average airborne dust concentration is obtained for the sampling period. The second method involves using an instrument that gives a direct reading of the dust concentration at any instant of time, usually on the basis of scattering of light from the aerosol or some other process.

Filtration systems are lightweight enough to be worn by employees and the equipment can then be used to determine their personal exposure to the airborne dust, i.e. 'personal' monitoring. If the worker moves in and out of dust clouds or if the emission varies in concentration over time then the result reflects the average exposure. The filtration method can also be used to monitor a working area throughout the sampling period – sometimes known as 'static' or 'area' monitoring. In this case, the equipment should, if possible, be attached to a tripod or fixed object in the area under study. To achieve sufficient reliability it is important to weigh the filters with a sensitivity of at least 0.01 mg. During the sampling the flow rates of the pumps must be checked with a calibrated flowmeter so that the total flow rate passing through the filter is accurately known.

An assembly of items is required to make up a sampling 'train' for aerosol sampling, consisting of

- An appropriate filter;
- An appropriate filter holder;
- A suction pump, which includes a rechargeable battery;
- Some connecting tubing;
- A harness.

In addition, a calibrated flowmeter is required to check airflow rates before, during and after sampling. A section on calibrating flowmeters is included later in this chapter.

The direct reading instruments are simple and can be used to track concentrations during tasks. Older instruments can be more bulky than filter sampling equipment and may not always be suited to personal monitoring, although newer instruments are light enough to be used to collect personal measurements. However, direct reading monitors are still often used to measure a working area (i.e. static sampling) rather than individual exposure. Their strength is often as an alarm monitor or as a tool to identify sources of dust, thus allowing better dust control. The measurement data can be logged using internal memory and later downloaded for analysis.

9.4.1 Filters

Filters need to collect the dusts or fibres efficiently and to allow the appropriate analysis to be undertaken.

They are made of a variety of materials with properties suited to different types of analyses. Filters are mainly 'fibrous' in structure. Most are made from glass, paper, polystyrene or from a 'membrane' of cellulose derivatives or PVC. Polycarbonate filters are flat membranes with visible, round pores of specified size. There are also sintered silver and PTFE filters available. The correct filter must be chosen to suit the airborne contaminant to be sampled and the subsequent analysis to be undertaken. For example, some filters can be dissolved in chemicals for further analysis of the collected dust, some can be made transparent for optical microscopic examination of the material collected, whilst others allow the collected dust to remain on the surface for scanning electron microscopic examination. Some filters are more sensitive to atmospheric moisture content than others, and need to be pre-conditioned before weighing. Some filters are particularly susceptible to the effects of electrostatic charge build-up, which can make weighing difficult.

Filters used for dust sampling are available in various sizes, although the 25-mm and 37-mm diameter sizes are most commonly used for personal sampling, with larger ones typically used for high-volume sampling.

Pore sizes, which are a measure of the 'porosity' of the filter and reflect the difficulty in drawing air through the filter material, vary between 0.1 and 10 μm – it is more difficult to draw air through small pore size filters. Note that the pore size does not limit the size of the dust to be collected; that is a 5-μm pore size filter is capable of capturing dusts smaller than 5 μm because the aerosol is captured by inertial and electrostatic forces that occur within the filter medium rather than a simple sieve mechanism. The 'pore size' is set with reference to liquid filtration rather than air filtration. Pore sizes in the range 5–10 μm are used, even for respirable dusts, to reduce the flow resistance and hence the power consumption of the battery in the sampling pump.

For fibre counting with a light microscope, it is useful to have the filter marked with a squared grid as it assists with focusing on the plane of view where the dust is deposited. Some filters are impregnated with a chemical to collect and react with chemically unstable airborne contaminants, e.g. isocyanates.

9.4.2 Filter holders and sampling heads

To accommodate the filter and to make a connection via tubing to the sampling pump a filter holder is required. These should be attached to a person as close to the nose as possible in an area known as the 'breathing zone', i.e. within about 30 cm of the nose. The holder usually has a clip so that it can be hung from a collar or from a harness, useful if the employee wears light workwear. Figure 9.2 shows sampling equipment being worn.

The filter holder is designed either to select inhalable dust on the filter or to separate the respirable fraction, discarding anything larger than about 10 μm. A special holder is also available for sampling asbestos. A range of holders is available for inhalable dust as shown in Figure 9.3. The seven-hole holder, also known as a multi-orifice head shown in Figure 9.3a has been in

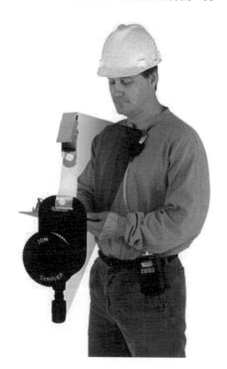

Figure 9.2 Dust sampling equipment worn by operator, with IOM inhalable sampler in blown-up inset. (© SKC Ltd. Reproduced with permission.)

use in Britain for many years but it is now preferable to use a sample holder specifically designed to collect inhalable dust such as the IOM holder, as shown in Figure 9.3b or the conical inhalable sampler, as shown in Figure 9.3c. Note that the IOM inhalable sampler takes 25 mm diameter filters whilst the conical holder takes 37 mm diameter filters. Some filter holders use an internal cassette to contain the filter. The advantage of using a cassette to hold the filter is ease of handling and fewer damaged or contaminated filters; the filter is protected once it has been weighed in the cassette and can be transported pre-loaded into the holder without further handling. Also, there may be some advantage in reducing bias from the dust deposited on the inner walls of the sampler. For measuring inorganic lead (Pb), a holder with a single 4-mm diameter hole was previously recommended, although an inhalable dust sampler is now advised.

Personal sampling of respirable dust is usually undertaken using a cyclone filter holder (Figure 9.4), which uses centrifugal force to remove the coarser dust particles. The dust-laden air spins within the cyclone throwing larger particles to the outside of the holder and thence down into a rubber 'pot' at the base; the contents of the pot are normally discarded. The finer respirable dust particles remain airborne and are collected on the filter. It is important to ensure the correct airflow rate through the sampling head to make the size cut-off follow the respirable curve in Figure 9.1. The cyclone filter holder illustrated in Figure 9.4 achieves this with a sampling flow rate of 2.2 L min^{-1}.

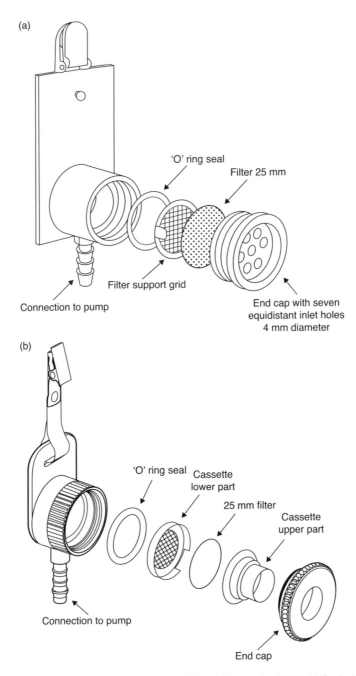

Figure 9.3 (a) Multi-orifice sampler (HSE). (b) IOM inhalable sampler (HSE). (c) Conical inhalable sampler (HSE). (Reproduced with permission *Monitoring for Health Hazards at Work*, 3rd edition, by Indira Ashton and Frank S. Gill, Blackwell Publishing Ltd., 2000. pp. 6–7.)

(c)

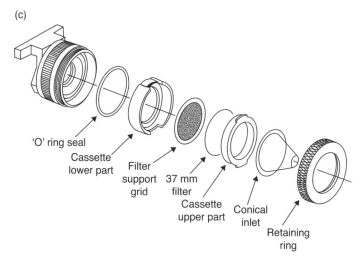

'O' ring seal

Cassette
lower part

Filter
support
grid

37 mm
filter

Cassette
upper part

Conical
inlet

Retaining
ring

Figure 9.3 (a) Multi-orifice sampler (HSE). (b) IOM inhalable sampler (HSE). (c) Conical inhalable sampler (HSE). (Reproduced with permission *Monitoring for Health Hazards at Work*, 3rd edition, by Indira Ashton and Frank S. Gill, Blackwell Publishing Ltd., 2000. pp. 6–7.) *(Continued)*

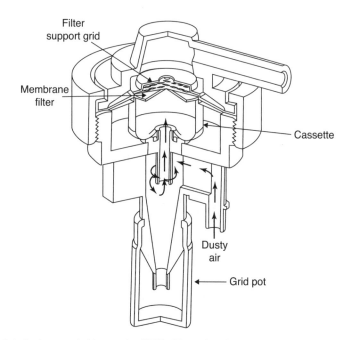

Filter
support grid

Membrane
filter

Cassette

Dusty
air

Grid pot

Figure 9.4 Cyclone respirable sampler (HSE). (Reproduced with permission *Monitoring for Health Hazards at Work*, 3rd edition, by Indira Ashton and Frank S. Gill, Blackwell Publishing Ltd., 2000, p. 9.)

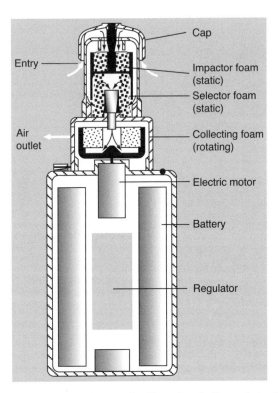

Figure 9.5 The CIP10-R respirable dust sampler. (Reproduced with permission from *Occupational Hygiene*, 3rd edition, edited by Kerry Gardiner and J. Malcolm Harrington, Blackwell Publishing Ltd., 2005, p. 194.)

Other types of personal sampler that give equivalent results to the cyclone respirable dust sampler are the CIP10-R respirable sampler with integral pump, which is operated at 10 L min^{-1}. This sampler is shown in Figure 9.5. The IOM dual-fraction respirable/inhalable sampler is also suitable for simultaneous respirable and inhalable dust sampling; this sampler is operated at 2 L min^{-1}.

For static sampling of respirable dusts some units have a combined pump and filter holder, for example the MRE 113 shown in Figure 9.6. In the past, the MRE sampler was commonly used in coalmines in Great Britain. In this sampler, size selection of respirable particles is achieved by means of an 'elutriator' where the larger sizes settle within a series of parallel plates between which the dust-laden air passes before reaching the 55 mm-diameter filter. As with all size-selection techniques the sampled airflow rate must remain constant at the recommended value for accurate sampling. The currently recommended method for sampling in British coalmines relies on personal sampling by using a cyclone filter holder with static sampling using the MRE 113 sampler.

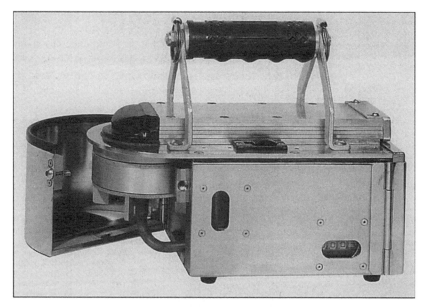

Figure 9.6 The MRE 113 respirable dust sampler (Reproduced with permission *Monitoring for Health Hazards at Work*, 3rd edition, by Indira Ashton and Frank S. Gill, Blackwell Publishing Ltd., 2000, p. 9.)

For asbestos and other fibrous dust sampling a cowl holder is used (see Figure 9.7). This is not size selective but the optical microscope fibre-counting technique used enables the respirable fibres to be selected and counted.

The sampling of welding fume (and gasses) is a little different from other occupational hygiene methodologies because the welder will always wear a visor in front of his face. Although there is an air gap between the visor and the face the barrier provides some small protection against welding fume exposure. To obtain a reliable assessment of the exposure of welders it is normal to place the sampling head behind the visor close to the side of the workers head. The methods are described in full in the standard BS EN ISO 10882. The conventional sampling heads are awkward to locate in the small gap between the face and the visor and some scientists have experimented with miniature sampling heads as an alternative approach (Liden and Surakka, 2009).

9.5   Measurement of flow rate

Flow rate through a filter sampler should be measured before sampling, periodically during the sampling and at the end of sampling. A calibrated flowmeter should be connected to the front face of the filter holder using an adapter provide by the equipment supplier and the flow rate recorded. Care should be taken to ensure that there is a tight connection as any small gaps will allow air to leak past the flowmeter and bias the measurement. At the start of

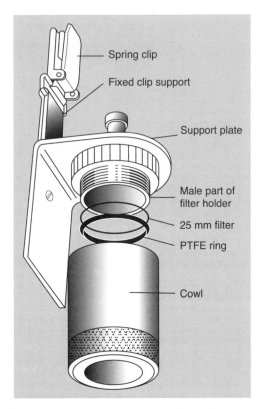

Spring clip

Fixed clip support

Support plate

Male part of
filter holder

25 mm filter

PTFE ring

Cowl

Figure 9.7 The cowl sampler used for asbestos and other fibrous dusts. (Reproduced with permission from *Occupational Hygiene*, 3rd edition, edited by Kerry Gardiner and J. Malcolm Harrington, Blackwell Publishing Ltd., 2005, p. 203.)

the sampling, the flow rate can be adjusted on the pump to match the rate required for the sampling method used. However, it is not recommended to readjust the flow rate partway through the sampling. If the flow rate changes by more than plus or minus 5% of the original value then the sample should be discarded.

9.6 Pumps

There are three basic types of pump unit that have been used: the dry vane rotary, the single-acting diaphragm and the double-acting piston. Rotary pumps produce the smoothest flow rates; the piston and diaphragm pumps produce a pulsating flow and require a flow 'smoother' to be added to the sampling train if particle size selective sampling is being undertaken. Although most modern sampling pumps have a diaphragm mechanism they also have an integrated flow smoother. Note that pulsating flow can cause errors in flow measurement with some types of flowmeter.

For personal sampling, portable battery operated pumps are used, some of which can achieve flow rates of up to 15 L min^{-1}. Some pumps have built-in flow sensors or rotameter-type flowmeters, although it is still necessary to measure the flow with an external flowmeter. Sampling pumps are battery-powered using rechargeable batteries and the suppliers provide suitable chargers. Personal sampling pumps should have automatic constant flow control and may have timers to start and stop the sampling at pre-set times and to record the elapsed sampling time.

Constant mass flow or constant volume flow pumps are used to achieve flow control. Two approaches are generally used to compensate for variations in flow: the critical orifice, where a constant pressure differential is achieved throughout the sampling, or a sensor is used to maintain a constant speed of rotation of the motor (i.e. constant volume flow). In practice either approach will provide adequate flow control.

9.7 Direct-reading aerosol monitors

Compared with the filter method, which requires calculations and the use of accurate weighing techniques, direct-reading instruments are simpler to use. They also have the advantage that localised peaks of concentration can be identified and remedial measures immediately put into effect. Direct-reading monitors may have a range of pre-selectors that can be fitted to enable them to measure respirable dust or some other pre-defined fraction of the aerosol. They are normally coupled to a data-logging system that records real-time exposures and gives time-weighted average concentrations and other relevant statistics. Manufacturers of direct-reading dust monitors calibrate their equipment to a specific type and size of particles, often a relatively coarse mineral dust. It should be assumed that, without further calibration by you, the readings on a direct reading dust monitor could be inaccurate by a factor of as much as three times high or low. To obtain accurate results it is necessary to calibrate the instrument to the specific type of dust in the environment where it will be used. This can be done by running filter-based samplers alongside the direct reading monitor on a number of occasions in different situations (i.e. a side-by-side comparison of the results of filter-based sampling and the direct reading monitor). Some direct-reading instruments incorporate a facility for collecting a sample of the dust on a membrane filter so that calibration can be achieved by comparing the average recorded dust concentration with that calculated from the weight gain of the filter. Direct-reading monitors are more expensive to buy than the equipment required for the filtration methods.

For their operation, these direct-reading instruments rely upon one of the following physical principles: the scattering of light by airborne dust particles; the β-ray absorption of a deposit of dust on a plastic film or variation in the oscillation frequency of a crystal of quartz when laden with dust (this latter technique is known as a 'piezo-electric' microbalance). Most of the instruments have a digital display that gives a reading of dust concentration in mg m^{-3}. However, there are a number of monitors that provide a particle count per unit volume of air rather than a mass concentration, some will sense only very fine particles, i.e. with diameter less than 1 μm.

One of the important advantages of direct reading monitors is their ability to show change in air concentrations over time. They can be used to investigate the relative importance of different tasks in contributing to overall dust exposure or to estimate the effect of a control measure on worker exposure.

Note that it is important to be aware that connecting any plastic tubes to the inlet of a direct reading aerosol monitor will remove a proportion of the aerosol due to electrostatic or inertial effects inside the tube. The longer the length of tubing, the greater the losses will be.

As the number of direct reading instruments available is increasing and their design is continually being improved, it is advisable to discuss your requirements with a technical representative from the main suppliers before making a choice. Examples of direct-reading dust monitors are shown in Figure 9.8a–c together with a figure showing the real-time dust concentrations measured by one such device (Figure 9.8d).

Further information about dust and vapour direct reading monitors is available to download from the British Occupational Hygiene Society at http://www.bohs.org/resources/res.aspx/Resource/filename/197/tg15.pdf

9.8 Calibration of a rotameter or electronic flow calibrator by using the soap-bubble method

When sampling for dust in a work situation, it is necessary to check the flow rate of air being drawn through the sampling train by the pump. A portable rotameter, which consists of a graduated tube containing a small float, is often used. The indicated flow rate is read from the graduation level with the top of the float. Alternatively, an electronic soap film flowmeter or mass flowmeter can be used. All of these flowmeters must be calibrated – the soap-bubble technique is a cheap and reliable method for doing this. Alternatively, the manufacturer of the equipment can undertake the calibration.

9.8.1 Equipment required
A steady flow rate sampling pump capable of supplying air at the required flow rate, a calibrated glass burette graduated in millilitres, the rotameter, electronic flowmeter or mass flowmeter to be calibrated, a rubber bulb, a glass T-piece, some flexible tubing of suitable size to connect the items, two stands, clamps, tubing clips, liquid soap, cotton wool, stopwatch or timer, and a beaker. The size of the burette will depend upon the range of the flow rates to be used in the calibration; for medium-flow-rate pumps, that is 1.0–4 L min^{-1}, a burette of 250–500 mL capacity is most suitable but for lower flow rates a 100 mL size is sufficient.

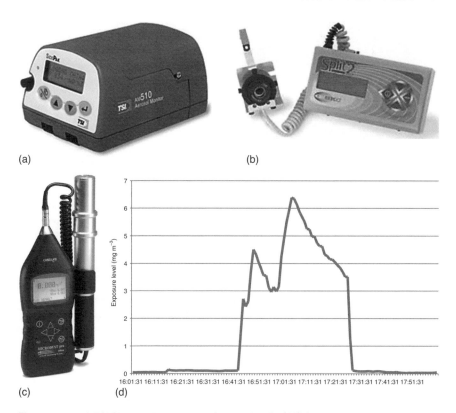

(a)

(b)

(c)

(d)

Figure 9.8 (a) A TSI Sidepak direct-reading dust monitor (b) SKC Split 2 sampler (a and b reproduced with permission from *Occupational Hygiene*, 3rd edition, edited by Kerry Gardiner and J. Malcolm Harrington, Blackwell Publishing Ltd., 2005, p. 197.) (c) Casella Microdust sampler. (© Casella Measurement Ltd. Reproduced with permission.) (d) Output from a Sidepak sampler showing variation in aerosol concentration during work task.

Some pump manufacturers supply their electronic flow calibrators which, although more expensive than assembling the equipment above, are self-contained and may be less trouble (Figure 9.9).

9.8.2 Method

1. Wash the burette with water and then wet the inside surfaces with a thin film of the liquid soap. This can be done by pouring in a little of the soap and washing it down with water from a beaker or wash bottle.
2. Assemble the apparatus as shown in Figure 9.10 and place a small plug of cotton wool at the top of the burette to prevent soap from being drawn into the pump.
3. Place some of the liquid soap in the rubber bulb.
4. Clamp the rotameter in a vertical position by using the retort stand and fittings.
5. Start the pump to draw air through the system.

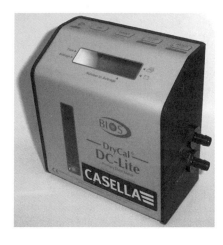

Figure 9.9 An electronic flow calibrator. (© Casella Measurement Ltd. Reproduced with permission.)

6. Squeeze the rubber bulb gently to release some soap into the airstream so that a bubble will be formed.
7. Time the bubble passing between the 0 and 250 mL marks on the burette and repeat this five times for one particular setting of the flow. Note that when observing the position of the bubble for timing, it is important to keep one's eye level with the mark.

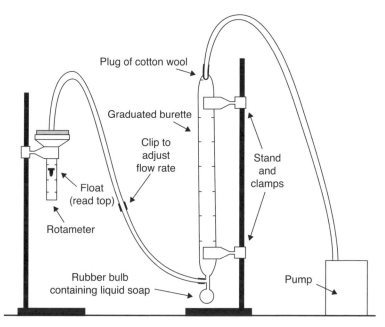

Figure 9.10 Apparatus used to calibrate a rotameter. (Reproduced with permission *Monitoring for Health Hazards at Work*, 3rd edition, by Indira Ashton and Frank S. Gill, Blackwell Publishing Ltd., 2000, p. 16.)

Table 9.1 Example results sheet for the calibration of a rotameter.

Indicated flow on rotameter (L min^{-1})	0.5	1.0	1.5	2.0	2.5	3.0
Average time taken for bubble to travel between marks (s)	27.0	15.5	10.4	7.2	6.0	5.1
Flow rate (L min^{-1})	0.6	1.0	1.4	2.1	2.5	2.9

8. By means of a tubing clamp or by altering the pump flow rate, the position of the float in the rotameter can be altered and steps 6 and 7 can be repeated. This should be done for several flow rates throughout the range of the rotameter.

9.8.3 Results and calculations

Using a chart similar to Table 9.1, record or plot the results as they are taken.

To calculate actual flow, F_a, use the expression

$$F_a = \frac{60 \times V}{t}$$

where V is the swept volume of the bubble in litres (1 L = 1000 mL), and t is the mean time in seconds.

Plot the calculated mean flow rates against the rates marked on the stem of the rotameter as shown in the graph in Figure 9.11. This graph should always be carried with the rotameter for checking the pump flow rates during surveys or tests.

The data from the table are plotted on the chart in Figure 9.11 by using the Excel software package.

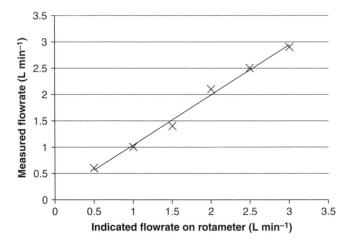

Figure 9.11 Typical rotameter calibration chart.

9.8.4 Possible problems

1. The rotameter float may be pulsating due to the pump having a pulsating flow characteristic. To reduce this, either fit a flow smoother into the line or change to another pump.
2. The soap bubble may burst before reaching the end of its travel, due to the sides of the burette being too dry. The burette should be removed from its clamps and the sides wetted with liquid soap and water as in step 1 in the method section.

9.9 The measurement of inhalable airborne dust

This, the most basic of airborne dust measuring techniques, is used to obtain a measurement of inhalable dust concentration in the breathing zone of an employee or at a particular fixed location in the workplace. It is normal to place the sampling head on the lapel of the worker within about 30 cm of the nose, i.e. in their breathing zone. If the individual is right handed then place the filter holder on their right lapel, if left handed then put the filter holder on the left side. It may be that the concentration is slightly higher on the person's dominant side. Care must be taken since in some operations airborne particles may impinge on the filter from the process being undertaken and in so doing cause overestimation of the true inhaled concentration. If this occurs, then it is preferred to locate the sampling head closer to the nose, which may require a special headband to hold the apparatus. Alternatively, the filter holder could be attached to protective clothing worn on the head such as a welder's visor or a hard hat.

9.9.1 Equipment required

For each person to be sampled simultaneously, a sampling pump capable of a flow rate of approximately 2 L min^{-1}; an Institute of Occupational Medicine (IOM) type sampling head capable of holding a 25 mm diameter filter; 1 m of 7-mm internal diameter plastic tubing; a calibrated rotameter or flowmeter; 25 mm glass fibre filters; cassette; forceps; harness or headband to carry filter holder; a balance with a sensitivity of at least 0.01 mg; labels; small metal tins; and, if static samples are to be collected, a tripod stand or similar and some means of attaching the holder and pump to it such as adhesive tape or string.

9.9.2 Method

1. Because the weight of filters tends to vary with the humidity of the air, it is necessary to allow them to become pre-conditioned by placing each one in a metal tin to stand overnight in the room in which they are to be weighed. The tin should be loosely covered by the lid to allow air to circulate but covering the filter to avoid contamination from dust in the air.
2. Always handle filters with forceps and avoid damaging the filter material. Place the filter into the IOM cassette. Weigh the filter and cassette to 0.01 mg. Wait a further 24 h and repeat the weighing – use the average of these two measurements as the initial weight. Weigh more filters than are

required for sampling so that some can be used as controls and the others are spares in case of accidental damage or contamination. If a filter is accidentally dropped or touched then it must be discarded or re-weighed as the weight will be altered. If another type of filter holder is used, each filter should be weighed prior to inserting them into the holder.

3. Transport each of the weighed IOM cassettes to the measuring site. If an alternative sampler is to be used then separately labelled metal tins may be used to transport the filters.

4. Unscrew the front of the filter holder and using forceps or tweezers carefully place the cassette inside and replace the front. Do not overtighten as the filters can easily be damaged. It is important to number and label each filter holder.

   Note: It may be more convenient to place the filter cassette in the holder immediately after weighing and transport it to the site in the holder with a suitable cover.

5. Make up the sampling train by connecting the filter holder to the pump by means of the plastic tubing and place in the sampling position. If the measuring position is on an employee then it may be convenient to have the whole assembly held in position by means of a harness.

6. Attach the filter holder face forwards as close to the worker's face as possible on the front of the shoulder strap or her/his lapel, and hang the pump on the belt. If a static measuring position is to be taken, then attach the filter holder securely in place on the tripod.

7. Switch on the pump noting the time, and by means of the calibrated flow meter measure the flow rate of air passing through the sampling train and adjust if necessary to the desired flow rate. To check the flow rate, place the face of the filter holder tightly down on to the sponge seal of the flow meter and record the reading. If using a rotameter, the mark level with the top of the float indicates the flow rate. Keep the rotameter vertical at all times or it will give an erroneous reading. Rotameters are unsuitable for use with pulsating flow.

8. It will be necessary to check the pump flow rate from time to time during the sampling period but do not attempt to adjust the pump to try to maintain a constant flow rate. Some pump designs have an automatic flow adjuster, which maintains a constant flow throughout the monitoring period. Pumps may also have a timer whose value can be noted at the beginning and end of the period. The length of time of sampling will depend upon circumstances, but measurement sensitivity will be lost if an insufficient volume of air is drawn through the filter. Recommended minimum sampling times (t_{min}) should be calculated using the following expression:

$$t_{min} = \frac{1000 \times m_{min}}{C_{min} \times f}$$

where m_{min} is the smallest mass that can be reliably measured with the balance in milligrams (if you use an analytical laboratory to weigh your filters then they can tell you this value), f is the sample flow rate in L min^{-1}

and C_{min} is the minimum concentration to be measured. This value will depend upon the dustiness of the workplace sampled and the type of dust but it is suggested that if there is any doubt then set C_{min} at 1/10 of the OEL. Should it be necessary to stop and restart the pump at any time during the test then all times must be noted and flow rates checked.

9. At the end of the sampling period stop the pump and record the finish time.
10. In a clean environment, remove the cassette and cap for return to the laboratory or alternatively transport the filter cassette and holder back to the laboratory for processing.
11. A period of pre-conditioning in the balance room similar to that used for the initial weighing should elapse before re-weighing, which should be done on two separate occasions 24 h apart. The control filters should also be pre-conditioned and re-weighed. Some control filters should be taken to the sampling site and handled in exactly the same manner as the actual samples but no air should be drawn through them – these are known as 'field blanks'. Other blanks are retained in the laboratory – i.e. 'laboratory blanks'. If any contaminant is detected on either of these types of blank filter then the problem can be isolated to either the laboratory or field procedures.
12. Record all readings and results as they are made. Remember that during the sampling it is very important to make notes of the relevant contextual information.

9.9.3 Calculations

The first step is to determine the total volume of air (V) that has passed through the filter by using the expression:

$$V = f \times t$$

Note: If the flow rate (f) has changed during the period this calculation must be carried out for each change of rate and all the volumes added together.

To calculate the true weight gain of the filter it is necessary to have measured the average weight of the cassette and filter before exposure monitoring (x_1 in mg), the average weight of the cassette and filter after the sampling (x_2 in mg), the average weight of laboratory control cassette and filter before (z_1 in mg) and the average weight of laboratory control cassette and filter after (z_2 in mg).

Then the weight of dust on filter (M_a in mg) can be calculated as follows:

$$M_a = (x_2 - x_1) - (z_2 - z_1)$$

Next the concentration of dust in air (C_a in mg m^{-3}) is calculated by dividing the mass of dust sampled by the volume of air that has passed through the filter.

$$C_a = \frac{M_a}{V}$$

9.9.4 Possible problems

1. Care must be taken to ensure that the filters and cassette holders are not contaminated either accidentally or deliberately by extraneous dust. They must always be handled with forceps or tweezers in a clean environment.
2. If the pump flow rate alters by more than 5% during the sampling period then the sample should be rejected.
3. Damaged filters must be discarded and those samples discounted.
4. Filters can be overloaded if the sampling rate is too high or if the dust concentration is very high. If this is suspected a shorter sampling period should be adopted. Do not use a lower flow rate as this will alter the sampling characteristics of the equipment.
5. Overloaded filters can lose dust during handling and transport. Always handle filters with care and avoid jarring motions. It is not advised to send samples by post or courier, particularly heavily loaded samples.

9.10 The measurement of airborne respirable dust by using a cyclone sampler

To separate the respirable fraction of airborne dust from the inhalable dust a modification of the previous method is adopted. The filter holder most commonly used is a cyclone separator, which will separate dust according to the respirable curve shown in Figure 9.1 when operated at the correct flow rate. The technique is similar to sampling for inhalable dust except that it is important to maintain a smooth steady flow rate throughout the sampling period.

9.10.1 Equipment required

For each place to be sampled simultaneously, a cyclone separator and a pump capable of a smooth flow rate of at least 2.2 L min^{-1} are required. There are several designs of cyclone sampler available, but the one commonly used in Britain is the SIMPEDS type cyclone, which takes a 37 mm or 25 mm cassette (the smaller cassettes are more difficult to handle but provide greater sensitivity for mineral analysis in the laboratory). The sampling head is shown in Figure 9.4. The remaining equipment required is the same as listed in Section 9.9.1.

9.10.2 Method

1. Filters should be weighed in the same way as steps 1 and 2 described in Section 9.9.2. The filter should be selected depending on any subsequent laboratory analysis to be undertaken, e.g. assessment of the mass of quartz on the filter. If there is any doubt about the type of filter to be used then the laboratory that will analyse the samples should be consulted.
2. Loading the filters into the cyclone varies with the type of separator used. With the SIMPEDS cyclone the filter is assembled into a cassette.

3. The sampling procedure is the same as for the open face filter, steps 5–11, except that the sampling rate for the SIMPEDS type cyclone must be maintained at 2.2 L min^{-1}, which should be checked regularly during the sampling period by using a calibrated flow meter. It is necessary to connect the flowmeter to the inlet nozzle by means of tubing.

9.10.3 Calculations
These are exactly the same as with the inhalable dust sampling method outlined in Section 9.9.3.

9.10.4 Possible problems
1. If the pump flow rate has changed by more than 0.1 L min^{-1} or 5% above or below the nominal flow rate then the filter has not collected a representative sample of respirable dust. If the flow rate has reduced then dust larger than respirable size will have been collected, perhaps giving an exaggeratedly high result. The opposite would have occurred if the flow rate was above that specified for the sampling head.
2. The sampling duration should be as long as possible, ideally more than about 6 h.
3. Damaged filters must be discarded as it is impossible to obtain a meaningful weight gain from them.
4. In some workplaces, dust is emitted in a concentrated stream and in a predictable direction, for example in grinding or sawing. Care must then be taken to ensure that it is not projected directly on to the filter holder. It may be necessary to move the holder to an alternative position to avoid this.

9.11 The sampling and counting of airborne asbestos fibres

The measurement of airborne asbestos is described in detail in the HSE publication *The Analysts Guide* (HSE, 2005). It is necessary to have detailed training in these methods before collecting this type of sample and it is advisable to use a laboratory that is accredited by UKAS for this type of sampling and analysis to the standard ISO17025; for some work it is legally required. Asbestos analysis in Britain is now highly regulated and should only be undertaken by experienced, trained individuals. The methods are described in this section to provide an understanding of the approaches used.

Asbestos is still present in many work situations, for example, as thermal insulation on pipes, as an acoustic absorbent material on walls, ceilings and silencers; as a building material used in roofs, walls, pipes and gutters; in vehicle brake linings; and in many other places. As the health hazard of inhaling fibres from the manufacture, use, fabrication and removal of this material has been clearly demonstrated, and because legislation in Britain requires the monitoring and control of airborne fibres, it is necessary to establish the airborne concentrations in work situations where asbestos-containing materials are disturbed.

In Britain, the OEL for asbestos is still known as a 'control limit', although it is used in much the same way as the limits for other hazardous substances. The main difference is that measurements should be made over a 4-h duration. There is also a short-term exposure limit over 10 min, which is used to help demonstrate whether exposures are 'sporadic and low intensity' in relation to the requirements of the Control of Asbestos regulations. There is a 'clearance' indicator level of 0.01 fibres mL^{-1} that is used to help identify when it is acceptable to re-enter an area after work with asbestos has been completed.

Personal sampling may be required:

- To assess exposure;
- As a check of the effectiveness of control measures;
- To find out whether a control limit is exceeded so that appropriate respiratory protection can be selected;
- To confirm that the respirator being used is capable of providing the appropriate protection;
- For medical surveillance records;
- To help make a risk assessment.

Static sampling is used:

- For background sampling before asbestos-containing materials are disturbed to check airborne fibre levels are not elevated above background;
- During work to ensure there is no leakage from an enclosure around the work with asbestos – often called 'reassurance sampling';
- For 'clearance testing' on completion of asbestos removal work to ensure the area is suitable for reoccupation.

9.11.1 Equipment required for sampling

For each place or person to be sampled simultaneously: for personal sampling, a sampling pump capable of a flow rate of between 1 and 4 L min^{-1}; for static sampling in asbestos clearance work, a pump capable of up to 16 L min^{-1}; a 25-mm diameter cellulose acetate membrane filter with a gridded surface to assist in focusing on the correct plane for counting; a cowl-type filter holder as shown in Figure 9.7; 1 m of 7 mm internal diameter plastic tubing; a harness for personal sampling or a tripod for static sampling; Petri dish or metal tin and forceps or, if the filters are loaded into the holders prior to leaving base, a cover for the filter holder.

9.11.2 Equipment required for counting

Microscope slides and cover glasses; a binocular microscope having phase contrast Koehler illumination and an eyepiece of magnification ×12.5, one eyepiece to contain a Walton–Beckett eyepiece graticule as illustrated in

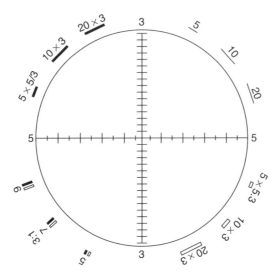

Figure 9.12 The Walton–Beckett eyepiece graticule. (Reproduced with permission *Monitoring for Health Hazards at Work*, 3rd edition, by Indira Ashton and Frank S. Gill, Blackwell Publishing Ltd., 2000, p. 28.)

Figure 9.12; a phase contrast test slide, an acetone vapouriser, see Figure 9.13; glycerol triacetate (triacetin); two push-button digital counters.

9.11.3 Method for sampling

The procedure for sampling follows the same principles as for inhalable or respirable dust, as described earlier, although it is not necessary to weigh the

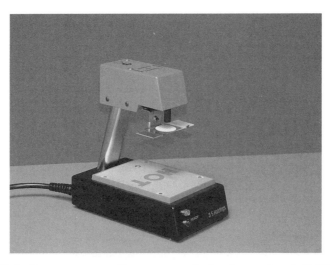

Figure 9.13 Acetone vapouriser used to prepare samples for microscopic analysis. (© JS Holdings. Reproduced with permission.)

membrane filter before or after use. The flow rate of the pump will depend upon the volume of air to be sampled and the time available for monitoring. Note that unlike respirable or inhalable dust sampling, the inlet characteristics of the cowl sampler are not really dependent on the air flow rate, so the flow rate can be varied over a wider range of values and still produce a valid sample, although during sampling the flow rate should be controlled within 5% of the original setting. However, for assessment against the control limit the sample flow rate should be 1 L min^{-1}.

9.11.4   Method of evaluation

1. Carefully remove the membrane filter from the holder by using blunt forceps and place centrally with the gridded side uppermost on a suitably labelled clean microscope slide. Try to have the grids parallel to the side of the slide.
2. Place the slide into the vapouriser according to the manufacturer's instructions and inject the appropriate amount of acetone. The white membrane should now be seen to become transparent as the structure of the membrane disappears under the action of the vapour.
3. Wait for a few minutes before adding a few drops of triacetin on the cleared membrane and cover with a 25–mm diameter cover glass. The triacetin provides for a good optical connection between the filter and the cover glass.
4. The slide should be left for 10–20 min before evaluation on the microscope.

To estimate the number of respirable fibres on the membrane, proceed as follows:

1. Set up phase contrast lighting conditions on the microscope according to the manufacturer's instructions and check the dimensions of the eyepiece graticule at magnification ×500 by means of a stage micrometer; it should be 100 μm.
2. Ensure the microscope is set to ×500 magnification and check the performance by using a phase contrast test slide, making sure that block 5 on the slide can be seen. Adjust the microscope according to the manufacturer's instructions to achieve this.
3. Remove the test slide and place the slide to be counted on the microscope stage. Adjust to a low magnification and focus the microscope so as to observe to assess whether the fibres are evenly distributed over the filter – if they are not then the sample should be rejected. Re-adjust to ×500 magnification. Select a field of view at random and count the number of respirable fibres present in the circle of the graticule. It may be necessary to slightly alter the position of the focus up and down to ensure that any fibres out of focus can be seen. Rules for counting fibres that lay across the boundaries of the graticule, for split fibres and fibre bundles, are detailed in HSE guidance, which should always be consulted before sampling and counting.
   Note: A respirable fibre is defined as one that is greater than 5 μm in length and having a length/breadth ratio of at least 3:1 and a diameter less than

3 μm. The blocks and lines around the outside of the Walton–Beckett graticule assist in selecting the correct fibres to count.

4. Having decided upon the number of fibres present in the field, use one of the digital counters to record the fibres, randomly change the field of view by using the second digital counter to record the number of fields observed, and repeat. Normally 100 fields of view should be counted unless 200 fibres have been seen in fewer than 100 fields. However, at least 20 fields must be counted whatever the number of fibres counted.

9.11.5 Calculations

D (mm) = effective diameter of the membrane (i.e. the actual diameter less the overlap due to the retaining ring of the filter holder)

d (μm) = the diameter of the Walton–Beckett graticule

n = the number of fields examined

N = the number of fibres counted

V (L) = the volume of air sampled.

V = flow rate of pump (L min^{-1}) × duration of sampling (min)

C is the fibre concentration (fibres mL^{-1}), and is given by the equation:

$$C = \frac{1000 \times N \times D^2}{V \times n \times d^2}$$

The results obtained should be compared with the *Control Limits* published in the Control of Asbestos regulations. The Control Limits previously depended upon the type of asbestos that was present; the limits were more stringent if amosite, crocidolite or other amphible asbestos types were present than if they were not. However, there is now a single Control Limit for all asbestos types.

9.11.6 Possible problems

1. Always use a trained and experienced laboratory for fibre counting. Accreditation for these tests is offered by UKAS (www.ukas.com).
2. The filter may be heavily contaminated with other dust, thus making it difficult to see the fibres. In this case repeat the sampling and reduce the sampling flow rate and/or reduce the sampling time.
3. Care must be taken to ensure absolute cleanliness throughout to prevent unwanted contamination of the sample by fibres.

The measurement method for man-made mineral fibres (MMMF) is similar to that described for asbestos and is described in the HSE publication MDHS59.

9.12 The choice of filter and filter holder to suit a specific dust, fume or mist

When sampling for a specific dust of known composition it is important to consult the analyst before starting as the method of analysis will vary depending on the chemical composition of the dust. Each method will require the dust to be presented in a particular way and the analyst should be able to advise as to the best filter to use to suit the technique being applied. Table 9.2 gives some of the more commonly encountered dusts and the recommended filter to use.

To take a sample, proceed as with the inhalable dust or the cyclone separator methods described previously but using the type of filter and holder detailed in Table 9.2.

9.13   To trace the behaviour of a dust cloud by using a Tyndall beam

Many particles of dust are too small to see with the naked eye under normal lighting conditions, but when a beam of strong light is passed through a cloud of particles they reflect the light to the observer and as a result can become visible. This phenomenon is observed when a shaft of sunlight shines into a dark

Table 9.2   Details of filters and filter holders to be used for various types of dust.*

Type of dust	Method of analysis	Filter required	Filter holder required
Asbestos fibres	Optical microscopy	Cellulose ester	Cowl type
	Scanning electron microscopy	Nucleopore	Cowl type
Man-made fibres	Optical microscopy	Cellulose ester	Cowl type
	Gravimetric	Glass fibre	Inhalable
Crystalline silica	X-ray diffraction	PVC or Silver membrane	Respirable
	Infrared	Polyvinyl chloride or PVC-acrylonitrile co-polymer	Respirable
Lead, heavy metals, their oxides and salts	Atomic adsorption spectroscopy	Cellulose ester	Inhalable
Low toxicity dust	Gravimetric	Glass fibre	Inhalable or Respirable
	Optical microscopy	Cellulose ester	Inhalable or Respirable
Unknown mineral dusts	X-ray diffraction	PVC or Silver membrane	Respirable
Coal	Gravimetric	Glass fibre or Cellulose ester	Respirable
	X-ray diffraction	PVC or Silver membrane	Respirable
Oil mists	Gravimetric	Glass fibre	Inhalable
	Fluorescent spectroscopy	Cellulose ester	Inhalable
Welding fume	Gravimetric	Cellulose ester	Welding
	Atomic adsorption spectroscopy	Cellulose ester	Welding
Pharmaceuticals	HPLC	PTFE	Inhalable or respirable

*Note that where cellulose ester membranes are used the pore size should be 0.8 or 1.2 μm.

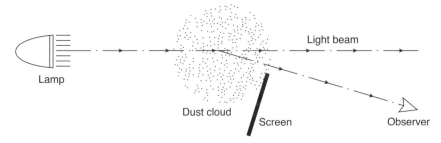

Figure 9.14 Layout of Tyndall beam apparatus (A&G Marketing). (Reproduced with permission *Monitoring for Health Hazards at Work*, 3rd edition, by Indira Ashton and Frank S. Gill, Blackwell Publishing Ltd., 2000, p. 33.)

building highlighting the airborne particles. The nineteenth-century Irish scientist John Tyndall studied the reflection of light by airborne dust and large molecules, and his name has been associated with the technique from that time on. Thus, if a portable lamp having a strong parallel light beam is set up to shine through an environment suspected of being dusty the movement of the particles can be observed. Although no numerical measurements are normally made, the performance of local ventilation systems associated with dust-emitting processes can be examined and design corrections made if unsatisfactory capture is observed. It may be useful to use a video or still camera to record the occurrence. Of the Tyndall effect, this technique is particularly useful for training workers to understand that airborne dust may be present even if it is not normally visible.

9.13.1   Equipment required

A strong mains or battery-powered parallel-beamed lamp (a car spotlight is suitable; a fog light is not), a tripod stand for mounting the lamp and a black screen. There is a Tyndall beam apparatus commercially available in a portable kit form, which has a lamp reflector designed to provide a strong parallel beam of light (Figure 9.14).

9.13.2   Method

Set up the lamp and screen as shown in Figure 9.14 with the observer in the position indicated. When the lamp is switched on the dust cloud should be clearly seen and the movement of the particles observed, photographed or filmed. The best position of the lamp and screen may have to be adjusted by trial and error but it is important to shield the lamp from the eyes of the observer or the camera to prevent glare.

References and further reading

Mark D. (2005). The sampling of aerosols: principles and methods. In: *Occupational Hygiene*, 3rd edition (Gardiner K Harrington JM, eds).Oxford, UK: Blackwell Publishing.

HSE (2005). *Asbestos: The Analysts' Guide for Sampling, Analysis and Clearance Procedures*. Sudbury, UK: HSE Books. (Note: The CA regulations were published after the Analysts' Guide and some of the details of the regulations described there are incorrect.)

HSE Methods for the Determination of Hazardous Substances (MDHS) guidance. Available at http://www.hse.gov.uk/pubns/mdhs/. These include methods for measuring most common airborne contaminants, including the following:

MDHS 14/3: General methods for sampling and gravimetric analysis of respirable and inhalable dust.

MDHS 39/4: Asbestos fibres in air sampling and evaluation by Phase Contrast Microscopy (PCM) under the Control of Asbestos at Work Regulations.

MDHS 42/2: Nickel and inorganic compounds of nickel in air (except nickel carbonyl). Laboratory method using flame atomic absorption spectrometry or electrothermal atomic absorption spectrometry.

MDHS 52/3: Hexavalent chromium in chromium plating mists. Colorimetric field method using 1,5:diphenylcarbazide.

MDHS 59: Man-made mineral fibre. Airborne number concentration by phase-contrast light microscopy.

MDHS 82: The dust lamp. A simple tool for observing the presence of airborne particles.

MDHS 84 Measurement of oil mist from mineral oil-based metalworking fluids.

MDHS 101: Crystalline silica in respirable airborne dusts.

There are a number of British and international standards that are relevant to sampling workplace air, although it is normal to refer to the HSE methods described above. Standards that are relevant are

BS EN ISO 10882-1:2001. Health and safety in welding and allied processes. Sampling of airborne particles and gases in the operator's breathing zone. Sampling of airborne particles.

PD ISO/TR 27628:2007. Workplace atmospheres. Ultrafine, nanoparticle and nano-structured aerosols. Inhalation exposure characterization and assessment.

PD CEN/TR 15230:2005. Workplace atmospheres. Guidance for sampling of inhalable, thoracic and respirable aerosol fractions.

Thorpe, A. (2007). Assessment of personal direct-reading dust monitors for the measurement of airborne inhalable dust. *Annals of Occupational Hygiene* 51(1): 97–112. Available at http://annhyg.oxfordjournals.org/cgi/reprint/51/1/97.

Kenny LC, Aitken R, Chalmers C, Fabriès JF, Gonzalez-Fernandez E, Kromhout H, Lidén G, Mark D, Riediger G, Prodi V. (1997). A collaborative European study of personal inhalable aerosol sampler performance. *Annals of Occupational Hygiene* 41(2): 135–153. Available at http://annhyg.oxfordjournals.org/cgi/reprint/41/2/135

Liden G, Surakka, J (2009) A Headset-Mounted Mini Sampler for Measuring Exposure to Welding Aerosol in the Breathing Zone. *Annals of Occupational Hygiene;* 53(2): 99-116. http://annhyg.oxfordjournals.org/cgi/reprint/53/2/99.

WHO (1999). *Hazard Prevention and Control in the Work Environment: Airborne Dust*. Protection of the Human Environment Occupational Health and Environmental Health Series, Geneva: World Health Organization. Available at http://www.who.int/occupational_health/publications/airdust/en/index.html.

10 # Gases and Vapours

10.1 Introduction

The range of gases and vapours that occur in industry, commerce, medicine, agriculture, in the home and street is vast. Many industrial processes as well as natural or biological degradation processes use or produce gas, often under pressure. Containing these gases is important since many are toxic or may cause asphyxia in enclosed environments. Leaks may occur around joints, valves or through piping, and access covers when opened can release gas into the atmosphere. Suitable precautions must be taken to contain these gases and their presence in the atmosphere around these containers should be monitored.

Vapours are gaseous materials that have been generated from the evaporation of substances that are liquids or solids at room temperature. Solvents are an important class of materials that may generate vapours. They are liquids chosen for their ability to dissolve a particular material and often for their ability to evaporate and dissociate themselves from the solute. Many solvents have narcotic effects, acting upon the central nervous system slowing down nerve responses; others are extremely toxic or are sensitising agents; and some are mutagenic and/or carcinogenic.

The physical and toxicological properties of gases and vapours mean that they can rapidly build up to concentrations that can immediately damage health or even kill. Long-term exposure to many gases or vapours can also progressively damage health. This vast range of gases and vapours, together with the mixture of chronic and acute effects on health, requires a wide variety of monitoring and detection techniques. A number of methods of sampling and detection are described in this chapter. The techniques available fall into two basic types: (1) indirect analysis of the pollutant from air collected in the workplace and analysed in a laboratory and (2) direct measurement of concentrations or indication of presence with instruments or detection devices. The satisfactory use of some of the more complex instruments available requires a good knowledge of chemistry. However, some more simple devices such as colorimetric detector tubes and some specific gas monitors can provide low-cost measurement systems that provide a quick indication of the airborne gas or vapour concentration.

As with airborne dust measurement, if a long-term average concentration is required then it is usual to collect a sample of the gas- or vapour from the air

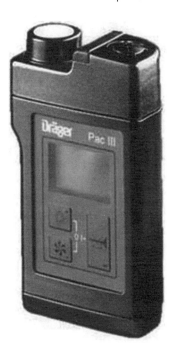

Figure 10.1 A single-gas detector with optional datalogger. (© Draeger Safety UK Ltd. Reproduced with permission.)

over the working period rather than use a direct-reading instrument, which is often used to make an instantaneous measurement and may not permit characterisation of the pollutants in the air sampled. Most direct-reading instruments, however, do have electronic data-logging capabilities so that the variation in concentration over time can be seen and the average concentration calculated after the data is downloaded to a computer. If these instruments are relatively large then they can only be used to measure general workroom gas or vapour concentrations because of the difficulty in attaching them to employees to estimate their personal exposure. However, for a number of gases, specially designed long-term detector tubes that can be used as personal samplers are available to measure concentrations over a work shift. Furthermore, there are many, very portable personal gas detectors on the market capable of detecting gases, such as carbon monoxide or hydrogen sulphide. They produce a real-time direct-reading display that can be stored on a data-logger. Both long-term average and peak concentrations can be retrieved from the data-logger. One such device is illustrated in Figure 10.1.

There are basically three ways of sampling gases or vapours for subsequent laboratory analysis:

- By collecting continuously a small amount of the workroom atmosphere into an airtight container, gradually filling the container over the test period;

- By allowing workroom air to pass through an adsorbent material such as activated charcoal, which can later be desorbed for analysis; or
- By drawing air through a solution in a bubbler or impinger where the contaminant reacts with the liquid.

Where the sample is collected into a container then it is important that the gas or vapour will not chemically react with the walls of the container or adsorb onto them, which means that this method is only applicable to a very small number of non-reactive gases, e.g. nitrous oxide.

The adsorbent method is commonly used for vapours and requires the adsorbent material to be matched to the vapour being sampled. Samples can be collected by diffusive or passive techniques, where the contaminant is collected by diffusion onto an adsorbent substrate or by drawing air through the adsorbent by using a pump. For example, not all vapours will be effectively adsorbed onto activated charcoal and other vapours are adsorbed but either react chemically when adsorbed or are not readily removed by desorption. A range of alternative adsorbent materials is therefore available.

Bubblers and impingers were historically used for many gases and vapours but their inconvenience and instability means that these procedures are used now primarily for reactive gases and vapours, such as isocyanates and sulphur dioxide.

In some circumstances, there may be a chance that the environment could contain high concentrations of gases or vapours that could be explosive, e.g. within a petrochemical refinery. In this type of environment, there are generally severe restrictions on the type of electrical equipment that can be used and most direct-reading or pump-based monitoring systems would not comply with these restrictions. It is necessary to use measurement equipment that is certified as 'intrinsically safe'. Some environments with fine dusts also have the potential for explosion and require monitoring equipment to be intrinsically safe.

10.2   Collection devices

Before embarking upon any form of air sampling it is important to discuss with the analyst which method of collection best suits questions being asked of the measurement. Considerations include the sensitivity required, the sampling period, the capacity of the adsorbent and the analytical technique to be employed when the samples are returned to the laboratory. The method of analysis dictates the type of container or collection device to be used, as the final sample has to be introduced into the analytical instrument.

10.2.1   Adsorption methods

Certain gases and vapours are readily adsorbed by solid materials such as silica gel, activated charcoal and various types of porous resins. When air containing these gases or vapours is passed through the material in a powder or granular form, they will be adsorbed. Tubes of metal or glass can be purchased containing one of these materials. The tubes should remain sealed until ready for use. (Note: It is important not to confuse adsorbent tubes with colorimetric detector tubes, which are described later.) Air is drawn through the adsorbent tube by means of an air pump, and the granular material will adsorb those gases or vapours that have an affinity for the adsorbent. Provided that the volume of air passed through the tube has not overloaded, the adsorbent then the amount of pollutant collected can be determined in the laboratory by chemical analysis and the average concentration calculated knowing the amount of air that has passed through the monitoring device.

One advantage of this technique is that the pumps and tubes are small and can be attached to an employee in a similar way to the airborne dust samplers. Another advantage is that the pollutant is collected in a concentrated form, thus analytical techniques need be less sensitive than with the container methods, and in most cases several gases or vapours can be collected and analysed from the same tube.

Not all gases or vapours can be collected by means of the adsorbent tube. Another technique available is to bubble the workroom air through water or some liquid in which the gas is soluble. The pollutant can then be chemically analysed from the solution. The container for the liquid is known as an impinger or 'bubbler' (see Figure 10.2) because the sampled air is introduced via a tube whose end is below the surface of the liquid; thus the air is bubbled through it. Unfortunately, most bubblers need to be kept upright to prevent the reagent from spilling out. This limits their use for personal sampling because employees wearing them are limited in their ability to bend or stoop. Another disadvantage of this technique is that it is difficult to guarantee that all the gas passing through the bubbler will be absorbed, as bubbling does not ensure 100% contact between the gas and the liquid. To improve contact 'fritted bubblers' are used, which have an inlet tube whose end is made of porous glass that produces very small bubbles.

When drawing air through adsorbent tubes, a low airflow rate is required. Pumps are available that provide rates as low as 2 mL min^{-1}) but the range for this type of sampling is usually between 20 and 500 mL min^{-1}, depending on the nature of the adsorbent, the analyte, the size of the tube, the sampling period and the sensitivity that is required. These pumps operate under the same principles as the dust sampling pumps, that is, diaphragm, piston and rotary, and, with certain exceptions, are supplied by the same manufacturers. Bubblers tend to require higher flow rates and so the medium-flow pumps as used in dust sampling are preferred in these situations. Flow rates of any pump should always be checked against a soap bubble flowmeter or other suitable flowmeter as described in Chapter 9. Note that some of the low-flow samplers in the market have pulsating flow and for that reason rotameter style flow meters may not be appropriate.

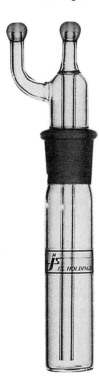

Figure 10.2 Typical impinger samplers (SKC Ltd). (Reproduced with permission *Monitoring for Health Hazards at Work*, 3rd edition, by Indira Ashton and Frank S. Gill, Blackwell Publishing Ltd., 2000, p. 54.)

To hold the adsorbent tube and to attach it to an employee, a tube holder is available from the suppliers of the low flow-rate pumps. A piece of flexible plastic tubing connects the holder to the pump.

10.2.2 Adsorbent tubes

There is a wide range of adsorbent tubes available (Figure 10.3). The materials that are used for adsorbing gases and vapours are listed as follows: charcoal, silica gel, alumina, various porous materials including polyurethane foam (PUF), Poropak N, P, Q, R and T, Chromosorb 102 and 106, XAD 2, 4 and 7, Anasorb 708, 727, 747, CMS and C300, Florisil and Tenax GR and TC. Some of these are available with chemical coatings to collect specific gases or vapours. They each have the ability to adsorb various gases and vapours but charcoal is the most widely used as it has an adsorbent affinity with more substances than any other material. The materials are contained in either glass or metal tubes, depending upon the method of desorbing the gas in the laboratory. One method of desorbtion involves breaking the tube so that the adsorbent material falls into a liquid that leaches the gas out of the material into solution. Glass tubes are used in this application. Another method, known as thermal desorbtion, involves heating the tube to drive off the collected vapour into a detection system and metal tubes are used for this technique. Charcoal adsorbent is not generally suitable for thermal desorption.

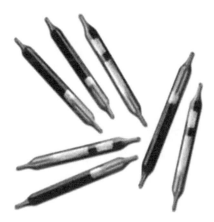

Figure 10.3 Adsorbent tubes. (© SKC Ltd.
Reproduced with permission.)

The tubes designed for solvent desorption are made up in two sections to indicate what is known as 'breakthrough'. This occurs when the sorbent material is completely saturated with the sampled gases; i.e. there is no more adsorbent capacity left. If the second section of the tube is free of the sampled vapours then breakthrough has not occurred in the first section and the total sample collected on that section can be used in the calculation of airborne concentration. Breakthrough occurs when the sample volume is too high, either because the sample duration is too long to suit the airborne concentration or the flow rate has been set too high.

With metal tubes used for thermal desorption, no second section is available, thus breakthrough must be carefully guarded against by calculation of breakthrough volumes and ensuring these are not exceeded during sampling. If there are concerns about breakthrough, a second tube can be used behind the first.

It cannot be emphasised too strongly that, when sampling for airborne gases and vapours, the chemist who undertakes the analysis of the collected samples and the hygienist must work together to select the best sampling method. If adsorbent tubes are to be used, she/he will advise on the sorbent material and sample volumes that should be used. Some suppliers offer guidance on tube selection.

10.2.3   Passive samplers

Techniques are available whereby diffusion is used to drive airborne pollutants onto an adsorbent without using a pump. The adsorbent material, which can be liquid or solid, is contained in a holder designed to allow the gases to diffuse to the adsorbent surface. These holders are small enough to be worn like a lapel badge (Figure 10.4) or tube (Figure 10.5) and are free of any pump or tubing. At the end of the sampling period the holder is returned to the laboratory where the amount of gas or vapour collected can be analysed as with adsorbent tubes. The concentration can be calculated using an 'effective' sampling flow rate provided by the sample supplier.

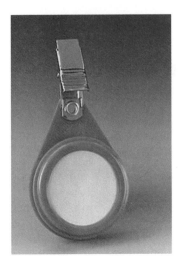

Figure 10.4 Badge type diffusive sampler. (© 3M United Kingdom PLC. Reproduced with permission.)

The advantages of this type of sampling are:

- It removes the need for a costly pump, with the associated problems of monitoring flow rates and maintaining battery charge in the sample pump;
- The samplers are light and unobtrusive, overcoming worker resistance to use;
- There is a constant sampling rate;
- The samplers can be used in environments where flammable or explosive gases may be present.

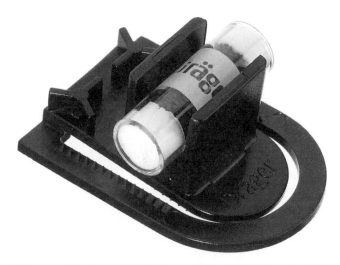

Figure 10.5 Tube-type diffusive sampler. (© Draeger Safety UK Ltd. Reproduced with permission.)

10.2.4   Colorimetric detector tubes

A comparatively simple method to detect airborne gases uses the colorimetric detector tube – it is a direct reading method but is included here because it shares a lot with the other pump-based sampling methods. The monitor consists of a glass tube containing crystals treated with a chemical reagent that will react with a particular gas or vapour and change colour as a result. As contaminated air is drawn through the tube a colour change occurs from the inlet end, and extends along the tube, depending upon the concentration of the contaminant present. A scale is printed on the side of the tube and the measured concentration is indicated by the length of stain. A hand-operated suction pump or calibrated syringe ensures the appropriate sample volume passes through the tube, provided the sample has been collected in accordance with the maker's instructions. The tubes are sealed at each end, and both ends must be broken before inserting into the pump. An example of this type of sampler is shown in Figure 10.6. Two companies specialise in these devices – Dräger and Gastec – and between them detector tubes for over 200 substances are available. The tubes supplied by these companies are not interchangeable, that is, Gastec tubes cannot be used with a Dräger pump or vice versa.

Whilst the technique appears simple there are certain difficulties that can lead to error in the results obtained. The detector tubes deteriorate with time and have a shelf life of no more than 2 years if stored at normal room temperatures. The presence of other gases can interfere with the gas or vapour to be measured and result in an erroneous measurement. The manufacturer will advise in these cases. Also, it is important that the designed sample volume passes through the tube at the defined sample flow rate otherwise the result will be invalid. Any damage to the pump or syringe causing a leak in the airflow will reduce the volume of air passing through the tube. It is important, too, that the air is sampled at a suitable point, either at a fixed location or close to the breathing zone of the operator being monitored.

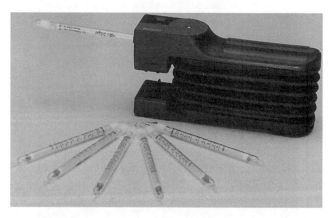

Figure 10.6 Colorimetric detector tube sampler and a range of tubes. (© Draeger Safety UK Ltd. Reproduced with permission.)

It is possible to obtain a long-term average concentration by means of a colorimetric detector tube for certain gases or vapours. The technique involves using a battery-powered sampling pump and drawing air through the tube, which is placed in the breathing zone of the worker. Sampling must be undertaken with purpose-made long-running tubes, as short-term tubes cannot be used for this type of sampling.

10.3   Containers

If a sample of the workroom air is required for analysis for the normal constituents of fresh air, oxygen, nitrogen and carbon dioxide; and for certain other pollutants such as nitrous oxide or methane, then it can be collected in a container to be returned to the laboratory. This method is not suitable for solvent vapours or for reactive gases such as nitrogen monoxide. Therefore, there are important limitations with this method, and detailed knowledge of the behaviour of the gases to be sampled and the materials used in the construction of the container is required.

Samples can be collected in metal cylinders, syringes, glass or plastic pipettes and certain special plastic bags (Figure 10.7). For short-term, i.e. 'grab, samples, they can be filled by hand pump. For long-term samples, bags should be used as they can be filled slowly over the sampling period using a small battery-powered pump.

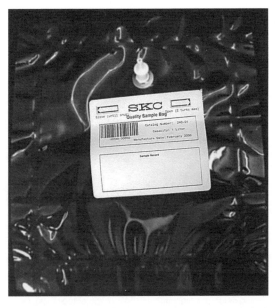

Figure 10.7 Gas-tight sampling bags. (© SKC Ltd. Reproduced with permission.)

One disadvantage with the container method of sampling is that it is difficult to obtain a personal sample as most receptacles are rather bulky or are only suited to grab sampling. As a result these methods are not widely used in occupational hygiene.

10.4   Direct-reading instruments

There are many direct-reading instruments on the market that are specific to a particular gas or vapour, e.g. carbon monoxide, sulphur dioxide or mercury vapour. The range of instruments available is so large that it is impossible to cover them in a book of this nature and so we have just highlighted a few of the more commonly used instruments.

Most direct-reading monitors either have an integrated data-logger or can be coupled to an external logger to obtain a continuous record of the variation in gas or vapour concentrations, which can be very useful for relating the job being undertaken with the concentration at any moment. Several modern instruments are small enough to use as personal samplers and they have the added advantage of having exposure alarms fitted, e.g. for where toxic gases could reach concentrations that are immediately threatening to life.

If several gases require to be measured by direct means it can become quite expensive to buy an instrument for each one. However, there are several types of direct-reading monitor available that can be used to measure a range of gases and vapours. One of these, the organic vapour analyser (OVA), is a portable battery-powered gas chromatograph. This will either indicate total hydrocarbon concentration or, if fitted with a suitable column, can indicate the concentrations of specific vapours. The Gasmet monitor is a portable Fourier-transform infrared (FTIR) gas analyzer, which is located in backpack worn by the person undertaking the sampling (Figure 10.8). The The MultiRAE monitor (Figure 10.9) is another device that can measure multiple gases and vapours. This device combines a photoionisation detector with sensors for the lower explosive limit (LEL), oxygen and two 'specific' toxic gas sensors. They can also be set up as 'total VOC' monitors, i.e. to

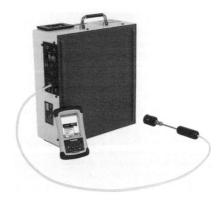

Figure 10.8 A portable Fourier-transform infrared analyser. (© Quantitech Ltd. Reproduced with permission.)

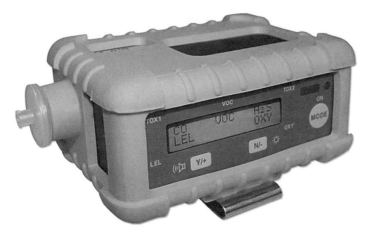

Figure 10.9 A MultiRAE photo-ionisation monitor. (© RAE Systems UK. Reproduced with permission.)

measure total volatile organic compounds. The MultiRAE IR can be used as a personal monitor or as a continuous area monitor.

10.5 To measure personal exposure to solvent vapours using an adsorbent tube

To obtain a time-weighted average concentration of the exposure of an employee to solvent vapours it is necessary to collect a representative sample of the air from their breathing zone over the period of exposure. This can be achieved by collecting the vapour onto an adsorbent medium such as charcoal. Other media are available but the analytical chemist can advise as to the most suitable for the vapours in question. Note that you will need to have identified a competent laboratory to undertake the analysis – search www.ukas.com to identify a suitable organisation.

10.5.1 Equipment required
A low flow-rate pump; an adsorbent tube; a tube holder with a length of plastic tubing to connect to the pump and a calibrated portable soap bubble calibrator. A harness to hold the equipment may also be useful.

10.5.2 Method
1. Label the tube for identification purposes with a unique number that is linked to the sampling records and details of the worker being sampled. Break the glass seals or remove the covers at each end of the tube packed with adsorbent and insert into the holder. Connect the other end of the tube to the pump. Make sure that air will be drawn through the tube in the correct direction, i.e. through the larger section of charcoal first.

2. Attach the tube holder to the worker within the breathing zone on the lapel or clothing, close to the collarbone being the most acceptable place. Place the pump in a convenient pocket or hang from the worker's belt.
3. Turn on the pump and note the time of starting.
4. Set the flow rate to the appropriate level (after taking into account the concentration of vapours expected and the length of the sampling period). Check the flow rate with a calibrated soap bubble flowmeter, as described in Section 9.8, and note the value.
5. From time to time during the sampling operation check the flow rate for constancy by using a soap bubble flowmeter. Remember to make a record of the contextual information relevant to the measurement.
6. At the end of the sampling period stop the pump and note the time.
7. Remove the apparatus from the worker and place seals over the open ends of the adsorbent tube.
8. Send the tube to the chemical analyst with information concerning the substances likely to be adsorbed on the medium and which require analysis.
9. It is prudent to collect a small number of 'field blanks' and have these analysed in the same way as the actual samples; i.e. field blanks are sample media that have been handled in the same way as the samples but no air has been drawn through them.

10.5.3 Calculations

It is first necessary to establish how much air has passed through the tube. Calculate the average flow rate (mL min^{-1}) throughout the sampling period and multiply by the sample duration (min) to give the sample volume in millilitres. Convert to cubic metre by dividing the answer by 10^6.

After the adsorbent tube has been analysed the total amount of each vapour tested will be given in milligrams (mg) or micrograms (µg). Divide the mass of each contaminant given by the total sampled volume to give the concentration in milligram per cubic metre or microgram per cubic metre.

10.5.4 Example

A charcoal-adsorbent tube connected to a pump running at 5 mL min^{-1} sampled an atmosphere for 6 h and 40 min. The workplace atmosphere contained solvents from a spray painting task. The analyst reported that the sample contained the following amounts of solvent: 1-butanol, 0.156 mg; xylene, 0.298 mg; styrene, 0.187 mg. Calculate the airborne concentrations of each.

Total time of sampling $= (6 \times 60) + 40 = 400$ min

Total airflow through tube at 5 mL min^{-1} $= 5 \times 400 = 2{,}000$ ml $= 0.002$ m^3

Note that the most inaccurate part of this or any similar measurement lies with the determination of the flow rate of the pump, which could be as much as $\pm 10\%$ in error. Therefore, it is unwise to be pedantic about the number of significant figures in the calculation. Results should generally only be quoted to two significant figures, e.g. 273.563 mg m^{-3} should be presented as 270 mg m^{-3}.

Concentrations derived by dividing the mass of solvent extracted from the tube by the volume of air sampled through that tube.

$$\text{1-Butanol} = \frac{0.156 \text{ mg}}{0.002 \text{ m}^3} = 78 \text{ mg m}^{-3}$$

$$\text{Xylene} = \frac{0.298 \text{ mg}}{0.002 \text{ m}^3} = 150 \text{ mg m}^{-3}$$

$$\text{Styrene} = \frac{0.187 \text{ mg}}{0.002 \text{ m}^3} = 94 \text{ mg m}^{-3}$$

Note that the concentration of gasses and vapours are sometimes quoted in milligram per cubic metre and sometimes in ppm, i.e. parts of gas by volume per million parts of air. It is possible to convert from one set of units to the other with a simple calculation.

$$C \left(\text{mg m}^{-3}\right) = \frac{M \times C \text{ (ppm)}}{24.45}$$

and

$$C \text{ (ppm)} = \frac{22.45 \times C \left(\text{mg m}^{-3}\right)}{M}$$

where M is the molecular weight of the compound – this can be calculated knowing the chemical formula and there are various websites that facilitate the calculation, e.g. http://www.chemeurope.com/tools/mm.php3? language=e.

There are also calculators that will make the conversion between the two units, e.g. http://www.cdc.gov/niosh/docs/2004-101/calc.htm.

These formulae can be used when measurements are made at 25°C and the air pressure is 760 mm Hg, i.e. 1 atm.

10.6 Sampling for gases by using a bubbler

Some gases are not readily adsorbed by or are unstable on solids but dissolve in liquids or form chemical reactions with certain reagents. One method of sampling this type of workplace contaminant is to bubble the workroom air through the appropriate liquid using a device called a bubbler or impinger. The success of this technique depends upon the readiness of the pollutant in question to react with the solution or reagent.

Clearly, devices such as these are unwieldy and there is a risk that the liquid may be spilled if the bubbler is not kept upright. A spill-proof bubbler is available; nevertheless, obvious resistance from the workforce to wearing devices containing liquids is likely to be encountered. Bubbling techniques are therefore usually of limited use in occupational hygiene measurement.

10.6.1 Equipment required

A bubbler containing the correct amount of appropriate liquid as advised by the analytical chemist, a suction pump, connecting tubing, a tripod stand, adhesive tape, a calibrated flowmeter, and, if the atmosphere to be sampled is dusty, then an open-face filter holder containing a glass-fibre filter should be added at the entrance to the sampling train.

10.6.2 Method

To establish the required pump flow-rate it is important to have a trial run beforehand by using clean water in the bubbler, the amount being the same as that required for the test. This is to ensure that no liquid is unintentionally drawn into the pump causing damage and also to judge whether there is a chance of significant loss of liquid during sampling because of evaporation. If the bubbler is filled beforehand and carried to the site it must be kept upright and the open ends sealed. It may be more convenient to fill on site but that involves carrying a measuring device to dispense the correct amount of liquid.

1. Connect the bubbler to the pump, that is, connect the pump to the tube not in contact with the liquid. *Do not connect the pump to the central tube as this will result in the liquid being drawn into the pump.*
2. At the sampling site attach the assembly to a tripod stand by means of adhesive tape or suitable clamps. Alternatively, fit the sampler to the worker to be sampled, locating it as close to the breathing zone as is practicable. Make sure the bubbler is labelled with a unique sample identifying code. It is unwise to use bubblers for personal sampling if the liquid is flammable, toxic or corrosive.
3. Start the pump at the pre-set rate of flow, noting the time.
4. By using a calibrated flowmeter or rotameter check and note the airflow rate passing through the sampling train and repeat periodically throughout the test. Take care to note whether there is any significant loss of liquid (it is sometimes possible to top up the liquid during sampling).
5. At the end of the sampling period stop the pump and note the time.
6. Disconnect the tubing from the bubbler, seal the ends.
7. Return the bubbler to the laboratory immediately so that the analysis can proceed without delay as some chemicals can react in a relatively short period of time. The chemical analyst will advise whether any special precautions are needed such as avoiding exposing the liquid to sunlight or keeping the liquid cold.

10.6.3 Calculation

Establish the total amount of air that has passed through the sampler by multiplying the elapsed time by the flow rate. Convert to cubic metres (m^3). The analyst will report the amount of pollutant collected in milligrams (mg) or micrograms (μg) and from that the airborne concentration can be obtained in milligram per cubic metre or microgram per cubic metre by dividing the sample amount by the total volume of air sampled.

10.6.4 Example

A bubbler was run for 20 min at a flow rate of 1.5 L min^{-1} in an atmosphere containing formaldehyde. The analyst reported that the sample contained 0.048 mg of formaldehyde. Determine the airborne concentration.

Total airflow through the bubbler $= 20 \times 1.5 = 30\,l = 0.03\ \text{m}^3$

Airborne concentration of formaldehyde $= \dfrac{0.048\ \text{mg}}{0.03\ \text{m}^3} = 1.6\ \text{mg m}^{-3}$

10.7 To measure the short-term airborne concentration of a gas by using a colorimetric detector tube

It is often necessary to obtain a quick indication of an airborne concentration of a gas or vapour. This may be required in a situation such as checking the concentration in an enclosed space, such as a sump or a large empty vessel, before permitting persons to enter. This type of measurement is also useful in a workplace or workroom to check the general concentration of a specific gas or vapour. Short-term detector tubes can be used for this purpose but it must be remembered that these devices give an indication over a short period of time, usually a few minutes. The exact time taken to produce the result depends upon the type of gas or vapour to be detected and type of tube being used and is governed by the flow resistance of the tube. In occupational hygiene this type of sample is known as a 'grab' sample and does not provide an estimate of the long-term average concentration. Colorimetric tubes should not be confused with an adsorbent tube used for short-term sampling.

10.7.1 Equipment required

A colorimetric sampling kit containing a hand-operated suction pump and, from the same manufacturer, a box of detector tubes for the vapour or gas to be measured and for the range of concentrations likely to be found. If sumps, enclosed vessels, or difficult-to-access places, are to be sampled then an extension hose is also required. Remember, you need to take care in confined spaces and must make a risk assessment before undertaking such work.

There are two basic types of suction pump available, the bellows type as shown in Figure 10.6 and a syringe pump. Each pump is designed to draw a measured volume of air for an operating stroke, e.g. bellows type draw 100 mL.

The type of detector tube available depends upon the gas/vapour to be measured. This dictates the chemical reaction that occurs within the tube to produce the indicating stain. With some types the concentration is indicated by means of the length of a coloured stain measured against a single scale inscribed on the glass wall of the tube, although a double scale may be provided to accommodate two different numbers of pump strokes. Less commonly, indication of concentration may be by colour change rather than length of stain;

in these cases a means for colour comparison will be available, either built into the tube or as a separate item.

The construction of the tubes also varies for different gases, depending upon the chemical reaction producing the stain. For example, it may be necessary to activate the tube by breaking an ampoule of reagent within the tube. Alternatively, it may be necessary to employ a pre-tube before the indicator thus placing the two tubes in sequence with a short connection between them. Instruction on the method of use will be given in a leaflet enclosed with the box of tubes.

10.7.2   Method – using the bellows pump

Before making a test it is necessary to undertake some preliminary checks on the pump.

1. Check for a leak in the bellows: without breaking the ends of the glass detector tube insert it into the pump orifice and squeeze the bellows to the closed position and release immediately. If the bellows remain closed then no leaks exist; a leaking pump would open during this test.
2. Check for a blockage in the suction channels: squeeze the bellows to closed and with no tube in position the bellows should spring open immediately on release. If the channels are blocked the bellows would open relatively slowly. Remember to make a record of these preliminary checks.

   Note: Before undertaking a test with colorimetric detector tubes read the instructions supplied with the box of detector tubes, and if they have been stored check the expiry date.
3. Break both glass end seals on the detector tube by using the tip breaking device. If an internal ampoule is provided, break that as per instructions. *Take care, the ends of these tubes are very sharp and accidental injuries are possible.*
4. Insert the tube into the suction orifice of the pump making sure the arrow on the tube points towards the pump. If a pre-tube is required, break its seals and connect it to the assembly according to the instructions.
5. Squeeze the bellows and release immediately. They will open at a rate governed by the flow resistance of the tube. Do not hinder this operation by trying to control the rate of opening. If sufficient gas or vapour is present in the air sampled a dark stain will appear from the zero and extend up the tube in response to the concentration of the gas present.
6. If the scale on the tube requires one stroke then read the indicated concentration corresponding to the end of the stain, as inscribed on the wall of the tube.
7. If the scale requires more pump strokes repeat operation 5, carefully counting the number of strokes until the required number is reached (most models incorporate a stroke counter to assist with this). The range of some tubes can be extended by increasing the number of strokes but this must be done

according to the maker's instructions. At the end of the test, read the concentration, as described earlier, and make a record of the result.

It is important to make good notes of the conditions when the test was carried out and where the measurement was made. This will help with the subsequent interpretation of the data.

10.8 To measure a vapour concentration using a diffusive sampler

Measuring exposure to a vapour by using a diffusive sampler is relatively straightforward. As with other measurements based on chemical analysis, you will first need to find a laboratory to undertake the analysis. It is important to discuss with your analyst whether your planned measurement strategy is appropriate and will provide the necessary sensitivity, i.e. that you can reliably measure the lowest concentrations you expect to encounter, and specificity, i.e. that you can detect those chemical compounds that are of interest. Identify the type of badge or tube you want to use; in this example we want to sample for styrene in a plastics factory. Diffusive samplers have a relatively low effective sampling rate so you must be careful to ensure that you have sufficient sensitivity, i.e. that you sample for a sufficiently long time to obtain detectable levels. They can, however, become saturated or otherwise lose efficiency if you sample for too long.

10.8.1 Equipment required
Several 3M 3500 diffusive samplers (details of the sampler are available on the 3M website) are required.

10.8.2 Method – Collecting a sample using a diffusive sampler
1. Calculate the minimum sampling time to measure a concentration of 40 mg m^{-3}. Use the equation from Chapter 9

$$t_{min} = \frac{1000 \times m_{min}}{C_{min} \times f}$$

where m_{min} is the minimum mass of styrene detectable in the chemical analysis, which your analyst will be able to tell you (in this case 5 μg or 0.005 mg).

C_{min} is 40 mg m^{-3} and f is the effective flow rate, which you can either obtain from your analyst or from HSEs publication MDHS88 (for styrene on 3M 3500 samplers it is 28.9 mL min^{-1} or 0.0289 L min^{-1}).

$t_{min} = (1000 \times 0.005)/(40 \times 0.0289) = 4$ min.

Therefore in this case there is no problem in sampling for the duration of the task involving styrene (i.e. 30 min) or for 15 min if comparing with a short-term exposure limit.

2. Make sure that you collect at least one field blank, i.e. a sampler that is handled in exactly the same way as the real samples but is never exposed to the contaminated atmosphere.
3. Immediately before sampling, take the sampler from its protective metal can. Record the sampling details on the reverse of the sample holder. Clip the sampler on the lapel or some other suitable location in the worker's breathing zone, ensuring it is not obscured by clothing or other objects. Record the time sampling started and other relevant contextual information.
4. At the end of the sampling period, retrieve the sampler and note the time sampling stopped. Take the sampler to an area uncontaminated with styrene and remove the white membrane and retaining ring. Push the closure cap securely onto the top of the sampler. Replace in tin for transport to the laboratory.
5. The laboratory will take care of the analysis and should provide you with a report detailing the measured concentrations. The sample would be analysed by gas chromatography.

References and further reading

Brown RH. (2005). The sampling of gases and vapours: Principles and methods. In: *Occupational Hygiene*, 3rd edition, (Gardiner K, Harrington, JM, eds). Oxford, UK: Blackwell Publishing.

Eriksson K, Liljelind I, Fahlén J, Lampa E. (2005). Should styrene be sampled on the left or right shoulder? An important question in employee self-assessment. *Annals of Occupational Hygiene* 49(6): 529–533. Available at http://annhyg.oxfordjournals.org/cgi/reprint/49/6/529.

Rosén G, Andersson IM, Walsh PT, Clark RD, Säämänen A, Heinonen K, Riipinen H, Pääkkönen R. (2005). A review of video exposure monitoring as an occupational hygiene tool. *Annals of Occupational Hygiene* 49(3): 201–217. Available at http://annhyg.oxfordjournals.org/cgi/reprint/49/3/201.

Van Rooij JG, Kasper A, Triebig G, Werner P, Jongeneelen FJ, Kromhout H. (2008). Trends in occupational exposure to styrene in the European glass fibre-reinforced plastics industry. *Annals of Occupational Hygiene* 52(5): 337–349. Available at http://annhyg.oxfordjournals.org/cgi/reprint/52/5/337.

HSE Methods for the Determination of Hazardous Substances (MDHS) guidance. Available at http://www.hse.gov.uk/pubns/mdhs/.

These include methods for measuring most common airborne contaminants, including the following:

MDHS16/2. Mercury and its inorganic divalent compounds in air. Laboratory method using Hydrar diffusive badges or pumped sorbent tubes, acid dissolution and analysis by cold vapour atomic absorption spectrometry or cold vapour atomic fluorescence spectrometry.

MDHS53/2. 1,3-Butadiene in air. Laboratory method using pumped samplers, thermal desorption and gas chromatography.

MDHS71. Analytical quality in workplace air monitoring.

MDHS 88. Volatile organic compounds in air. Laboratory method using diffusive samplers, solvent desorption and gas chromatography.

MDHS 96. Volatile organic compounds in air. Laboratory method using pumped solid sorbent tubes, solvent desorption and gas chromatography.

The Diffusive Monitor is a free publication of the Health and Safety Executive – Committee on Analytical Requirements, Working Group 5. This Working Group is concerned with workplace and environmental applications of diffusive sampling for assessing air quality. Available at http://www.hsl.gov.uk/publications/diffusive-monitor. html.

The NIOSH Manual of Analytical Methods (NMAM) is a collection of methods for sampling and analysis of air contaminants that are used in the United States. The methods have been developed or adapted by NIOSH. NMAM also includes chapters on quality assurance, sampling and direct-reading instrumentation. Available at http://www.cdc.gov/niosh/nmam/.

CHAPTER 11

11	**Bioaerosols**

11.1 Introduction

Biological agents comprise microorganisms along with a range of associated toxins and allergens that originate from animals and plants. These materials may be found in some manufacturing processes, in products used at work, as contaminants in work products or as contaminants in the environment. Most microorganisms are harmless viruses, bacteria or fungi that pose no threat to human health, but there are a few microorganisms that are highly infectious, produce endotoxins or other hazardous chemicals or can trigger an immunological response in humans.

As with most aerosols the principal route of entry into the body is by inhalation. For some microorganisms there is a possibility of skin infection (e.g. anthrax) or the transfer of the material into the body by ingestion from hand-to-mouth contacts, e.g. for *Escherichia coli* or Hepatitis A virus. Some microorganisms may result in infection if introduced into open wounds. However, in this chapter we focus exclusively on monitoring inhalation exposure to bioaerosols.

The main types of workers who may be at significant risk from bioaerosols are staff involved in recycling activities, sewage workers, staff in biological laboratories in industry and research institutions, health care workers, staff in diagnostic laboratories in hospitals and production areas where biological materials are handled or processed. Risks may arise from handling animal or human tissue such as post-mortem materials, blood, cultures, solutions, reagents and other materials containing harmful infectious agents. Farmers, foresters, veterinary staff, mortuary attendants, abattoir workers, refuse collectors, cleaners, engineering workers (from contaminated metalworking fluids) and many other jobs may involve exposure to bioaerosols.

Bioaerosols are classified as hazardous substances by the Health and Safety Executive (HSE) under the Control of Substances Hazardous to Health (COSHH) regulations in the Britain. This implies that employers have a responsibility to carry out a risk assessment to identify whether risks are acceptable and as part of this process they may wish to rely on the results from an exposure monitoring survey, although in laboratory or manufacturing situations reliance is often placed on clearly defined containment measures.

11.2 Classification of microorganisms

In Britain, the Advisory Committee on Dangerous Pathogens (ACDP) classify microorganisms into one of four hazard groups, depending on their ability to cause infection in humans. The ACDP comprises experts in occupational and public health biosafety from Government departments and academia. The four hazard groups are defined as follows:

- Hazard Group 1 – Unlikely to cause human disease. Usually the precautions taken to avoid contamination and ensure purity of the product, known as good manufacturing practice (GMP), are sufficient to protect employees in manufacturing processes using biological agents.
- Hazard Group 2 – Can cause human disease and may be a hazard to employees, but agents in this category are unlikely to spread to the community and there is usually effective prophylaxis or treatment available.
- Hazard Group 3 –Can cause severe human disease and these agents may be a serious hazard to employees; they may also spread to the community, but there is usually effective prophylaxis or treatment available.
- Hazard Group 4 –Causes severe human disease and are a serious hazard to employees; these agents are likely to spread to the community and there is usually no effective prophylaxis or treatment available.

The HSE has published a list of biological agents belonging to groups 2, 3 and 4. There is general advice available about the design and operation of facilities handling agents in groups 2–4, for example the degree of physical containment required, use of personal protective equipment (PPE) and the level of bio-security needed.

11.3 Viruses

Viruses range in size from about 20–450 nm in diameter. They consist of the genetic materials deoxyribonucleic acid (DNA) or ribonucleic acid (RNA) surrounded by a protein coat and possibly other components, and they can reproduce and replicate only in other living cells. Viruses are not considered to be living. Although viruses may be present in the work environment, they will die or remain dormant until a suitable living cell is available for their reproduction to commence and progress. The virus genetic material is enclosed in virions, varying in size from 100 to 1000 nm, which are capsules or coats of protein and/or lipids. Viruses can be the cause of occupational diseases in certain specialised industries, for example in farming, veterinary work and the pharmaceutical industry.

Because of their small size it is difficult to collect air samples to determine the concentration of viruses. Some researchers have developed systems to collect airborne viruses by using complex bubbler systems, but they generally have a low efficiency for collection. Sampling of airborne viruses is not routinely undertaken.

Airborne or water-droplet borne viruses such as influenza can be transferred by person–to-person contact, person-to-surface contact or by inhalation. Blood-borne viruses are a particular occupational hazard for those in healthcare professions. Needle-stick injuries, where a contaminated needle pierces the skin of a worker dealing with a patient who carries a virus such as HIV or hepatitis B, should be considered in particular settings. Assessment of the risk, appropriate training and implementation of specialised handling and transfer protocols are the main methods of preventing needle-stick injuries.

11.4 Bacteria

Bacteria are free-living single cells with an average size of about 500 nm and are capable of reproducing themselves in conditions that provide sufficient nutrients and water. They do not need other cells for their survival. They are found in different forms or colonies that are visible as:

- Cocci (spheres), which form clumps, pairs or chains;
- Bacilli (rods);
- Spirochaetes (spirals or filamentous);
- Actinomycetes (long rods that may show branching).

Bacteria have two types of cell wall, which affects their capacity to retain stains (Gram positive and negative), and this offers a method for their identification (Table 11.1). Many bacteria form spores or resistant dormant forms. This has a bearing on their ability to survive under various environmental conditions and contributes to their identification and classification. *Mycoplasma* are bacteria that have no defined cell walls.

Bacteria do not have a defined nucleus and the genetic material is not seen clearly under a microscope, as distinct from cells in higher forms of life, which have a definite nucleus inside a nuclear membrane. They are ubiquitous in many environments and reproduce asexually by dividing into two (binary fission). Bacteria need water to reproduce so they do not reproduce in air, although they may be transported through the air and consequently inhaled by workers. Some bacteria have flagella (whip-like appendages), which enable them to move through liquids.

Table 11.1 Examples of types of bacteria.

	Cocci	Bacilli
Gram positive	Staphylococcus aureus Streptococcus faecalis Micrococcus luteus	Bacillus Lactobacillus Corynebacterium
Gram negative	Neisseria vaginalis	Salmonella Escherichia coli Pseudomonas aeruginosa Legionella

Each environment or habitat supports specialised types of bacteria, adapted to make the best of that situation and this can help in their identification. For example, Gram-negative bacilli are sensitive to drying so are usually found only in moist or wet habitats. Gram-positive cocci, on the other hand, are associated with animal skins and mucous membranes.

Tuberculosis is mainly caused by *Mycobacterium tuberculosis,* which most commonly attacks the lungs but can also affect other organ systems. Tuberculosis is a serious potential risk for healthcare workers and other occupations that come into contact with people with tuberculosis, e.g. prison officers or welfare workers.

Legionella pneumophila is a Gram-negative bacterium that is common in low levels in water, but given the right conditions of nutrients and elevated temperature can multiply into large numbers. When made airborne, it is infectious via inhalation, which makes it a serious potential risk in occupations where workers may be exposed to water systems, such as process cooling waters.

An endotoxin is an insoluble structural component of bacteria that is toxic, endotoxin is released when bacteria are lysed, i.e. when the bacteria dies and the cell wall breaks down. *Pyrogens* are fever-producing compounds that increase body temperatures when inhaled or ingested. The bacterial substance lipopolysaccharide (LPS), which is a cell wall component of Gram-negative bacteria, is an example of a pyrogenic endotoxin.

11.5 Moulds and yeasts

Moulds are microscopic plants (fungi) with projections called mycelia. These can be broken into pieces that will grow and reproduce. They also produce spores that may become airborne and then be inhaled by workers. Moulds vary in their resistance to adverse conditions such as low pH and exposure to disinfectant.

Some of the more commonly identified moulds found in occupational environments are

- *Penicillium species;*
- *Cladosporium species;*
- *Aspergillus species* – commonly *Aspergillus flavus, Aspergillus terreus* and *Aspergillus fumigatus;*
- *Fusarium species;*
- *Stachybotrys chartarum* (also known as *Stachybotrys atra*).

Many moulds also produce 'mycotoxins', which are metabolites that have been identified as being toxic to humans. Aflatoxins, which are carcinogenic, are mycotoxins produced by many species of *Aspergillus.*

Moulds are generally found in soil, water and decaying material, and exposure to them via the respiratory route mostly does not cause ill health. However, they can produce respiratory disease among people whose immune system is compromised, primarily pneumonia, by inhalation of contaminated aerosols. Long-term exposure may result in asthma or other allergic respiratory diseases.

Yeasts are fungi that are usually bigger than bacteria and have their nuclear materials in a cell nucleus, whereas bacterial nuclear material is free in the cytoplasm. Yeasts usually reproduce by budding. There are a small number of yeasts that are pathogenic, including the *Candida* species of yeast that can cause a 'thrush' infection. Inhalation of yeast can very occasionally cause occupational asthma.

11.6 Allergens

There are a number of bioaerosols that are known to cause asthma or other allergic diseases. These include biological enzymes obtained from bacteria or fungi (used in detergent washing powders amongst other things), latex, and animal proteins from rats, mice, shell food, dust mites, and many other sources of high molecular weight substances.

In the 1960s, when the first powdered protease was introduced into detergent manufacture processes, high rates of asthma in the workforce were recorded. To solve this problem, the enzymes used in the products were encapsulated to reduce the emission of respirable dust and better engineering controls were introduced. More recently other encapsulated enzymes, such as amylases, cellulases and lipases have been added to detergent powders, with some of these agents being more potent sensitizers than protease. Occasional outbreaks of sensitization amongst workers have been attributed to higher exposures when encapsulated powders are inadvertently crushed to produce respirable size dust. The industry guideline level for exposure to enzymes is $0.015\ \mu g\ m^{-3}$.

Workers involved in processing of crabs, prawns and other shellfish are exposed to aerosolized protein that can cause sensitisation. The allergen aerosol exposure can range from 0.001 to about $5\ \mu g\ m^{-3}$. The prevalence of occupational asthma in such workplaces can be as high as a third of the workforce. Sensitised individuals may react to other fish species within a major seafood grouping.

Laboratory animal allergy (LAA) results from exposure to mouse and rat urinary proteins dispersed into the air on bedding etc. Up to a third of workers may become sensitized and one in ten may then go on and suffer from occupational asthma. The air concentrations of the sensitizing proteins in animal facilities are generally very low, with animal technicians experiencing personal inhalation exposures typically in the 10 to $100\ \mu g/m^3$, with protein exposures 10 to $100\ \mu g/m^{-3}$ range. Dermal exposure may be more important in these circumstances.

11.7 Principles of containment

To prevent microorganisms used in industry from entering into or infecting a worker various levels of barriers need to be set up:

1. Primary barriers are used to confine the organisms so that they cannot escape from the containers in which they are produced or handled. This is done by the use of appropriate equipment including microbiological safety cabinets, by the use of effective disinfection and sterilisation procedures and by good laboratory and/or industrial practice.
2. Secondary barriers are the barriers that are placed between the worker and the organisms. These include protective clothing, medical surveillance and immunisation and a high level of personal hygiene.
3. Tertiary barriers are placed around the work areas, which includes security and limited access, supervision of invitees and visitors. They also include procedures such as autoclaving of infected waste before it leaves the work area and waste management.

Deliberate processing or handling of harmful biological agents is normally confined to specifically designated work areas. Ideally these work areas should be provided with a ventilation system for which the air supplied to the corridors always flows into the work areas and in which there is a slight excess of exhaust over supply, which creates 'negative' pressure. Although circumstances vary according to needs, the air is often filtered both at the inlet and exhaust ends of the system and where necessary, forced by a fan through high-efficiency particulate air (HEPA) filters.

When working with contaminated materials in buildings or the outside environment then it is important to plan the work carefully. Reliance should be placed on work methods that minimise aerosol generation, e.g. wet vacuuming, and in the use of PPE, particularly respiratory protection. In some instances biocides or fungicides may be used and it is important to consider the risks from using these chemicals in addition to the biological hazards.

11.8 Handling microorganisms

Microorganism cultures must always be handled carefully, and treated as if they contained pathogens. Work with microorganisms can be performed safely if the following safety rules are observed:

- Wash hands thoroughly before and after working;
- Do not eat or drink in the work area;
- Do not touch known microorganisms with unprotected hands;
- Never pipette suspensions containing microorganisms with the mouth – always use mechanical aids to pipette;
- Prior to and after use, sterilise inoculating loops and wires by flaming until they glow red-hot, and if possible, substitute their use by disposable plastic inoculating loops;
- Sterilise all equipment that comes in contact with microorganisms;

- Ensure that everything that leaves the work area, such as contaminated waste, discarded agar plates etc., is not infectious by disinfecting, autoclaving or incineration;
- Ensure that the decontamination methods used are effective against the microorganisms being handled.

11.9 Monitoring bioaerosols

Monitoring for bioaerosols, like other forms of monitoring, entails collecting a representative sample, examining or analysing it and interpreting the results before any conclusions can be drawn.

Sample collection can be carried out by a health and safety professional under the guidance of a microbiologist or other expert, although it should be realised that this area of measurement is complex and requires particular knowledge and expertise. Those who take the samples must be trained in aseptic techniques, and should understand the routes by which samples can become contaminated and hence invalid.

In general, the equipment that is available for routine monitoring of bioaerosols is bulky and unsuitable for personal sampling. Microorganisms are placed under a great deal of stress during the sampling process, and if the analysis requires that the biological agent is viable, i.e. living, then it is normal practice to keep the sampling time quite short, typically less than 20 min and often just a minute or two. Another reason for short sampling times is to avoid overloading the sampling media, which would lead to an underestimation of the number of viable aerosol particles collected. The sampling technology for microorganisms has developed separately from mainstream occupational hygiene air sampling and so most samplers available for bioaerosols are not compatible with the modern inhalable, thoracic and respirable sampling conventions.

It is often difficult to predict in advance the range of biological agents that will be present in the air at a workplace and it is therefore difficult to choose the growth medium for the sampler to enable the agent of interest to grow effectively. Storage conditions of the sample after collection are again critical. Ensuring that samples are kept at the correct temperature and humidity will ensure that the biological agents remain viable. There may also be differences in the analysis between laboratories and between analysts from the same laboratory. Appropriate laboratory quality assurance procedures are key to getting reliable results.

Air sampling for microorganisms either assesses the *viable and culturable* or *total* microorganism load. Not all microbial cells within a bioaerosol will be capable of being cultured, the remainder being either dead but intact cells, or 'viable but non culturable' (VBNC), i.e. live cells that cannot be cultured either because they are metabolically dormant or because the collection media used will not support their growth. Because these intact cells may still represent an immunological challenge, they are measured in some human health

Table 11.2 Examples of active sampling for culturable bioaerosols.

Method of sampling	Typical instruments	Free bacteria or fungi diameter $<4\,\mu m$	Clumped diameter $4\,\mu m$
Impactors	Casella Airborne Bacteria Sampler (ABS)	May undersample smaller spores	Suitable
	Anderson Microbial Sampler (6-stage)	Suitable for concentrations <5000 CFU m^{-3}	Suitable for concentrations <5000 CFU m^{-3}
	Surface Air Sampler (SAS)	Not suitable	Good collection efficiency
Impingers	SKC BioSampler	Good collection efficiency	Good collection efficiency
	Burkard May-Type Sampler	Good for very high or very low concentrations. May underestimate concentration.	May overestimate concentration due to break up of clumps.
Membrane filters		Good for very high or very low concentrations. Only for desiccation resistant bacteria or fungi	Good for very high or very low concentrations.

impact studies, but for the most part bioaerosol sampling focuses on assessment of culture-based analysis. Active sampling (Table 11.2) involves drawing a measured volume of air through a collection device and subsequently analysing the sample. The results from these analyses for culturable bacteria are expressed in terms of colony forming units (CFU), based on the number of bacterial colonies counted on the sampling substrate or in an analytical system, and expressed as CFU m^{-3}.

Size selection can be achieved by means of a cascade impactor or multistage liquid impinger as shown in Figure 11.1. After collection the sample is inoculated onto agar plates (if the method does not involve direct inoculation) and incubated at an appropriate temperature. Microbial growth as colonies are then counted visually or using an automated image analysis system. Impactors rely on the airflow being directed towards a flat plate that then collects the aerosols based on the inertia of the particle, i.e. as the air is diverted past the plate the particles, if they have sufficient momentum, continue until they strike the plate. Impingers are similar to impactors except that the air is directed through a thin tube towards a liquid where the larger particles deposit as they impinge on the liquid surface.

Slit impactors. These samplers are designed to collect on culture media any organisms that are present in the air. In some samplers, such as the Casella Airborne Bacteria Sampler (ABS), shown in Figure 11.2, the air is drawn through

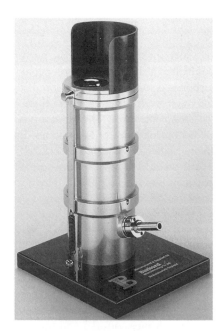

Figure 11.1 A multi-stage liquid impinger.
(© Burkard Manufacturing Co. Limited.
Reproduced with permission.)

slits and the microorganisms impact on rotating agar plates. The dimensions of the slits and the distance from slits to the agar surface and the airflow are controlled to minimise the damage to the organism, while effectively collecting the aerosol. For example, the Casella sampler draws air at the rate of 700 L min^{-1} and the recommended sampling time is 5 min. The sampling time may be extended by coating the agar with hydrophilic wax. The plates are incubated and the numbers of colonies counted.

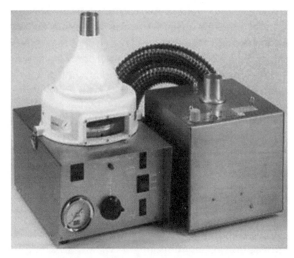

Figure 11.2 Cascade impactor for bioaerosols. (© Casella Measurement Ltd. Reproduced with permission.)

Single-stage impactors. The air sample is drawn through slits and the particles impinge on an agar plate. An example is the SAS Microbial Air Sampler in which the distance from the perforations to the agar surface is not as highly controlled as in the slit sampler, making this sampler less efficient at capturing airborne contaminants. The sampling volumes will be large enough to examine most environments where there is some concern about exposure.

Cascade impactors. The air sampled is drawn through a series of perforated plates onto a stack of agar plates. Each agar plate is separated by perforated metal plates, the size of the perforations decreasing from the top to the bottom of the stack. Larger particles impact on the top agar plates and the smaller particles pass through until they impact on the appropriate plate lower in the stack. An example of this type of device is the Andersen sampler, where the sampling rate is 28 L min^{-1} and the device can have between one and eight stages.

Centrifugal sampler. These are usually battery operated and hand-held, making them useful for fieldwork. The air is drawn into the sampling head by means of an impeller that directs the aerosol onto an agar strip fitted around the circumference of the sampling head. An example is the Biotest Folex sampler in which the sampling rate is 40 L min^{-1}. The strip is incubated, the numbers of colonies counted and the viable count estimated. Strips containing selective and non-selective culture media are available.

Liquid impingement. The air sampled is drawn through an aspirator bottle containing a suitable medium. After the specified sampling time the solution is serially diluted, plated, incubated and examined to determine the number of colony forming units. An example of an impinger is the All Glass Impinger – 30 (AGI-30), where the end of the tube is 30 mm above the base of the impinger. The SKC BioSampler is a specially designed impinger with three curved tubes that cause the liquid to swirl around inside the vessel. It has high collection efficiency and can be used to sample over long periods when a low volatility liquid is used in place of water. An advantage of impingers is that the collected sample is relatively easy to dilute prior to analysis.

Filtration. The air sampled is drawn through a membrane or gelatine filter. The filter is then plated out, incubated and examined. Microorganisms will dry out on a filter surface and become non-viable or non-culturable, and so this method is not particularly suitable for assessing viable bioaerosols.

11.10 Measurement of endotoxins and allergens

Conventional air sampling techniques are generally used for most non-viable allergen aerosols. For example, sampling for endotoxin is normally undertaken by using conventional filter-based monitoring techniques, although it is possible to analyse endotoxin in the liquid of impinger samples and this can allow determination of microorganism content and endotoxin from the same sample. A wide range of filters is used to collect samples for endotoxin analysis and it is best to consult with the laboratory that will undertake the analysis about the exact choice for your situation. Analysis of these samples is normally based on the LAL (*limulus amebocyte lysate*) assay, which measures how the extract from blood cells of the horseshoe crab responds to the presence of endotoxin from Gram-negative bacteria. Because this is a biological assay it is necessary to standardise the results to a reference material – currently *E. coli*-6. The measurements are expressed in terms of endotoxin units, i.e. EU m^{-3}.

Laboratory animal allergens can be sampled onto Teflon filters in inhalable sampling heads. Analysis is normally carried out using a sophisticated immunoassay. One of the difficulties with these analyses is the lack of standardisation of the assays between laboratories and so one must be careful in interpreting differences between measurements made by different laboratories.

11.11 Interpretation of sample results

There is no general scientific consensus about the maximum permissible levels of exposure to airborne bacteria or fungi to protect health, although a number of organisations have issued guideline levels that can be used in the interpretation of measurements. In general, airborne fungi levels are higher outdoors compared with indoor environments. The Bioaerosol Committee of the American Conference of Governmental Industrial Hygienists (ACGIH) states that the outdoor concentration of airborne fungi routinely exceeds 1000 CFU m^{-3} and may be higher than 10,000 CFU m^{-3}. They also note that concentrations above about 100 CFU m^{-3} may be unhealthy in immunosuppressed individuals. Indoor bacterial aerosols may range up to 4500–10,000 CFU m^{-3} due to ubiquitous bacterial contamination.

Clearly, the identity of the bacteria or fungi may help to indicate an unexpected contamination. For example *actinomycetes* are often found outdoors in agricultural areas, but according to NIOSH Thermophilic *actinomycetes* at levels above about 70 CFU m^{-3} should provide an indication that further control measures are necessary.

The National Health Council of the Netherlands originally proposed a health-based limit for endotoxin of 50 EU m^{-3}, but after completing a feasibility study where it was clear that levels in the agricultural sector were generally higher than the proposed limit and they finally adopted a pragmatic limit of 200 EU m^{-3}. This is not yet implemented as a statutory exposure limit, but is used in that country as an industry guidance standard.

References and further reading

Douwes J, Thorne P, Pearce N, Heederik D. (2003). Bioaerosol health effects and exposure assessment: progress and prospects. *Annals of Occupational Hygiene* 47(3): 187–200. Available at http://annhyg.oxfordjournals.org/cgi/content/full/47/3/187.
Spaan S, Schinkel J, Wouters IM, Preller L, Tielemans E, Nij ET, Heederik D. (2008). Variability in endotoxin exposure levels and consequences for exposure assessment. *Annals*

of Occupational Hygiene 52(5): 303–316. Available at http://annhyg.oxfordjournals.org/cgi/reprint/men024v3.

Jensen PA, Schafer MP. (2003). Sampling and characterization of bioaerosols. In *NIOSH Manual of Analytical Methods*, 4th edition. NIOSH Publication Number 2003-154 (3rd Supplement). Washington, DC: CDC NIOSH. Available at http://www.cdc.gov/niosh/docs/2003-154/pdfs/chapter-j.pdf.

HSE (2001). *The Management, Design and Operation of Microbiological Containment Laboratories.* Sudbury, UK: HSE Books.

Advisory Committee on Dangerous Pathogens websites:
http://www.hse.gov.uk/aboutus/meetings/committees/acdp/index.htm
http://www.advisorybodies.doh.gov.uk/acdp/index.htm.

HSE infections website:
http://www.hse.gov.uk/biosafety/index.htm.

On the HSE infections web site there is the guidance Infection at Work – Controlling the risk (http://www.hse.gov.uk/pubns/infection.pdf), which is a very good general document.

Also, guidance on blood-borne viruses such as HIV and hepatitis. Available at http://www.hse.gov.uk/biosafety/diseases/blood-borne-virus.htm.

The Approved List of Biological Agents is available at http://www.hse.gov.uk/pubns/misc208.pdf.

Working with highly pathogenic avian influenza virus at http://www.hse.gov.uk/biosafety/diseases/avianflu.htm.

HSE legionnaires website: http://www.hse.gov.uk/legionnaires/index.htm.

US NIOSH Asthma and Allergies topic page: http://www.cdc.gov/niosh/topics/asthma/.

3 Dermal and Ingestion Exposure

12   Dermal and Ingestion Exposure Measurement

12.1   Introduction

As we have seen, interest in protecting health from exposure to hazards in the workplace has traditionally focused on the inhaled route. Breathing in too much of a particular gas, vapour, dust or fibre often leads to acute health effects that can either be immediately life threatening or can damage an individual's health over time. Historically, this resulted in many respiratory physicians working in occupational medicine. Over the last 20 or 30 years there has been an increasing awareness of the health effects that can arise from dermal exposure to chemicals in the workplace, both in terms of uptake through the unbroken skin and entry to the systemic blood circulation as is the case of chemicals such as solvents, and from local effects that can damage the skin and lead to dermatitis or more serious conditions. Much of our understanding of dermal exposure, particularly in relation to the development of exposure measurement methods and in assessing the effectiveness of protective clothing, has arisen from research on pesticide use. Assessment of inadvertent ingestion exposure, for example from hand-to-mouth contacts, is still at an early stage of development. In this chapter, we outline some of the issues associated with measurement of dermal and ingestion exposure, although it should be realised that these techniques are not routinely applied in occupational hygiene practice.

12.2   Occupations where dermal exposure is important

Dermal exposure to chemicals is found in a wide variety of jobs. The agricultural sector includes many workers who either apply pesticide formulations to crops, veterinary medicines to the skins of animals or who become indirectly exposed by handling treated animals or harvesting crops. Fruit pickers, despite not being involved in the application of pesticides, may receive high dermal exposure due to 're-entry' and 'harvesting' tasks, where they are in contact with pesticide residues on fruit surfaces. Engineers involved in tool-setting, cutting and lathe operations also regularly have high dermal exposure to metalworking fluids, oils and cleaning solvents. Painters,

Table 12.1 Some key occupations where dermal exposure may arise.

Occupation	Typical substances where dermal exposure may need to be assessed
Farm workers	Pesticides, solvents, diesel, wood preservatives, wet-work
Bakers	Flour dust, wet-work
Hairdressers and barbers	Hair dyes, wet-work
Chefs and cooks	Acids, alkalis, detergents, wet-work, garlic and many other food stuffs
Electronic equipment assemblers	Solder flux, epoxy resins, isocyanates
Nurses	Detergents, disinfectants, latex rubber, drugs, wet-work, wearing gloves
Laboratory technicians	Various chemicals, wearing gloves
Metal workers	Metals (nickel, chromium), metal working fluids (wet-work)
Florists	Plants, pesticides, wet-work
Construction workers	Cement, epoxy resins, solvents, isocyanates, metals, wet-work

especially those involved in spraying, can often receive widespread paint and solvent coverage of their skin depending on their working environment and the protection afforded by their clothing. Other occupations less obviously have dermal exposure problems. However, hairdressers, cleaners, catering staff and nursery nurses all have an increased risk of developing skin disease due to their frequent contact with chemicals or simply as a result of repeated wet-work; water being one of the most frequently overlooked irritant chemicals in the workplace. Table 12.1 provides a list of some key occupations where dermal exposure is likely to require some degree of assessment to ensure tasks are properly controlled.

The top ten agents causing occupational skin disease in Britain are the following:

- Rubber;
- Soaps and cleaners;
- Wet-work;
- Impervious gloves;
- Petroleum and petroleum products;
- Nickel;
- Metalworking fluids;
- Epoxy and other resins;
- Solvents and alcohols;
- Aldehydes.

12.3 Local and systemic effects

Before measuring or assessing dermal exposure to chemicals it is important to consider the type of skin–chemical interaction taking place. First, the chemical may pass through the skin and contribute to the amount of that substance in the blood and other organs; adding to the mass of the same chemical absorbed into the body through the lungs. This percutaneous uptake of chemicals is seen with many lipophillic substances including pesticides, solvents and polycyclic aromatic hydrocarbons (PAHs). Systemically absorbed chemicals can then go on to have health effects in many target organs such as the liver, brain, reproductive organs and other sites remote to the original dermal contact.

The second type of interaction occurs when chemicals cause local skin damage. Some chemicals such as acids, alkalis, soaps, disinfectants and water are irritants and may cause damage at the point of contact. Note that that the wearing of impervious gloves causes the hands to be moist from sweat and this can also cause irritant dermatitis. Some solvents can de-fat the skin, and hence cause irritation, while also undergoing percutaneous absorption. Other chemicals can cause skin cancer; sometimes the risk is increased because of co-exposure to sunlight, e.g. mixtures containing polycyclic aromatic haydrocarbons.

The third skin–chemical interaction involves immune responses to a chemical's contact with the skin. These can trigger allergic skin reactions both at the site of contact and on other areas of the body. There is also evidence that some substances may produce respiratory sensitization from dermal contact, e.g. aromatic isocyanates.

12.4   How do we know if dermal exposure is an issue?

There are three main ways of identifying if dermal contact has the potential to cause problems in the workplace: from details of 'skin notation' for a substance, from risk phrases on the product safety data sheet (SDS) or product label and from observation of prolonged wet-work or prolonged use of impervious gloves. Skin notation is assigned to chemical substances by many national regulatory authorities when they set occupational exposure limits (OELs). The purpose of the notation is to alert users to the fact that the material can contribute substantially to total body burden by uptake through the unbroken skin. In Britain, the Health and Safety Executive (HSE) has assigned a skin notation to over 120 chemicals. Details of current skin notations can be found in HSE guidance note EH40.

Risk phrases, as required by the chemicals (Hazard Information and Packaging for Supply) regulations, can also provide information useful in assessing the risk from dermal exposure to a given material. Table 12.2 provides details of some of the risk phrases relevant to dermal exposure and skin disease. If a task or process involves some skin contact with chemicals that have one or more of these risk phrases then an assessment of exposure should be made and, if necessary, appropriate control measures should be introduced.

Water and wet-work are probably the cause of the majority of occupational irritant contact dermatitis in jobs such as catering, health care and cleaning. There is no specific guidance on limiting wet-work exposure in Britain, but

Table 12.2 Risk phrases relevant to dermal exposure and skin diseases.

Risk phrase	Description
R21	Harmful in contact with the skin
R24	Toxic in contact with the skin
R27	Very toxic in contact with the skin
R34	Causes burns
R35	Causes severe burns
R38	Irritating to the skin
R43	May cause sensitization by skin contact
R66	Repeated exposure may cause skin dryness or cracking

The introduction of the United Nations Globally Harmonised System of Classification and Labelling of Chemicals (GHS) will result in changes to these phrases by 2015.

the German authorities have introduced the guidance TRGS 531, which recommends limiting the duration of wet-work to 2 h daily, avoiding more than 20 wet-dry cycles per shift and prohibiting the wearing of gloves for more than 4 h. Work outside these parameters should be considered to present a risk for irritant dermatitis.

12.5   What do we measure?

Dermal exposure can be assessed by considering four parameters:

- intensity of skin exposure (mass or concentration on skin M_{sk} or C_{sk});
- area of skin exposed (A_{sk});
- duration of exposure (t) and
- frequency of exposure.

Dermal uptake of chemicals occurs when the substance diffuses through the outer layers of the skin. It is the concentration of the chemical on the outer skin surface that drives this diffusion process but in the absence of methods to measure concentration, the mass of contaminant is often used as a surrogate. Measurement of mass can then be further divided into 'potential' or 'actual' exposure. 'Potential' exposure refers to the material that deposits on the worker's overalls, clothing and gloves while 'actual' exposure refers to the substance that comes into contact with the skin.

The second parameter required to assess dermal exposure is the surface area of the body that is exposed to the chemical. Methods for measuring this are described later in this chapter but it should be remembered that the area exposed is likely to be subject to a high degree of day-to-day and between-worker variation, especially where dermal contact results from random or uncontrolled processes such as splashes or spills.

The duration and frequency of contact are also important in characterizing dermal exposure. The length of time that the worker handles a material may not be relevant when the substance soaks onto her clothing and overalls and then continues to be in contact with the skin long after the end of the task. In such cases the length of time until removal of the clothing is likely to be the more relevant factor.

For wet-work the duration and frequency of contact are likely to be the keys to understanding and controlling a worker's risk of developing skin disease. Observation of the tasks is the primary method of assessment but there can be significant difficulties in identifying times when a worker's hands are wet or dry. Immersion and hand-washing events are clearly visible and obvious occasions when there is exposure, but other tasks such as using a damp cloth to wipe surfaces or incomplete drying of the hands can make it problematic to identify wet-work frequency and duration. Work is underway to develop a wet-work monitor attached to the finger that uses two small thermocouples sensors to record the temperature on the skin and just above it to objectively measure the times that the skin surface is wet. This monitor may be commercially available in the future.

12.6 Methods for dermal exposure measurement

Unlike inhaled exposures there are very few standard methods for dermal exposure assessment. Protocols for dermal exposure measurement have developed in a piecemeal manner and have often been targeted at particular chemicals or tasks. Many of the methods are based on, or are adaptations of, techniques used to measure dermal exposure to pesticides.

Dermal sampling methods can broadly be divided into three classes:

- interception methods
- removal methods and
- in situ visualisation methods.

Interception methods use whole body overalls or patches of absorbent or adsorbent materials to capture the chemical under study at various locations on the body. These methods are often referred to as 'surrogate skin' methods and have the advantage of directly capturing the contaminant and also providing detail on the distribution of the exposure over different areas of the body. The two most commonly used interception methods are those published by the World Health Organisation (WHO) and the Organisation for Economic Cooperation and Development (OECD). The type of sampling material should be matched to the chemicals being monitored, with cotton, polyester, cellulose paper and polyurethane foam all commonly used. Whole body suits obviously have the advantage of capturing exposure across the whole body surface but extraction of the chemical from about 2 m^2 of material can be both analytically complex and expensive. Patches can limit these problems but as they typically cover only 3–8% of the body surface they have the disadvantage of possible under- or overestimation of exposure due to the necessary scaling up of results from small areas to estimate the whole body exposure. The information to scale up the results from patch samples depends on the body part the patch is attached to, and Table 12.3 shows the standard skin surface areas

Table 12.3   Area of various body parts for dermal exposure assessment.

Body part	Area (cm²)
Head	1075
Neck	230
Back	1536
Thighs	3456
Calves	2592
Feet	1229
Shoulder	1306
Chest	1536
Hips	1747
Hands	1075
Forearms	1286
Upper arms	1862
Whole body surface	19,200

Note: The data in the table are based on the 50th percentile male, height 175 cm, weight 78 kg.

for various sections of the body that can be used to extrapolate results from patch samplers.

The number and location of patches used can vary but generally range from 6 to 16 locations with sizes from 5 × 5 cm to 10 × 10 cm. A typical arrangement of patch samplers is illustrated in Figure 12.1.

Unlike interception methods, removal methods aim to sample the mass of the material remaining on a worker's skin at a particular point in time. Removal methods use wipe sampling, tape stripping or washing techniques to physically extract the contaminant from the skin surface. Often sequential washes, wipes or tape strips are taken to maximise recovery. It should be noted that recovery efficiencies can show considerable variability particularly between different operators using different pressures of wiping or due to subtle difference in skin-stripping technique, but in some cases it is just difficult to recover the substance from the skin. Removal methods are of limited use for materials that are volatile and likely to evaporate from the skin surface or for materials that are very quickly absorbed through the skin; in these situations it is necessary to use patches containing activated charcoal or some other adsorbent, or a skin-stripping methodology.

Washing methods are most often used for the hands and typically use water or some water/detergent mixture to remove material from the skin surface. Hand washing is often performed inside a bag to prevent loss of fluid. Alternatively, the wash can be carried out with a known volume of fluid poured over the hands above a collecting funnel directed into a sample jar. These techniques have been used for pesticide exposure measurement, but not more extensively.

Wiping typically uses a wetted cloth or proprietary moist wipe, which is applied with uniform pressure over a pre-determined area of skin that may

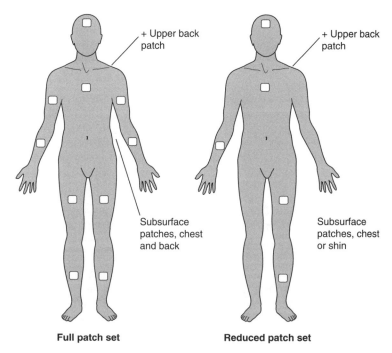

Full patch set   **Reduced patch set**

Figure 12.1 Typical arrangement of patches used in patch-sampling methods. (Reproduced with permission *Occupational Hygiene*, 3rd edition, edited by Kerry Gardiner and J. Malcolm Harrington, Blackwell Publishing Ltd., 2005, p. 395.)

be marked out using a 5 cm × 5 cm or 10 cm × 10 cm template, depending on the preference of the investigator. Similarly, tape stripping uses small sections of adhesive tape to physically remove the outer layers of the skin and any contaminant material that has already been adsorbed.

With all removal methods it is important to have detailed discussions with the laboratory responsible for the sample analysis to ensure that they will not encounter problems with interference between the materials used in the wipe or tape substrate or wash and the chemical under study. Pilot work to determine recovery efficiencies from spiked samples is advisable as is good training of those performing the sample collection to reduce operator variability.

The third type of measurement method is in situ visualisation, which generally involves the addition of a fluorescent tracer to the material being studied. The fluorescent marker binds to skin proteins on contact and allows visualisation of the areas of skin contaminated and some measure of the mass of contaminant by using the correlation between the fluorescent image intensity and a calibration standard image. Visualisation typically involves the use of complex software and ultraviolet lighting to capture data in three dimensions from the body surface. Two similar systems exist for visualisation: the fluorescent interactive video exposure system (FIVES) and the video image technique to assess dermal exposure (VITAE). Although the systems are portable, they require specialist knowledge to operate, plus detailed calibration and the agreement of the workplace management to add the fluorescent marker to the material under study. The use of visualisation techniques has tended to be limited to research special applications, but they can be a powerful tool to educate workers about dermal exposure. Images of contamination at the end of a work-shift can help workers identify where and how their skin was exposed.

A summary of the main types of dermal exposure measurement is provided in Table 12.4.

12.7 Sampling strategy

The collection of dermal exposure samples is not straightforward. Design of a sampling strategy that will maximise the amount of useful information obtained will require consideration of how the task is performed, the number of workers exposed and the variability in exposure between workers and over time. In addition, the strategy should examine the timing of sample collection and the degree of substance evaporation, absorption and removal during the time between exposure and collection. Using a hand wash method at the end of the work day to measure pesticide contamination from a short mixing task that occurred some 7 h previously will yield very different results to the same method targeted at the period immediately after completion of the mixing. Task-based sampling or frequent collection of samples at regular times during the work-shift may be the most appropriate answer, but this approach will inevitably increase collection and analysis costs. When using removal methods in particular, it is very important to explain to the worker the timing of the sampling strategy in relation to the work-breaks to prevent personal hand washing taking place prior to sample collection. Collection of contextual information about the worker's tasks, such as the number of times contaminated surfaces are contacted and accidental splashing onto the skin, plus information on hand cleaning or removal of gloves or clothing is of particular importance.

12.8 Liquids and solids

Most dermal exposure research has focussed on exposure to liquids but there is increasing interest in dermal exposure to solids including fine particulate matter and even nanoparticles, for example used in pharmaceuticals or sun protection creams. Metals such as nickel and chromium can cause local irritant or allergic effects by dissolving in the sweat and sebum layer on the skin surface and then being absorbed across the unbroken skin. Studies suggest that intact sub-micrometer particles of beryllium metal may penetrate into the skin and then initiate an immune response leading to chronic beryllium disease, although in almost all cases, solids must dissolve in sweat before they can be absorbed through the skin. Measurement of dermal exposure to other metal

Table 12.4 Methods for measuring dermal exposure.

Method type	Description	Advantages	Disadvantages	Measurement of the key parameters				References
				M_{sk}	A_{sk}	t	C_{sk}	
Interception: patches	Small square cotton or other cloth patches attached to the body	Standard method for pesticides	Only low volatility substances, only small proportion of body sampled	✗	✗	✓	✗	Soutar et al. (2000)
Interception: suit sampling and gloves	Workers wear lightweight cotton overalls with hood.	Whole body sample	Only low volatility substances, practical difficulties in sampling and analysis	✗	✗	✓	✗	Soutar et al. (2000)
Removal: washing or wiping	Defined areas of skin washed with a solvent or wiped with a moist cloth.	Low cost, easy to use	Only for low volatility substances that don't quickly penetrate through the skin	✓	✗	✓	✗	Brouwer et al. (2000)
In situ: Fluorescence	Fluorescent compound added to the source and then the intensity of fluorescence on the workers body.	Accurate assessment of area exposed, whole body sample	Requires specialist equipment, must add fluorescent agent to source	✓	✓	✓	✗	Cherrie et al. (2000)

dusts has been undertaken using removal techniques including washing and wiping. Understanding dermal exposure to solids is particularly important in cases of inadvertent ingestion exposure in the workplace; hand and face contamination can then result in hand-to-mouth transfer of the contaminant and result in ingestion. Measurement of dermal exposure coupled with data on behaviours including hand-to-surface, tool-to-mouth and hand-to-mouth contacts can then be used to provide information on the possible contribution of the ingestion route to total body burden. We consider inadvertent ingestion in 'Inadvertent ingestion exposure' section.

12.9   Biomonitoring and modelling of dermal exposure

Measurement of dermal exposure is a labour-intensive process and due to the complexities of sample collection and analysis can be prone to error. Where you have some information about the level of exposure from other routes and where a suitable method is available, biomonitoring can provide a useful way of quantifying dermal exposure and uptake. Such methods require an understanding of the toxicology and pharmacokinetics of the material being studied; i.e. how it is transported around the body.

Using a model to estimate dermal exposure has many advantages over measurement. Using a simple conceptual model, similar to that shown in Figure 3.1b, it is possible to consider how dermal exposure is taking place and therefore to target controls at the most important compartments and transfer processes. A detailed conceptual model of dermal exposure was developed by Thomas Schneider and other scientists in the late 1990s and has been used as the basis for many research studies examining occupational dermal exposure. This source–receptor model involves a series of sources and compartments linked to each other by transport processes and can be used to describe how a chemical passes from the source to the skin of the worker. Emissions from the source can travel to the air compartment, to surfaces in the work environment, to the outside of the worker's clothing or to the worker's skin. Material may then be transferred between these compartments by transfer, removal, evaporation or deposition. When deposited on the outer clothing compartment a substance can permeate, i.e. diffuse through the intact material, or penetrate, i.e. pass through gaps in the material, to the skin compartment.

In addition to the use of the conceptual model to target control methods, it can also be used to inform dermal sampling strategies. For example, the measurement of a contaminated work surface as a surrogate for dermal exposure may be possible given a conceptual analysis using the model. Such a strategy would require consideration of evaporation of the material from the surface, the frequency and nature of the worker's hands with the contaminated surface and the spatial variability of both the contamination and the worker's contact. The model can also be used to identify which items of contextual information you should collect when measuring dermal exposure; e.g. is the number of contacts with a particular surface important?

12.10 From exposure to uptake

The relationship between inhaled exposure and uptake into the body is well understood, with the biological effect of inhaled exposure generally well correlated with the concentration measured in the breathing zone. Unfortunately, the same cannot be said for dermal exposure. The mass of material absorbed by the body is linked to that measured on the skin surface by the ability of the substance to pass through the outer layers of skin, i.e. the *stratum corneum*. The uptake rate of the chemical is dependent on the following parameters:

- The substance molecular weight;
- The substance solubility in water;
- Substance solubility in oils and
- Its chemical structure.

These factors can be used to predict the K_p or permeability coefficient (measured in cm h^{-1}) of the substance, which can then be combined with the concentration of the material on the skin to estimate a flux rate of the chemical through the skin, i.e. the mass of contaminant passing a unit area of skin per unit time, which could be measured in mg cm^{-2} h^{-1}. By using data on the area of the skin exposed and the duration of exposure, the flux rate can then be used to calculate the mass of material absorbed through the skin in a given situation. Permeability coefficients differ greatly between substances and preparations containing those substances and hence the uptake of two different chemicals with the same dermal exposure can be several orders of magnitude apart.

In comparing dermal uptake to inhalation uptake it is worthwhile to look at a simple example of a painter who washes his/her hands in neat xylene thinners for about 1 min at the end of a task lasting 1 h, where the concentration of xylene in the air was measured at 10 ppm (equivalent to 44 mg m^{-3}). The mass of xylene absorbed by inhalation is given by the following calculation:

$$U_{inh} = C_{air} \times B \times t$$

where C_{air} is the concentration in the air (mg m^{-3}); B is the breathing rate (m^3 h^{-1}); t is the duration of exposure (h).
The inhalation uptake therefore is

$$U_{inh} = 44 \text{ mg m}^{-3} \times 1.5 \text{ m}^3 \text{ h}^{-1} \times 1 \text{ h}$$

$$U_{inh} = 66 \text{ mg}$$

The dermal uptake can be estimated from the equation:

$$U_{sk} = K_p \times C_{sk} \times A \times t$$

where K_p is the permeability coefficient (cm h^{-1}) [0.012 cm h^{-1} for xylene]; C_{sk} is the concentration of the material on the skin (mg cm^{-3}) [900 mg cm^{-3} for xylene thinners]; A is the area of skin exposed (cm^2) [1075 cm^2 for hand washing in this example]; t is the duration of exposure (h) [0.0167 h in this example].

So the dermal uptake therefore is

$$U_{sk} = 0.012 \text{ cm h}^{-1} \times 900 \text{ mg cm}^{-3} \times 1075 \text{ cm}^2 \times 0.0167 \text{ h}$$

$$U_{sk} = 194 \text{ mg}$$

In this case, it is possible to see that the contribution to the total body burden from the short dermal exposure from the painter washing their hands in thinners is almost twice that from the inhaled exposure during the 1 h of spray painting.

12.11 Controlling dermal exposure

Personal protective equipment has often been recommended to control dermal exposure. While overalls and gloves can help reduce the deposition of material on the skin and/or the area of skin exposed the use of personal protective equipment should, for both inhaled and dermal exposure routes, not necessarily be considered the best or most appropriate approach to control. Elimination of the exposure should be the primary aim and often this can be achieved by automation or changes to work practices. A simple example of this would be the provision of a dishwashing machine in a catering establishment, thereby removing the need for staff to hand-wash crockery and cutlery. Engineering controls to prevent the generation of mist or vapours in a workplace will reduce the amount of contamination on work surfaces, with consequent reductions in dermal exposure from contact with material previously deposited there. Separation of the worker from the exposure can also take place with the use of simple tools to prevent the need for immersion of the hands into sinks and sumps. Selection of personal protective equipment should be carried out with care – no material is completely impervious to chemicals. Provision of the wrong type of gloves may allow liquid contaminants to 'break through' the glove material within very short time periods and as the worker then wrongly believes they are protected it can lead to even higher dermal exposures than would have been experienced without the gloves. Wearing gloves also leads to occlusion of the skin, which may increase the uptake of any chemical that gets inside the glove due to increased blood flow and sweating of the hands within the glove plus removal of the opportunity for evaporation from the skin surface.

12.12 Inadvertent ingestion exposure

While dermal exposure measurement has become increasingly common in the past 30 years the importance of the oral route and of ingestion exposure has tended to be ignored in relation to exposure measurement. For certain substances such as lead (Pb), pharmaceuticals and pesticides, there is awareness of the possibility of inadvertent ingestion in the workplace and consequently, occupational hygiene programmes in industries handling these materials tend to be designed to minimise and control the spread of contamination. There may be potential for uptake into the body by hand-to-mouth contact, contamination of food and drink, or from ingestion of inhaled particles deposited in the upper airways of the lungs. However, there are complex personal behaviour patterns involved in these routes of exposure and such exposures may be interrelated with other exposure routes, thereby complicating further the assessment procedure.

A recent review suggested that approximately 4.5 million workers in Britain undertook tasks that placed them at risk of significant inadvertent ingestion of hazardous substances. The main materials identified in this review as being of importance were the following:

- Pesticides and biocides;
- Metals;
- Pharmaceuticals;
- Radionuclides;
- Pathogens;
- High molecular weight allergens.

Jobs in the agricultural sector, engineering and metal processing and health care are among the main areas where inadvertent ingestion exposure may be particularly common.

Some specific activities that workers engage in that can influence ingestion exposure include:

- Eating and drinking at the work station without prior hand washing;
- Speaking with a respirator face mask resting on the lip;
- Removal of gloves by using the teeth;
- Removal of gloves to perform work tasks such as writing on report boards.

There are many serious difficulties in the measurement of inadvertent ingestion exposures. Biological monitoring of chemicals or metabolites is possible but may be intrusive, expensive and only gives an indication of total exposure, not necessarily the fraction received by ingestion. Recent work has focussed on the development of a conceptual model of ingestion exposure similar to that used for dermal exposure scenarios, and a simplified version of this model is shown in Figure 3.1c. This source–receptor model again looks to determine the relationship between different compartments and transfer processes.

In many environments the primary drivers of ingestion exposure will be the level of surface contamination, the transfer of material from surfaces to hands and then the frequency of hand-to-mouth contacts. A simple qualitative assessment of the potential for ingestion exposure and whether it will importantly contribute to the total body burden can be obtained using the checklist outlined here:

- Is the substance used or produced in a fine particulate or liquid form or does direct handling of the material by the worker occur?
- Is there potential for the material to contaminate surfaces that the worker comes into contact with?
- Does the worker have the opportunity to engage in hand-to-mouth or hand-to-perioral contact, i.e. contacts in the area around the mouth?
- Are there particular workplace or behavioural factors that might increase the frequency of mouth and peri-oral contacts?
- Can the internal surfaces of respiratory protective equipment become contaminated due to storage conditions or handling?
- Is there a high degree of awareness among the workforce of the potential for ingestion exposure?
- Are there suitable washing facilities?
- Is there a sufficient level of de-contamination procedures and physical separation between exposed and clean areas when workers take breaks and eat?

We can consider the example of a worker in a well-run hospital pharmacy preparing cytotoxic drugs for delivery to patients undergoing chemotherapy. The pharmacist is involved in weighing and dispensing both fine particulate and liquid-drug formulations, although the procedures remove the need for any direct handling of the drugs. There is the potential for the material to contaminate surfaces although the use of a glovebox and double-bagging arrangements limit the potential for contamination considerably. During the task the worker's hands are contained in the glovebox and so the opportunity for hand-to-mouth or object-to-mouth contamination is removed. There is the possibility of hand-to-face contact when the hands are removed from the glovebox but at this point contaminated gloves should have been removed. In this scenario the pharmacy workers use disposable respiratory protective equipment. The workers are trained in the safe handling procedures, aware of the toxicity of the materials they handle and the potential for uptake via the ingestion route. Drug handling is carried out in a separate preparation room with restricted entry. Hand-washing facilities are available at the exit to this room and a well-defined de-contamination procedure prior to leaving the preparation room is in place. It is clear from our checklist that the potential for ingestion exposure exists in this workplace but also evident that there is a high level of control directed to limiting this exposure.

If we now use our ingestion checklist to consider a worker in a nickel refinery involved in the handling of nickel matte then we can see a much less controlled set of conditions. In this environment nickel metal and nickel compounds are produced by recovering elemental nickel from nickel matte by using an electrolytic process. Three operators control the production process, mainly from within a control room. They also carry out routine inspection of the plant and various cleaning tasks. The surfaces in the leaching area, particularly around the filter press are heavily contaminated with nickel sulphate residue and are hosed down regularly to remove any residual contamination from the floor and work surfaces. The operators do not wear respiratory protective equipment but they do wear gloves while carrying out inspection and maintenance tasks; the gloves are repeatedly used and often worn together with dirty overalls while in the control room, which is also where food and drinks are consumed. There is one sink that is used for both washing and food preparation. There is little awareness of the potential for ingestion exposure and the workers view the material as being of low toxicity so do not take any measures to control their ingestion exposure. The conditions are warm and dusty and so there is a high frequency of hand-to-mouth contact often, while wearing contaminated gloves. Clearly in this case there is a high probability of significant inadvertent ingestion exposure taking place and our checklist allows us to target specific behaviours and conditions to improve control.

Measurements of surface contamination and dermal exposure levels on the hands and peri-oral areas can be used as methods of determining the effect of training, procedural and engineering interventions and assessing progress towards effective control.

References and further reading

HSE (2004). *Medical Aspects of Occupational Skin Disease*. Sudbury, UK: HSE Books. Available at http://www.hse.gov.uk/pubns/ms24.pdf.

HSE (2001). *Assessing and Managing Risks at Work from Skin Exposure to Chemical Agents*. HSG205. Sudbury, UK: HSE Books.

HSE (2007). *Preventing Contact Dermatitis at Work*. INDG233. Sudbury, UK: HSE Books. Available at www.hse.gov.uk/pubns/indg233.pdf.

Cherrie, JW. (2005). Dermal exposure assessment. In: *Occupational Hygiene*, 3rd edition (Gardiner K, Harrington JM, eds). Oxford, UK: Blackwell Publishing.

Soutar A, Semple S, Aitken RJ, Robertson A. (2000). Use of patches and whole body sampling for the assessment of dermal exposure. *Annals of Occupational Hygiene* 44: 511–518.

Brouwer DH, Boeniger MF, van Hemmen J. (2000). Hand wash and manual skin wipes. *Annals of Occupational Hygiene* 44: 501–510.

Cherrie JW, Brouwer DH, Roff M, Vermeulen R, Kromhout H. (2000). Use of qualitative and quantitative fluorescence techniques to assess dermal exposure. *Annals of Occupational Hygiene* 44: 519–522.

Schneider T, Vermulen R, Brouwer D, Cherrie JW, Kromhout H, Fough CL. (1999). Conceptual model for the assessment of dermal exposure. *Occupational and Environmental Medicine* 56: 765–773.

Christopher Y, Semple S, Hughson G, Cherrie JW. (2007). *Inadvertent ingestion exposure in the workplace*. Bootle, UK: HSE Books. Available at http://www.hse.gov.uk/research/rrpdf/rr551.pdf.

Cherrie JW, Semple S, Christopher Y, Saleem A, Hughson GW, Philips A. (2006). How important is inadvertent ingestion of hazardous substances at work? *Annals of Occupational Hygiene* 50: 693–704.

Sithamparanadarajah R. (2008). *Controlling Skin Exposure to Chemicals and Wet-Work. A Practical Book.* Stourbridge, UK: RMS Publishing. Available at British Occupational Hygiene Society website www.BOHS.org.

Health and Safety Executive topic pages on skin. Available at http://www.hse.gov.uk/skin.

US NIOSH skin topic page. Available at http://www.cdc.gov/niosh/topics/skin/.

Where there is a translation of the German TRGS 531 for wet-work. Available at http://www.cdc.gov/niosh/topics/skin/pdfs/WetWorkTRGS531.pdf.

4 Physical Agents

13 | Noise

13.1   Introduction

Noise is a very common workplace pollutant and, depending on the level and duration of exposure, can cause a range of effects from annoyance, loss of concentration and sleep disturbance to permanent noise-induced hearing loss (PNIHL). Over a million people in Britain are exposed to occupational noise levels that put their hearing at risk and about 170,000 people suffer deafness or other ear conditions caused by excessive noise exposure at work. It is one of the key occupational health injuries that occupational hygiene aims to control. In this chapter, we provide a basic introduction to noise at work, and then focus on measurement methodology. We also briefly touch on noise control techniques.

Sound is a tiny oscillation in air pressure around atmospheric pressure. Sound has two main characteristics: the magnitude of the pressure variation and its frequency. The duration of exposure and the noise energy transmitted to the inner ear by the sound wave are important determinants of the risk of PNIHL. It is often said that noise is unwanted sound but this is not strictly correct since loud sound, regardless of whether it is music we enjoy or the din from a machine in our workplace, may damage our hearing.

13.2   Pressure and magnitude of pressure variation

Pressure is measured in pascal (Pa) where 1 Pa is a pressure of 1 N m^{-2}. The lowest sound pressure that can be detected by a young person with no hearing loss is about 0.00002 Pa (or 20 µPa). The normal ear can also respond to sound pressures to about 200 Pa, which might be measured about 25 m from a jet aircraft taking off. The ear can therefore respond to noise pressures that differ over a range of about 10^7, i.e. 10 million times. The energy transmitted by the noise, i.e. the intensity of the noise varies as the square of the pressure. The intensity range associated with the range of pressures that we can hear is therefore $(10^7)^2$ or 10^{14}. Given this wide range of intensities, these measurements are generally expressed using a logarithmic unit (to base 10) known as the bel (B), where 1 bel is a ratio of 10:1. Note that the bel is a ratio rather than an absolute level. As a bel is a large unit, it is usual to express sound pressures in decibels (dB), i.e. a tenth of a bel. For noise measurement, the decibel is used to compare the sound intensity being measured with a reference pressure.

Table 13.1 Typical sound pressure levels.

Source	Pressure (Pa)	Sound pressure levels (dB)
Threshold of hearing	0.00002	0
Quiet office	0.002	40
Ringing alarm clock at 1 m	0.2	80
Unsilenced pneumatic drill at 1.5 m (operator's ear)	6	110
25 m from a jet airliner at takeoff	200	140

The sound pressure level (SPL) or sound intensity is defined as

$$SPL = 10 \times \log_{10} \left(\frac{P_a}{P_r} \right)^2$$

where P_a is the sound pressure of the noise being measured, and P_r is the reference sound pressure, which is set at the threshold of hearing, i.e. 0.00002 Pa. SPL is measured in decibels.

The same equation can also be expressed as

$$SPL = 20 \times \log_{10} \left(\frac{P_a}{P_r} \right)$$

SPLs of typical noise sources are listed in Table 13.1.

Note that an SPL of about 80 dB will interfere with speech between people with normal hearing at about 1 m, at 90 dB they would have to shout to be heard and at 100 dB they would have to shout into each other's ear to be understood.

Given the logarithmic nature of the dB scale, an increase or decrease of 3 dB is a doubling or halving of energy and an increase or decrease of 10 dB is tenfold change in energy. If two noises, each at 90 dB are present together, the combined SPL is 93 dB. If one noise is 90 dB and the other is 92 dB, the total intensity is 94 dB; if one is at 90 dB and the other is 100 dB the total intensity is 100 dB. Note that if two sounds are ten or more dB different, the lower intensity can be ignored in calculating the total intensity.

It must be appreciated that intensity and 'loudness' are not the same. The normal ear can just detect a change of 3 dB in SPL in side-by-side sources and a SPL has to change by about 10 dB to give an apparent doubling or halving of subjective loudness. Significant changes in SPL can therefore occur before we are subjectively aware of the change.

13.3 Frequency

If we were to set up an experiment where we placed a microphone, which senses the sound pressure, at a fixed location and then switched on a sound source emitting a pure tone then the pattern of change in pressure would be as shown in Figure 13.1.

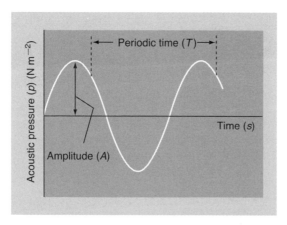

Figure 13.1 Change in acoustic pressure with time for a pure tone. (Reproduced with permission from *Occupational Hygiene*, 3rd edition, edited by Kerry Gardiner and J. Malcolm Harrington, Blackwell Publishing Ltd., 2005, Figure 17.1).

The gap between successive peaks or troughs on the trace is known as the periodic time and it is measured in seconds. The frequency of the sound wave (f) is the reciprocal of the periodic time and is measured in hertz (Hz), which is equivalent to 1 s^{-1}. The height of the wave is the amplitude.

In our experiment, if we had many microphones and we placed them in a line running away from the source and then at a single instant after the sound had started we measured the pressure on each we would get the graph shown in Figure 13.2. Notice in this case the horizontal axis is in units of distance rather than time.

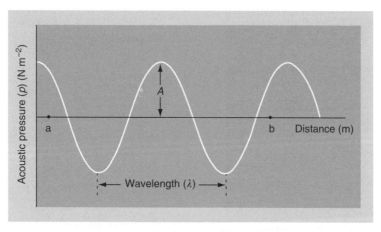

Figure 13.2 Change in acoustic pressure with distance for a pure tone. (Reproduced with permission from *Occupational Hygiene*, 3rd edition, edited by Kerry Gardiner and J. Malcolm Harrington, Blackwell Publishing Ltd., 2005, Figure 17.2).

On this occasion, the distance between the peaks is in units of metres and is known as the wavelength (λ).

Of course these two graphs are derived from the same wave and so there must be a way to convert from one to the other; i.e. knowing the wavelength it must be possible to calculate the frequency and vice versa. The equation to make this conversion involves the speed of sound in the particular circumstances where the experiment was carried out (c) in metres per second.

$$f \times \lambda = c$$

So to obtain the frequency knowing the speed of sound you would rearrange the equation as

$$f = \frac{c}{\lambda}$$

The normal ear can detect noises over a wide range of frequencies, from a very low pitch, about 20 Hz, to a very high pitch, about 20 kHz. Middle C on the musical scale is about 260 Hz. The ear is not equally sensitive across the audible frequency range, being most sensitive at about 4 kHz and least sensitive at the low and high frequency extremes of the range.

In practice, most noise measuring instruments electronically 'weight' the signals to approximate to the response of the ear. Four weightings are commonly used: the 'A' weighting that approximates to the ear's response at 'low' SPL, the 'B' weighting that approximates to the ear's response at 'moderate' SPL, the 'C' weighting that approximates to the ear's response at 'high' SPL and 'un-weighted' that applies no frequency correction. Figure 13.3 shows these three weightings, and as can be seen they have a zero correction value

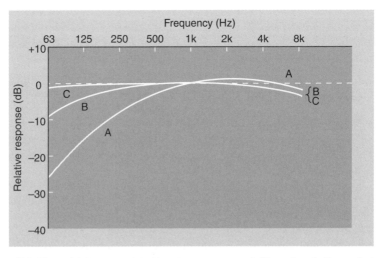

Figure 13.3 The weighting curves used in noise measurement. (Reproduced with permission from *Occupational Hygiene*, 3rd edition, edited by Kerry Gardiner and J. Malcolm Harrington, Blackwell Publishing Ltd., 2005, Figure 17.8).

at 4 kHz and that the 'A' frequency weighting applies relatively much greater significance to frequencies in the range 1–8 kHz and progressively discounts noise energy at frequencies below about 250 Hz. Some instruments also have a 'D' weighting, which was introduced for measuring noise levels from aircraft jet engines to assess noise nuisance. The major effects of the weightings are to discount the importance of lower frequency energy and to enhance the importance of frequencies around 4 kHz.

Weighted and un-weighted SPLs are expressed as dB(A), dB(B), dB(C) dB(D) or dB, as relevant. Current British legislation on occupational noise exposure defines OELs in terms of 'A' weighted measurements for continuous noise and un-weighted for instantaneous peaks or impact noises. Although the 'A', 'B' and 'C' weightings are specified in the relevant noise measuring instrument standards, no such specification has been defined for the un-weighted response. It is therefore now common for un-weighted measurements to be made using the 'C' weighting.

13.4 Duration

The critical factor in assessing the risk of noise induced hearing loss from continuous noise exposures is to determine the total noise energy to which the ear is exposed during a working shift; i.e. the hearing loss risk is given by the product of the noise intensity and the duration of exposure. For the purposes of convention, the 8-h time-weighted average is determined. For intense short-duration exposures, only intensity is important. Short duration 'spikes', such as from impact sources, are sometimes measured in terms of pascal only. Very intense short-duration noise can cause instantaneous damage to the ear, often called 'acoustic trauma'.

13.5 Occupational exposure limits

The Control of Noise at Work (CNAW) regulations contain three risk predictors:

(a) Peak sound pressure (P_{peak}) [dB re 20 µPa]: the maximum value of the 'C' frequency weighted instantaneous sound pressure.
(b) Daily noise exposure level ($L_{EP,d}$) [dB(A) re 20 µPa]: time-weighted average of the noise exposure levels for a nominal 8-h working day.
(c) Weekly noise exposure level ($L_{EP,w}$): time-weighted average of the noise exposure levels for a nominal week of five 8-h working days.

$L_{EP,d}$ is used to express noise exposure. It is defined as the equivalent continuous noise level that would give the same total amount of sound energy as the fluctuating noise. It is, in effect, a time-weighted average noise energy of the peaks and troughs of exposure over the period of time under consideration. Sound level meters and personal noise dosimeters are available that will record $L_{EP,d}$ and give the duration over which it was measured.

The CNAW regulations define the following limits:

Lower exposure action levels of:
- a daily or weekly personal noise exposure of 80 dB(A);
- a peak sound pressure of 135 dB(C);

Upper exposure action levels of:
- a daily or weekly personal noise exposure of 85 dB(A);
- a peak sound pressure of 137 dB(C);

Exposure limit values of:
- a daily or weekly personal noise exposure limit of 87 dB(A);
- a peak sound pressure of 140 dB(C).

13.6 Equipment available

There are effectively three main types of noise measuring equipment: sound level meters (SLM), integration sound level meters (ISLM) and personal noise dosimeters (PND).

The SLM and ISLM are generally held and operated by the person making the measurements and the PND is worn by the person carrying out the tasks to be measured. Both SLM and PND are available with datalogging facilities. Such datalogging instruments permit the time history of exposure to be examined and therefore allow periods of high intensity to be identified.

13.7 Sound level meters and personal noise dosimeters

A SLM or dosimeter comprises a microphone that converts the sound waves to electrical impulses, electronic circuitry that modifies and amplifies the signal according to the demands of the user, and an output section to store or display the signal in units of sound as required. Portable SLM and dosimeters are battery powered, thus the battery charge condition must also be displayed. The quality of SLM is governed by the requirements of several European Standards, particularly BS EN 61672-1: 2003. Meters are graded according to their accuracy from class 0 to class 2; for most instruments the main difference is the quality of the microphone, the electronics being effectively the same. The critical difference is the directionality of the microphone, as shown in Table 13.2. Class 0 instruments are really only for use in a laboratory or similar situation, Class 1 and 2 are used for noise surveys in industry.

From Table 13.2 it can be seen that in the range 1–8 kHz the directionality of a Class 2 microphone as compared with a Class 1 microphone is 1–4.5 dB poorer at 30° incidence to the source, 2 to more than 5 dB poorer at 90° and 2.7 to >6 dB poorer at 150°. Therefore, unless it is known that there is only a small single noise source, distant from reflecting surfaces with about 90% of the noise energy at frequencies below 1 kHz, then only Class 1 equipment can be used to get reliable measurements.

It should be noted that microphones are fragile, particularly those in the Class 0 and Class 1 categories, and they must be handled with great care. If

Table 13.2 Directional response limits including maximum expanded uncertainty of measurement, from BS EN 61672-1: 2003.

| | Maximum absolute difference in displayed sound levels at any two sound-incidence angles within ± degrees from the reference direction | | | | | |
| | 30° | | 90° | | 150° | |
Frequency (kHz)	Class 1	Class 2	Class 1	Class 2	Class 1	Class 2
0.25–1	1.3	2.3	1.8	3.3	2.3	5.
>1–2	1.5	2.5	2.5	4.5	4.5	7.5
>2–4	2.0	4.5	4.5	7.5	6.5	12.5
>4–8	3.5	7.0	8.0	13.0	11.0	17.0
>8–12.5	5.5	–	11.5	–	15.5	–

Note: Maximum absolute differences in displayed sound levels are extended by the expanded uncertainty of measurement for demonstration to the limits given in the table.

there is any indication that a microphone has been knocked against a hard surface or has signs of damage then it should be recalibrated as outlined later. If the instrument calibration has changed by more than about 0.5 dB, the microphone should be returned to the manufacturer for inspection and any necessary repairs.

A simple SLM, such as that shown in Figure 13.4, may only indicate dB(A) but others can provide a wide range of displays such as $L_{EP,d}$, octave and third octave band analysis (Figure 13.5), real-time spectral analysis and many other

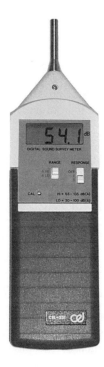

Figure 13.4 Simple sound level meters. (© Casella Measurement Ltd. Reproduced with permission.)

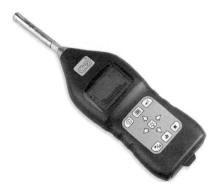

Figure 13.5 Octave band monitoring with a sound level meter. (© Casella Measurement Ltd. Reproduced with permission.)

useful measurements. The quality and facilities that a SLM offers are reflected in its cost. Prices start at around £100 for the simplest instruments and rise to several thousand pounds for the most accurate instrument providing a wide range of facilities. It is even possible for about £10 to download software to convert your mobile phone into a SLM (e.g. www.faberacoustical.com for software for the iPhone), although the final result is limited by the quality of the microphone.

Impulse noise and short-term transient peaks in sound level have an important effect upon noise exposure. Most traditional SLMs do not have sufficient dynamic range or a fast-enough response time to correctly record these short-duration events. International standards now specify requirements for Class 1 impulse SLM that respond very quickly. Care should be taken when purchasing new instruments to ensure that the class is suitable for the purpose required. Although, instruments with most facilities are the most expensive, Class 1 instruments should be used by an experienced and qualified person where important decisions are to be made based on noise measurements or if legal arguments are to be based on results.

Careful notes should be taken of the duration of all noise exposure measurements and the activities being undertaken at these times. Such notes should be kept, even if a datalogging instrument is being used, the notes constitute an independent check of the measurement data and help interpret the data in relation to the work.

A simple noise survey can be undertaken by measuring the SPL and noting the time when the operator entered and left the area where exposures occurred. However, in most workplaces noise fluctuates as different operations take place and various items of noise-producing equipment or machinery are turned on and off. Also, impact noise such as hammering, riveting and pressing cause short-duration peaks of high intensity. Thus, it is not easy to establish how long an operator has been exposed to each noise to estimate their total exposure unless an integrating SLM or PND is used. Good notes should always be kept about contextual information relevant to the noise exposure, such as the pieces of machinery operating during the measurements, the location of the operator in relation to the machine, the amount of time spent close to noise sources, the building dimensions and other factors that may determine exposure.

13.8 Personal noise dosimeters

The presence of the investigator standing beside the worker using a hand-held instrument to make measurements of noise exposure may cause the worker to change his or her behaviour, potentially affecting the reliability of the result obtained. The size and weight of an integrating SLM precludes its use for personal measurement. However, a small noise dosimeter can be easily carried by an operator throughout the shift, it will not hinder the task being performed and, once the wearer has become used to wearing the instrument, it should not affect their behaviour.

However, we have experience of personnel wearing dosimeters in a workplace for about 20 working days, where the average results from the first 3–5 days differed significantly, i.e. by over 3 dB, from the results over the remainder of the working month. The measurement results from a single day or a few days monitoring must therefore be treated with some care as they may overestimate the true long-term exposure.

Datalogging dosimeters will measure all noise levels to which the workers are exposed, making a record against time and storing the information for retrieval on demand. Dosimeters can either have an integral microphone, with for example the whole unit designed to be worn in the breast pocket, or they can have a separate microphone that can be clipped to the lapel with a lead carrying the signal to a small box containing the battery and electronics, which may be carried in a pocket or attached to a belt. An example of a noise dosimeter is shown in Figure 13.6. Some dosimeters can be used as an

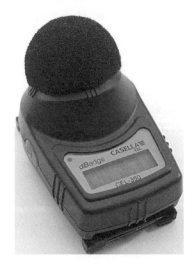

Figure 13.6 A noise dosimeter. (© Casella Measurement Ltd. Reproduced with permission.)

integrating SLM by attaching the microphone to a mast rather than attaching it to the worker lapel.

Noise dosimeters are generally fitted with Class 2 microphones and are therefore liable to have the directionality characteristics described earlier, and may over or underestimate actual exposure as a consequence.

The information from data-logging dosimeters can usually be downloaded to a computer to provide statistical analysis of the recorded sound levels. To avoid loss of data care should be taken to ensure that any logged data are recorded or downloaded before switching off the instrument or before proceeding to make new measurements.

It is good practice to occasionally use PNDs in parallel with a SLM so that the latter instruments provide a check on the validity of the dosimeter results.

13.9   Calibration

To ensure that the noise measurement instrument is reading correctly it is necessary to have a source of sound of a known intensity and frequency that can be introduced through the microphone, excluding all other sounds except the calibration tone. All instruments have a means of adjusting the settings to correctly indicate the noise level emitted by the calibrator.

Most calibrators for portable meters are battery powered, producing the calibration tone electronically. There must provide a tight fit around the microphone to ensure no other sounds are being received at the same time. To this end rubber '0' rings are used as seals and some have adapters to fit various microphone sizes. Calibration tones vary in intensity from one manufacturer to another, although 94 dB at 1000 Hz is the most usual. If dB(A) scales are to be checked then the calibrator must have a frequency of 1000 Hz. A 'pistonphone' calibrator is available, which can produce a wide range of frequencies. This type of calibrator must be used with an instrument set at a weighting other than 'A'.

It is essential to check the meter regularly with the calibrator, at least once before starting a series of readings and at the start and end of a working shift.

Both sound measuring instruments and calibrators should be stored in conditions of normal temperature and humidity. From experience, a calibrator that has been stored overnight in a vehicle in cold weather can take up to an hour to equilibrate to normal room temperatures. It is also important to ensure that the calibrator battery is in good order. Each manufacturer gives instructions as to how to achieve this. Calibrators are relatively easily damaged and should be inspected for any sign of physical damage before use.

If any calibration setting is found to vary by more than about 0.5 dB between calibrations, either during a shift or between sequential shifts or measurement periods, the instrument and the calibrator must be returned to the manufacturer. Sound-measuring instruments and calibrators need to be returned to the manufacturer at least biannually for servicing and re-calibration.

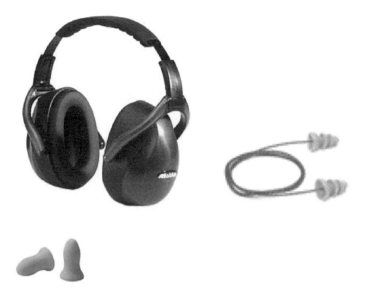

Figure 13.7 A selection of hearing protection devices (muffs, reusable inserts and disposable inserts). (From http://www.moldex.com/.) (© Moldex-Metric AG & Co. KG. Reproduced with permission.)

13.10   To measure workplace noise using a SLM

13.10.1   Aim

Workroom noise produced from machines or items of equipment can be a source of irritation, stress, can lead to hearing damage and/or can affect the intelligibility of speech. It is important to be able to measure noise levels at various workplaces to establish whether it is necessary to take remedial action to control the operators' exposure and to identify the main sources of noise, as required by the CNAW regulations. Following from that it may be necessary to designate certain areas of the workplace as hearing conservation zones, which people are forbidden to enter without wearing suitable hearing protection (Figure 13.7).

13.10.2   Equipment required

A SLM having a dB(A) weighting capability, one or more calibration devices defined by the instrument manufacturer as being suitable for the microphone on the meter. A tripod capable of holding the meter may also be useful. Notebook, pen and other general items are also required.

13.10.3   Method

Before commencing *always* check the manufacturer's instructions for both measuring instrument and calibrator. The steps described here do not apply to any specific instrument but may be part of the manufacturer's instructions, which should always be followed.

1. If an in-house secondary standard calibrator is available, check the calibrator to be taken on site against the in-house secondary standard calibrator.
2. Check the battery output by switching on both calibrator(s) and instruments on the 'battery test' setting. Each manufacturer has its own method of indicating the battery charge condition, as shown in their instruction manual. If the batteries do not have sufficient power they should be replaced. If the measurement site is distant from base it is good practice to fit new batteries even if the existing batteries indicate sufficient life as the cost of new batteries is small compared to the total cost of making the measurements.
3. Allow the instrument(s) and calibrator(s) to equilibrate to the temperature in the measuring environment.
4. Switch on the instrument(s) and allow it/them to warm up for at least 2 min.
5. Calibrate the instrument(s) as follows: remove the microphone cover, fit the calibrator gently over the microphone and set the reading to dB(A) for conventional electronic calibrators or to dB(C) for piston-phone calibrators and to the correct range[1] for the output of the calibrator. If the instrument has a 'fast' and 'slow' response switch set it to 'slow'. Use the calibrator to reset the instrument. However, if the adjustment is more than about 0.5 dB then the instrument and the calibrator should be returned to the manufacturer for checking.
6. Ensure that any data in the memory have been downloaded. Reset the memory before each measurement.
7. *For static measurements*: Remove the microphone cap, turn on, switch to 'slow' response, set the instrument to dB(A) for assessing daily exposure or dB(C) for measuring peak exposures, Hold the instrument at arm's length away from the body and keeping it at least 1 m above the ground at the location where you want to make the measurement.

   For personal measurements: Remove the microphone cap, turn on, switch to 'slow' response, set the instrument to dB(A) for assessing daily exposure or dB(C) for measuring peak exposures. Hold the microphone at least 300 mm sequentially from each ear of the operator, on the horizontal plane of the operator's ear and at the same distance from the source as the operator's ear but pointing towards the main noise source and note the readings. If any reading rises above or falls below the instrument measurement range then switch the range control to the appropriate value. To minimise the sound-blocking effect of the measurer's body, mount the instrument on a tripod if one is available and stand at least 0.5 m away from it when reading the meter. Some instruments have their microphone on a length of

---

[1] Instruments vary in the way they indicate the reading, although most modern instruments give a digital readout of decibels. However, it may be necessary to switch to the appropriate range, e.g. 70–90 dB(A).

cable or a flexible extension boom so that it can be mounted away from the meter for this purpose.

8. If there are multiple noise sources or hard reflective surfaces in the vicinity of the measuring location, rotate the instrument to check whether there are significant changes in the measured sound pressure levels. Take the result from the orientation with the highest reading as the 'correct' result. This is particularly important for an instrument fitted with a Class 2 microphone.

9. If the operator is working at a noisy source it may be useful to obtain a measurement of the background noise, therefore repeat steps 7 or 8 above with the main local source switched off. If there is little difference in the noise level between the background only, and the machine plus the background (i.e. less than 3 dB), then other sources of noise may be as important as the main source.

13.10.4 Results

From the results obtained, it should be possible to decide whether employees are subject to noise levels exceeding the limits set out in the CNAW regulations. If the noise is steady and above 80 or 85 dB(A) and the worker is present most of the day then certain actions need to be taken as defined in the regulations. Exposure above 87 dB(A) requires the employer to take steps to control exposure and implement other actions. If the levels fluctuate by more than 6–8 dB(A) or the work tasks vary from day to day, as for example may be the case with maintenance personnel, then you will probably need to measure over a whole working shift using a PND to ensure that you have a reliable assessment of exposure.

13.10.5 Possible problems

1. If the microphone is accidentally knocked during the measurement then the result must be disregarded. Check for damage to the microphone.
2. If the measurements are made outdoors on a windy day then the air movement over the microphone may give rise to an erroneously high reading. This effect can be minimised by using a porous foam shield over the microphone.
3. Reflection of noise from the worker's body towards the microphone will increase the reading. This should be avoided as far as possible.
4. Problems in assessing the contribution to exposure from noise close to the worker's ear and noise from hand-held tools may result in underestimation of exposure.

13.11 To measure workplace noise using a PND

To assess the degree of hearing hazard to which operators are exposed during the course of their job it is useful to monitor the operator rather than the workplace. This is particularly so if the operator moves about from one location to another where the levels of noise exposure differs or where the use of an ISLM is difficult or impossible due to the nature of the operations taking place. PNDs are designed to cause minimal interference when worn, as they are small and lightweight.

13.11.1 Equipment required

A PND and a suitable calibration device for the dosimeter are required.

Note that the readout displays of PND may vary. Some types give a numerical digital display, other models incorporate no integral readout but require to be connected to an external reading device or you must download the data to a computer.

The result of the measurement is generally expressed as either a percentage of the allowed $L_{EP,d}$; in Britain, an exposure of 87 dB(A) for 8 h would be 100%. Some instruments display a peak level warning that indicates when a specified dB(A) value has been exceeded during the measurement and/or that the microphone has been knocked during the measurement period.

As a PND is a device that stores information over a period of time it is important to ensure that all previous measurements are cleared from the memory. Thus, the manufacturer's re-setting procedure must be adopted if the readout is not showing zero.

Personal dosimeters from different manufacturers are so widely different that it is not possible to describe their use in a general way. Therefore, the user must closely follow the manufacturer's instructions. However, some general comments are provided here for guidance when using PNDs.

13.11.2 Method

Follow the instructions for SLMs plus the following:

1. The microphone should be placed as close to the ear as possible, either by clipping it to the lapel or by attaching it to the rim of a helmet. One ear of the operator may be exposed to a louder noise than the other and in this event the microphone should be attached on the "noisier" side of the operator's body. The microphone should also be pointed towards the most likely major noise source.
2. Care should be taken to ensure that the microphone could not be knocked in any way in the course of the operator's actions as artificially high readings may result.
3. Microphones should be protected by a dust cover when in use, although it is necessary to remove the cover during calibration.
4. The duration of dosimeter measurements should include all processes likely to be carried out by the operator, but it is preferable that the measurement period is a full working shift. Note that it may be necessary to recover the dosimeter at shift breaks.
5. It is prudent to check battery condition and noise readings at shift breaks.

6. Do not reset the memory or switch off the instrument until you have double-checked that the results have been recorded or data correctly downloaded.

13.11.3 Results

Some types of dosimeter display the result as $L_{EP,d}$, assuming that the measurement period corresponds to the full working day. If you are not measuring over a full day then you will need to obtain the result from the dosimeter in terms of $Pa^2\ h^{-1}$, percentage dose or L_{Aeq} to determine your $L_{EP,d}$. Consult the manufacturers literature to ensure that the output you have selected is appropriate for your purpose.

13.11.4 Possible problems

1. Operators can sometimes find that being asked to wear a noise dosimeter is a novelty and the device may also intrigue their colleagues. There can be a temptation to tamper with the instrument by shouting into it or, worse, by removing the microphone from the lapel to hold it close to a noisy machine. These actions will probably render the results useless.
2. Older instruments may display percent dose estimates against 90 or 85 dB(A). You should check the criteria that your dosimeter is set to.

13.12 To measure the spectrum of a continuous noise by octave band analysis

It is often useful to know something about the differences in intensity of the noise with frequency, particularly when selecting hearing defenders or when designing noise controls. The frequency spectrum is generally collected in an octave band analysis. The mid-point frequencies of the successive octave bands are double the previous one, typically: 62.5, 125, 250, 500, 1000, 2000, 4000 and 8000 Hz.

13.12.1 Aim

To select adequate hearing protectors for a given environment, it is necessary to ensure that the protectors are correctly matched to the frequency characteristics of the noise. It is therefore necessary to measure the intensity of noise in each octave.

13.12.2 Equipment required

A Class 1 SLM incorporating an octave band facility and a calibration device suitable for the microphone on the meter. For calibrating octave band analysis it is preferable to use a piston-phone calibrator. A tripod capable of holding the meter may also be useful but is not essential.

13.12.3 Method

Follow instructions for SLMs plus the following:

1. Calibrate the instrument as follows: remove the microphone cover, fit the calibrator over the microphone and set the instrument to 'filter' and set the response to 'fast'. Select the meter range and weighting to the correct ones for the output of the calibrator. If necessary, switch the octave band selector to the frequency of the calibrator. Turn on the calibrator and observe the reading on the meter. If it does not read exactly the calibration value adjust the instrument according to the manufacturer's instructions. Repeat for other frequencies.
2. Locate the meter at the position where the measurements are required to be taken. This may be at the place where the operator is stationed or, if the point of maximum noise level is required, then it will be necessary to ascertain this by using the SLM as described previously, and measuring in various places in the workroom until this point is established.
3. To obtain the sound spectrum: remove the microphone cover, turn on the instrument, switch to the 'filter' setting and to 'slow' response and hold the instrument at arm's length away from the body, pointing towards the noise source. Select the 62.5 Hz band and note the reading. Repeat for each filter band setting up to 8 or 16 kHz. Note most modern instruments display all of the octave band readings simultaneously. To minimise the shielding effect of the observer's body the instrument can be mounted on a tripod and read from a distance of at least 0.5 m.
4. As a check, turn off the external filter and set the instrument to dB(A) and measure the A weighting level.

13.12.4 Results

The octave band data are used to select hearing protectors as described in Appendix 2 and 3 of HSE (2005). Hearing protection should comply with the standard BS EN 352 and be provided along with information to describe the equipment performance at different frequencies. The information required includes

- The mean and standard deviation attenuation values at each octave band centre frequency from 125 Hz to 8 kHz, with data for 63 Hz being optional;
- The assumed protection values (APV) at each frequency, calculated as the mean attenuation minus one standard deviation.

The APV takes account of the variation in fit between individuals to ensure that most wearers should achieve that level of protection.

When hearing protection is used in the workplace the protection provided can be less than predicted from laboratory data provided by the manufacturer and so to give a more realistic estimate of the protection, allowing for fitting in the workplace and the actual condition of hearing protectors, it is recommended to add 4 dB to the calculated noise level to give a more realistic estimate for the level at the ear.

Table 13.3   Calculation of the noise level at the ear when wearing hearing protection.

Octave band centre frequency (Hz)	63	125	250	500	1000	2000	4000	8000	Overall dB(A)
Measured octave band noise levels (dB)	85	86	88	91	91	87	85	82	95
Mean attenuation from supplier (dB)	27	28	26	27	27	32	46	44	
Standard deviation of attenuation (dB)	8	8	7	9	7	8	7	13	

The HSE provides an Excel spreadsheet to calculate the noise level at the wearer's ear while wearing hearing protection, which is available at www.hse.gov.uk/noise/hearingcalc.xls.

For example, Table 13.3 shows the input data for the calculation of the protection from a hearing defender by using the 'octave band' tab on the spreadsheet.

The estimated level at the ear is 74 dB, and adding 4 dB to take account of actual fitting in a workplace would give an estimated level of 78 dB. Hearing protector should be selected so that daily exposure is reduced to less than 85 dB, and ideally between about 80 and 75 dB at the ear. Avoid selecting protectors giving less than 70 dB at the ear as this results in the wearer being 'isolated' from the general environment.

13.13   To determine the degree of noise exposure and the actions to take

From measurement results obtained it should be possible to establish whether operators are subjected to noise levels exceeding those defined in the CNAW regulations. If the noise is steady above 80 dB(A) and the operator is exposed to such noise level for more than about 25% of the day, then it should be assumed the lower action level is exceeded and certain actions have to be taken as defined in the regulations, including the provision of hearing protection on request. It should be noted that even if the lower action level is not exceeded some people are susceptible to hearing damage from levels below 80 dB(A) and annoyance and stress can be induced below 80 dB(A).

When the $L_{EP,d}$ exceeds 85 dB(A) the employer must delineate areas to be labelled as hearing-protection zones, where employees must wear suitable hearing protection. In the case of an assessment against the upper or lower action levels, it is not permitted to take any account of the protection afforded by any hearing protection.

Employers are required to eliminate noise at source or control exposure as low as is reasonably practicable. Control should be achieved by the following:

- Changing the working methods so as to reduce exposure to noise;
- Selecting appropriate work equipment that emits the least possible noise;
- Designing layout of workplaces, work stations and rest facilities;

- Providing information and training for employees, so that work equipment is used correctly and employees can work to minimise their exposure to noise;
- Reducing noise by technical means;
- Introduction of appropriate maintenance programmes for equipment, the workplace and workplace systems;
- Limitation of the duration and intensity of exposure to noise;
- Introduction of appropriate work schedules, including adequate rest periods.

The exposure of an employee, taking account of the likely effectiveness of any hearing protection worn, must not exceed the exposure limit, i.e. 87 dB(A).

References and further reading

Gardiner K. (2005). Noise. In: *Occupational Hygiene*, 3rd edition (Gardiner K, Harrington JM, eds). Oxford, UK: Blackwell Publishing.

Chang S-J, Chen C-J, Lien C-H, Sung F-C. (2006). Hearing loss in workers EXPOSED to toluene and noise. *Environmental Health Perspectives* 114(8): 1283–1286. Available at http://www.pubmedcentral.nih.gov/picrender.fcgi?artid=1552019&blobtype=pdf.

Ferrite S, Santana V. (2005). Joint effects of smoking, noise exposure and age on hearing loss. *Occupational Medicine* 55(1): 48–53.

Neitzel R, Seixas N, Goldman B, Daniell W. (2004). Contributions of non-occupational activities to total noise exposure of construction workers. *Annals of Occupational Hygiene* 48(5): 463–473. Available at http://annhyg.oxfordjournals.org/cgi/content/full/48/5/463.

Neitzel R, Somers S, Seixas N. (2006). Variability of real-world hearing protector attenuation measurements. *Annals of Occupational Hygiene* 50(7): 679–691. Available at http://annhyg.oxfordjournals.org/cgi/reprint/50/7/679.pdf.

Neitzel R, Daniell W, Sheppard L, Davies H, Seixas N. (2008). Comparison of perceived and quantitative measures of occupational noise exposure. *Annals of Occupational Hygiene* 53(1): 41–54. Available at http://annhyg.oxfordjournals.org/cgi/content/abstract/53/1/41.

HSE (2005). *Controlling Noise at Work. The Control of Noise at Work Regulations 2005.* L108. Sudbury, UK: HSE Books.

HSE (2000). *Noise in Construction. Further Guidance on the Control of Noise at Work Regulations 1989.* Sudbury, UK: HSE Books.

HSEs noise website with a range of advice and access to free leaflets. Available at http://www.hse.gov.uk/noise/. The site includes a range of noise control case studies. Available at http://www.hse.gov.uk/noise/casestudies/fullindex.htm. The HSE also published a short document entitled 'Top Ten Noise Control Techniques', available at www.hse.gov.uk/pubns/top10noise.pdf.

CHAPTER 14

Vibration

14.1 Introduction

Vibration is the mechanical movement of a solid or liquid to and from its resting position. Exposure to vibration is widespread in industry and is of concern because it may cause discomfort plus vascular, neurological or musculoskeletal disorders. In this chapter, we discuss some of the background to the measurement of vibration at work and then describe the measurement methodology.

Use of hand-held power tools, such as chisels, drills and pressure hammers, exposes workers to hand–arm vibration, which may cause the tips of the fingers to become white (blanching), with loss of feeling and dexterity. Excessive exposure over long periods can result in hand–arm vibration syndrome (HAVS). This disease is often diagnosed when it is too late to do anything. HAVS is reportable under the Reporting of Injuries, Diseases and Dangerous Occurrences regulations (RIDDOR) and is a prescribed disease. Sitting or standing on vibrating surfaces exposes the individual to whole-body vibration. Whole-body vibration may cause discomfort, pain and damage to the lower back.

About 5 million people are exposed to hand–arm vibration at work and there are perhaps 30–40% who are at risk of developing the disease. There are probably more people exposed to whole-body vibration. In 2000, Keith Palmer and colleagues from Southampton University estimated that 7.2 million men and 1.8 million women in Britain are exposed to whole-body vibration if work-related use of cars, vans, buses, trains, and motor cycles is included.

The risk of injury is dependent on the vibration level, frequency of vibration and on the duration of the exposure. Humans mainly respond to hand–arm vibration in the range 10 Hz to 1 kHz and to whole-body vibration mainly in the 1–100 Hz range. The human health effects appear to be most closely associated with the acceleration of the tool and so this is the basis of the exposure metrics for vibration, which is measured as the root-mean-squared sum (RMS) acceleration (m s^{-2}) for the x, y and z coordinate directions. Figure 14.1 illustrates the three orthogonal measurement directions (i.e. x, y and z) for hand–arm vibration. To minimize error, measurements should preferably be simultaneously made in the three directions by using a triaxial accelerometer.

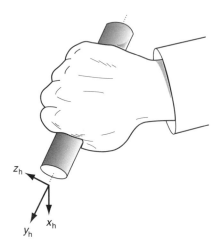

z_h

x_h

y_h

Figure 14.1 *x, y, z* coordinates. (Reproduced with permission from *Occupational Hygiene*, 3rd edition, edited by Kerry Gardiner and J. Malcolm Harrington, Blackwell Publishing Ltd., 2005, p. 252.)

There are frequency-dependent weightings that are applied to the acceleration measurements; separately for the x and y (W_d) coordinate directions and the z coordinate direction (W_k) for whole-body vibration, with a different frequency weighting (W_h) for hand–arm vibration. These weightings allow for differences in the way the body responds to vibration at different frequencies from different directions. Definitions for the whole-body frequency weightings are given in the standard BS ISO 2631-1. The definition for the hand–arm frequency weighting is given in British Standard BS EN ISO 5349-1.

Vibration at work is regulated by the Control of Vibration at Work (CVW) regulations. These regulations require you to:

- Assess the risk to health of your employees from vibration;
- Decide if they are likely to be exposed above the daily exposure action value (EAV) and if they:
  - introduce a programme of organizational and technical measures to eliminate risk at source, or where this is not reasonably practicable reduce exposure to as low a level as is reasonably practicable;
  - provide health surveillance for those employees who continue to be regularly exposed above the EAV or otherwise continue to be at risk;
  - provide information and training to employees on health risks and the actions you are taking to control those risks;
- Decide if they are likely to be exposed above the daily exposure limit value (ELV) and if they:
  - take immediate action to reduce their exposure below the limit value, identify the reasons for the limit being exceeded and change the control measures in place to ensure the ELV is not exceeded again.

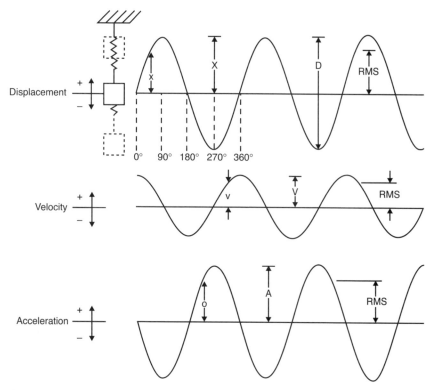

Figure 14.2 The relationship between displacement, velocity and acceleration for a simple mass and spring system.

14.2 Vibration

We can consider a simple analogy of a vibrating system to be a mass on the end of a spring. If we displace the mass from its resting position the system will oscillate up and down with a maximum displacement and if there is no energy lost in the change in displacement, measured in metres, with time follows a sine function as shown in Figure 14.2. We can also describe the velocity of the mass in m s^{-1}, which also follows a sine form but with the peaks and troughs shifted along the time axis in relation to the displacement so that the maximum velocity is reached at zero displacement and the velocity reaches zero at the maximum displacement. It makes sense that when the mass has reached the maximum extent of its travel, the velocity goes through zero, changing from positive to negative, i.e. the mass stops and then starts to move in the opposite direction. Finally, we can look at the acceleration of the mass (m s^{-2}), which follows the same form but is again shifted along the time axis. The displacement, velocity and acceleration are all related to each other; mathematically the velocity is the differential of the displacement with time and the acceleration is the derivative of the velocity with time.

The above-mentioned discussion is not such a stupid analogy to use to describe vibration because the human body can be simplified as a series of masses (the internal organs) held in place with elastic connections (the muscles and other connective tissue).

Going back to the mass and spring analogy, the frequency of the vibration will always be the same for the same combination of mass and spring; it will oscillate at its 'natural frequency'. If we change the mass to make it heavier then the natural frequency of the system will change to become lower. Similarly if we use a stiffer spring the system will oscillate at a higher natural frequency. The internal organs in the body all have different natural frequencies, and so the eye will tend to vibrate between 30 and 80 Hz if displaced while the stomach will vibrate at about 4–8 Hz. The natural frequency is also known as the resonant frequency of the system.

If we now connect the mass to a vibrating source then the combined system will vibrate at the forcing frequency from the source. However, the magnitude of the vibration will depend on how close the forcing frequency is to the natural frequency of the system; if it is close to the natural frequency then the displacement will be high and if it is further from this frequency then the displacement will be much lower. So someone standing on a surface vibrating at 4–8 Hz will probably feel a sensation in his or her stomach as it vibrates in sympathy to the forcing vibration. The maximum response to a forcing vibration occurs at the natural or resonant frequency of the system.

For vibration at work the daily exposure to hand–arm vibration over an 8-h period, designated as $A(8)$, is defined as follows:

$$A(8) = a_{hv}\sqrt{\frac{T}{T_0}}$$

and for whole body vibration:

$$A(8) = k \times a_w\sqrt{\frac{T}{T_0}}$$

where a_{hv} is the frequency-weighted RMS magnitude of the vibration in m s^{-2} and a_w is the corresponding vibration magnitude in one of the orthogonal axes at the surface where the person is supported, e.g. the seat. The term RMS is the square root of the average (or mean) of the square of the acceleration, and is particularly useful mathematical technique for estimating the 'average' value of a measure that can be both positive and negative.

The vibration is measured at the point where the body contacts the vibrating equipment. The acceleration for hand–arm vibration is based on the RMS of the frequency-weighted acceleration values from the three orthogonal axes:

$$a_{hv} = \sqrt{a_{hvx}^2 + a_{hvy}^2 + a_{hvz}^2}$$

14.3 Occupational exposure limits

Occupational exposure limits for vibration are contained in the CVW Regulations – there is an action value and an exposure limit.

The EAV is the daily exposure of hand–arm vibration averaged over 8 h at which employers are required to take action to control exposure. The EAV for hand–arm vibration is set at a daily exposure of 2.5 m s^{-2} $A(8)$ and at 0.5 m s^{-2} $A(8)$ for whole-body vibration.

The exposure limit value (ELV) is the maximum exposure of hand–arm vibration averaged over 8 h to which an employee may be exposed to on any single day. The ELV for hand–arm vibration is 5 m s^{-2} $A(8)$ and 1.15 m s^{-2} $A(8)$ for whole-body vibration.

The regulations have a transitional period for the ELV for hand–arm vibration until 2010 (2014 for some agricultural and forestry equipment), which is to allow, in certain circumstances, work tasks where older tools and machinery produce exposures above the limit value to continue.

14.4 Risk assessment

To carry out a risk assessment for vibration you should consider the work being carried out and:

- Identify those jobs where there may be a risk from hand–arm and/or whole-body vibration;
- Estimate the exposures and compare them with the EAV and ELV;
- Identify the sources of the vibration and the control measures that are available;
- If necessary, prepare a plan to control exposures; and
- Record the assessment, including any additional steps necessary to improve the controls.

To help you judge vibration level, a vibration of about 0.01 m s^{-2} is imperceptible and a level of more than about 0.3 m s^{-2} is strongly perceived. The Good Practice Guides on whole-body and hand–arm vibration published by the European Union (EU) have guidance on the range of vibration levels that are found with different types of tools. For example, the maximum hand–arm vibration from a saw is about 7 m s^{-2} and three quarters of such equipment produces vibration exposure below about 5 m s^{-2}, which suggests that exposure using a clearing saw will probably be less than the ELV. Manufacturers' data may also be used, although these data need to be used carefully because they may underestimate the exposure in actual use (see the EU Good Practice Guide for more information).

Knowing the duration of exposure will also help you make a good estimate of the exposure. It's worth doing this fairly carefully by using a stopwatch or video recordings to make the estimates. Use the formula in 'Vibration' section to adjust the vibration acceleration to estimate $A(8)$.

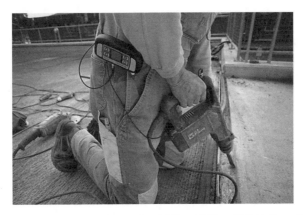

Figure 14.3 Vibration measurements in practice. (© Bruel & Kjaer UK Ltd. Reproduced with permission.)

14.5 Measurements and measurement equipment

Vibration measurements are complex to make and it is therefore likely that only a relatively small number of measurements will be made for a process or piece of equipment. It is therefore important to make sure that the tools and process conditions are typical of the actual work that is carried out. Where measurements are made of hand–arm vibration with a tool that is held by both hands the measurements should be made at both grip points and the higher value used in the exposure estimate.

The measurements are made using an accelerometer (the sensor) that is attached to the vibrating equipment and the associated electronics to process the signal. Examples of vibration measurement equipment are shown in Figure 14.3. There are several different types of accelerometer available, including: strain gauges, piezoresistive sensors and piezoelectric sensors.

For hand–arm vibration, the frequencies between about 8 Hz and 1 kHz are considered to be important in relation to the health risks. However, the risk of damage is not the same at all frequencies and so the measurements are 'weighted' to reflect the harm (W_h), with the weighted acceleration decreasing as the frequency increases. There is one frequency-weighting curve used for all three axes when measuring hand–arm vibration.

In the case of whole-body vibration, the harmful frequencies range from 0.5 Hz up to 80 Hz, again weighted to account for the relative risk. Two different frequency weightings are used: one for the x and y axes (W_d) and one for the vertical z axis direction (W_k). The acceleration measured in the lateral direction is multiplied by 1.4 to account for the health risks from this mode of vibration.

Vibration-measuring equipment should comply with BS EN ISO 8041. Accelerometers must be carefully selected for the particular application as, for example, the vibration from hand-held equipment can be very high and may overload unsuitable sensors. Fixing of accelerometers to equipment handles requires mounting systems that are rigid, lightweight and will not interfere with the operation of the tool. Guidance on the selection of accelerometers and their fixing to equipment is contained in BS EN ISO 5349-2.

All instruments should be assembled in accordance with the manufacturer's instructions. After assembly, a battery check should be carried out. The instrument must be checked against a field calibrator before and after use. The instrument and calibrator should be calibrated against a primary standard by an accredited organisation at least every 2 years. The equipment supplier will be able to assist.

14.6   To measure hand–arm vibration

14.6.1   Aim

Measurements are made to assess whether persons are likely to be exposed above the daily EAV or the ELV. Where measurements are being used to evaluate risk from the use of a particular type of tool, more than one operator should be measured as results can be highly variable between individuals, depending on many factors, including the operator's technique, the condition of the work equipment, the material being processed and the measurement method.

14.6.2   Equipment required

Hand–arm vibration meter and calibrator are required. In addition to the vibration measurement equipment, the following equipment should also be taken to site:

- Manufacturer's operating instructions;
- Clip board, squared paper, pencil and ruler.
- Camera;
- Electrical tape;
- Metal jubilee clips;
- Plastic cable ties;
- Scissors;
- Screwdrivers and Allen keys;
- Spare batteries.

14.6.3   Method

To evaluate daily vibration exposure, it is necessary first to identify the operations that are likely to contribute significantly to the overall vibration exposure. To identify potential exposures stop, look and listen! Walk around the site, stop frequently and observe what is going on; ask workers and supervisors about tasks that they believe produce the most vibration. Ask what equipment is used and whether there is information about the likely vibration levels from the manufacturer.

For each of these tasks identified, it is then necessary to measure the average vibration exposure. Where possible, the measurement period should start when the worker's hands first contact the vibrating surface, and should finish when the contact is broken. This period may include variations in the vibration intensity and may even include periods when there is no exposure. To accurately measure the average daily vibration exposure it is necessary to include all the following:

- Sources of vibration exposure;
- Modes of operation; and
- Changes in the operating conditions.

Where the normal work process is too short for measurement purposes it is recommended that measurements be made during simulated work to operations to produce longer uninterrupted exposures with work conditions as near to normal as possible. Simulated work procedures should be designed to avoid any interruptions that may disturb the measurement. Measurements made over a fixed duration should include as little time before, between and after bursts of vibration as possible. To carry out measurements it is necessary to do the following:

- Check that the accelerometer is: suitable with respect to the temperature, humidity, electrical fields and any other relevant environmental factors and not more than 5% of the mass of the object creating the vibration.
- Assemble the instrument following the manufacturer's instructions for the use of both the measuring instrument and calibrator.
- Check the battery output of instrument and calibrator. If the measurement site is distant from base it is good practice to fit new batteries even if the existing batteries indicate as having sufficient life.
- Check the instrument settings to ensure that the correct settings are being used. Care must be taken to ensure that the correct frequency weighting is chosen on the instrument for hand arm vibration or for the x, y or z component for whole body vibration.
- Ensure that any data in the memory have been recorded and/or downloaded. Reset the instrument memory.
- Check the instrument calibration against the field calibrator and record the results. Adjust the instrument if necessary.
- Watch the operator carrying out their tasks to identify locations and orientation of accelerometers. Photograph operator using the tool.
- Vibration measurements should be made where the vibration enters the body with the transducer preferably being located in the middle of the grip. Use a jubilee clip or plastic tie to mount the transducers so that the operator can work as normally as possible. Cables should be taped down. It is essential to ensure that transducers, mountings or cables do not interfere with the controls or with the safe operation of the tool.
- Record details of the following:

○ Task, including a description of activities and behaviours;
○ The operator;
○ The machine, tool or other sources of vibration;
○ Modes of operation of the equipment;
○ Operating and environmental conditions;
○ Positions of accelerometers;
○ Start and stop times for each measurement;
○ Acceleration measurements for x, y, z directions;
○ Shocks;
○ Observations of the work and the process equipment.
• At the end of each set of readings the instrument calibration should be checked against the field calibrator.

14.6.4   Possible problems

The most common problem with the measurement of hand-transmitted vibration is ensuring that a reliable connection is maintained between the accelerometer and the signal cable. Cables should be secured near to the accelerometer, using adhesive tape. Care should be taken to ensure that any cable connections are secure and that the cables have not been damaged in any way.

Exposing accelerometers to shocks, for example on percussive tools having no damping system, can cause the generation of DC shift, which produces a false reading with a sudden change in the accelerator reading. Any measurements showing signs of DC shift should be disregarded.

14.6.5   Results

The daily exposure to vibration ($A(8)$) of a person is given, using the formula in 'Vibration' section. Note that to avoid confusion between vibration intensity and daily exposure to vibration, it is conventional to express daily exposure to vibration in m s^{-2} $A(8)$.

Therefore the daily exposure from work with a chipping hammer used for 2.5 h with a measured vibration magnitude (a_{hv}) of 12 m s^{-2} is:

$$A(8) = a_{\text{hv}} \sqrt{\frac{T}{T_0}} = 12 \sqrt{\frac{2.5}{8}} = 6.7 \text{ m s}^{-1}$$

where both hands are exposed to vibration, the greater of the two magnitudes a_{hv} is used to ascertain the daily exposure.

If the work is such that the total daily exposure consists of two or more operations with different vibration magnitudes, the daily exposure for the combination of operations is given using the formula:

$$A(8) = \sqrt{A_1(8)^2 + A_2(8)^2 + A_3(8)^2 + \cdots}$$

where $A_1(8)$ is the daily vibration exposure from activity 1, $A_2(8)$ the corresponding value from activity 2 etc.

For work involving the chipping hammer and then a grinder used for 1 h giving a daily exposure of 1.3 m s^{-2} the overall daily exposure, assuming no other vibration exposure, would be:

$$A(8)_{\text{total}} = \sqrt{6.7^2 + 1.3^2} = \sqrt{46.6} = 6.8 \text{ m s}^{-1}$$

14.6.6 Reporting

The monitoring report should provide the following information:

- General information about the measurements and the situation being measured, including the date of the evaluation;
- The purpose of the measurements;
- The person carrying out the measurements and evaluation;
- Measurement instrumentation, including the type of instrument used and calibration traceability;
- The results from the onsite calibration checks;
- Environmental conditions at the workplace, including the air temperature and humidity;
- Location of measurements (e.g. indoor, outdoor, factory area);
- Information used to select the operations measured;
- Machines and inserted tools being used;
- Materials or workpieces being worked upon;
- The operators' personal details – name, age, gender etc;
- Daily work patterns for the workers being monitored;
- Exposure patterns (e.g. work rate or numbers of work cycles or components per day, durations of exposure per cycle or hand-held workpiece).
- Details of vibration sources, including a description of the power tool or machine, the type or model number, the age and maintenance condition of the tool or machine, the weight of the hand-held power tool or hand-held workpiece, the type of hand grip used, any vibration control measures on the machine or power tool and any additional relevant information;
- Acceleration measurement conditions, including the accelerometer locations and orientations (including a sketch and dimensions), the method of attaching transducers and the mass of the transducers;
- Arm posture and hand positions (including whether the operator is left- or right-handed) and any additional information (e.g. data on feed and grip forces);
- Any gloves worn, type and whether they are intended to offer any protection against vibration;
- Measurement results: x-, y- and z-axis frequency-weighted hand-transmitted vibration values for each operation;
- Measurement durations;
- If frequency analysis is available, the un-weighted frequency spectra;
- Daily vibration exposure evaluation results: vibration total values (a_{hv}) for each operation;

- The duration of vibration exposure for each operation;
- Partial vibration exposures for each operation;
- Daily vibration exposure, $A(8)$.

14.7 Control of vibration

When planning a control strategy for a particular job or workplace it is important to prioritize the equipment for action – targeting controls on the equipment that contributes most to daily exposure. This may not necessarily be the equipment with the highest vibration if the lower vibration equipment is used for a substantial part of the work shift. In the example already described it is clearly important to try to tackle the vibration from the chipping hammer first. Where employees are exposed above the daily exposure action value, take measures to:

- Investigate alternative ways of carrying out the tasks not involving vibration;
- Ensure there are purchasing policies and procedures to select and purchase low-vibration equipment;
- Use low-vibrating equipment or operate vibrating equipment remotely;
- Minimise individual exposure by rotating workers using vibrating equipment;
- Ensure that equipment is regularly and properly maintained;
- Provide regular health checks to those employees who are at risk;
- Instruct employees on the health risks of vibration, the signs of vibration injury and how to report early signs of ill health, the precautionary and preventative measures available and the procedures for reporting equipment defects.

Note that just wrapping some rubber or other elastic material around the handles of a vibration tool will have little impact on the vibration and may in fact make things worse. Similarly, 'anti-vibration' gloves do not normally provide any important reduction in hand–arm vibration risks. Gloves marketed as 'anti-vibration' should carry the CE mark and meet the requirements of BS EN ISO 10819.

Where employees are exposed above the daily exposure limit value take immediate action to reduce their exposure.

References and further reading

Palmer K, Griffin MJ, Bendalla H, Pannett B, Coggon D. (2000). Prevalence and pattern of occupational exposure to whole body vibration in Great Britain: findings from a national survey. *Occupational and Environmental Medicine* 57: 229–236.

Crocker MJ. (2007). *Handbook of Noise and Vibration Control*. New York: John Wiley and Sons.

Mansfield NJ. (2004). *Human Response to Vibration*. Boca Raton, FL: CRC Press.

Smith BJ, Peters RJ, Owen S. (1998). *Acoustics and Noise Control*, 2nd edition. London: Longman.

South T. (2004). *Managing Noise and Vibration at Work*. Oxford: Elsevier Butterworth-Heinemann.

HSE (2005). *Whole-Body Vibration. The Control of Vibration at Work Regulations 2005. Guidance on Regulations*. Sudbury, UK: HSE Books.

HSE. (2005) *Hand-arm vibration. The Control of Vibration at Work Regulations 2005. Guidance on Regulations*. Sudbury, UK: HSE Books.

British Standards related to vibration include the following:

BS EN ISO 5349-1:2001: Mechanical vibration – Measurement and evaluation of human exposure to hand-transmitted vibration – Part 1: General requirements.

BS EN ISO 5349-2:2002: Mechanical vibration – Measurement and evaluation of human exposure to hand-transmitted vibration – Part 2: Practical guidance for measurement at the workplace.

BS EN ISO 8041:2005: Human response to vibration. Measuring instrumentation.

BS ISO 2631-4:2001: Mechanical vibration and shock. Evaluation of human exposure to whole-body vibration. Guidelines for the evaluation of the effects of vibration and rotational motion on passengers and crew comfort in fixed-guideway transport systems.

The EU Guides to good practice on hand-arm vibration and the guide on whole-body vibration can be downloaded from http://www.humanvibration.com/EU/EU_index.htm.

Information from the equipment supplier Bruel & Kjaer is available on the internet.

Human Vibration published in 2002. Available at http://www.avt-sa.com/education/Human%20Vibration%20-%20ba7054.pdf.

Measuring Vibration from 1982 is available at http://www.bksv.com/pdf/br0094.pdf.

CHAPTER 15

15

Heat and Cold

15.1 Introduction

Heat is the energy that flows from one body to another because of a difference in temperature. The unit of energy is the joule and the rate of energy transfer is measured in watts (W), where 1 W is equal to 1 J s^{-1}. The watt is the unit of power. In this chapter we describe the basis for heat exchange, some of the simple measurement metrics for heat and cold stress and how to measure the thermal environment. Finally, we consider possible control strategies to mitigate thermal stress.

The human body converts energy from food into work, with typical energy conversion efficiencies ranging from about 25% for a fit person exercising with the major muscle groups down to almost zero when carrying out static work such as holding a weight above the head. The body also has to generate about 50–70 W of energy to maintain its own essential functions, for example to maintain core temperature at about 37°C. Energy derived from food that is not converted into useful work is converted to heat. For example, walking at 6.5 km h^{-1} on the level requires about 500 W; about 425 W of which is released into the body as heat. This energy must be lost to the environment to maintain the body's core temperature within about 1°C of its normal value. The higher the workload, the greater the amount of heat to be lost. For 'light' work, such as limited hand and forearm work, the body has to lose about 150 W of heat, for 'very heavy' manual work, such as shoveling or hand sawing, up to about 500 W of heat must be lost.

Heat can be lost from the body by convection, radiation, conduction or evaporation of sweat or humidifying inspired air. Heat is more easily lost in cold than in hot environments and when the person is clad in light open clothing than in air and/or vapour-impermeable protective clothing. It should be appreciated that only a few joules per gram of water are lost when sweat drips from the body whereas the evaporation of 1 g of sweat in contact with the body can result in about 2400 J being lost. Well-sealed garments with poor air and water vapour permeation can therefore substantially reduce heat loss by sweating as evaporation is much reduced in the high humidities within the garments. In this type of garment the body sweats copiously, but as the sweat cannot evaporate, little heat is lost. This type of well-sealed protective clothing can therefore cause significant heat storage for moderate or hard work in other than cold environments: particularly when such garments are worn together with gloves, respiratory protective equipment (RPE) and head coverings. Protective clothing ensembles that cause thermal discomfort may be worn incorrectly in an attempt to reduce discomfort; i.e. the fasteners may be opened to permit easier flow of air. This type of misuse can substantially reduce the protection provided by the clothing against hazardous substances. Also, it should be noted that wet skin may be more likely to absorb hydrophilic contaminants from the workplace environment and that the increased blood flow close to the surface of the skin in hot environments can enhance dermal uptake of chemical contaminants.

If heat cannot be dissipated fast enough then the deep body temperatures will rise, whereas if heat is lost too fast core temperature will drop. The rate of heat transfer between the body and its surroundings depends upon the thermal environment in contact with the skin. Convection and evaporation play a major role in dissipating body heat; therefore the temperature and the moisture content of the air are important parameters to measure when trying to assess risk. In addition, there may be heat loss or gain by conduction, e.g. through the feet for a standing person or through the back, buttocks and backs of the thighs for a seated person, such as a driver. Also, some parts of the body may be unclothed, e.g. the hands or the face, which may allow more effective conduction of heat from or to the body.

Heat exchange between the body and its surroundings by radiation can also play an important part in the regulation of body heat flow as the skin or clothing radiates heat to colder surfaces and receives radiant heat from hotter surfaces. The rate of radiant heat flow is proportional to the fourth power of the absolute temperature of the radiating surface, whether that is the human body or the surrounding environment. The exact equation for heat transfer between the body and its surroundings is difficult to establish because there are many surfaces at different temperatures, of different efficiency in emitting radiant heat (known as the emissivity) and orientation to the body. However, in the absence of significant radiant heat sources such as red or white-hot surfaces (excluding sunlight) the influence of radiant heat transfer is often minimal. A globe thermometer (Figure 15.2) can provide a good indication of the radiant heat exchange likely to be found at a point although it is affected by the speed of the air flowing over it and therefore does not provide the true mean radiant temperature of the surroundings unless adjusted for air movement.

The movement of air around the body also affects heat convection and evaporation; more heat being lost in high air speeds than in stagnant air. It is therefore important to measure the air speed over the body in the workplace. Thus the four parameters that must be tested to obtain a true indication of the stress from a thermal environment are the following:

- The air temperature;
- The water vapour content of the air;
- The radiant temperature;
- The air speed over the body.

If the heat transfer to the body is out of balance, either positive or negative, then the person may experience an uncomfortable or stressful situation. Many indoor workplaces display unsatisfactory thermal environmental conditions. For example, high temperature radiant sources can be found in steelworks and glass making, high humidity in laundries, kitchens and wet underground mines, and cold conditions in deep-freeze stores and warehouses. Extremes of heat and cold are experienced in many outdoor work situations, particularly with regard to radiant heat, hot and cold air temperature, high and low humidity, high wind speed and wet-working conditions. Whilst no legal standards exist in Britain for a satisfactory or safe thermal environment, Regulation 7 of the Workplace Health, Safety and Welfare regulations imposes the very simple duty that 'During working hours, the temperature in all workplaces inside buildings shall be reasonable'.

15.2 Heat stress

There are numerous heat stress and heat strain indices that have been developed: most of which have major limitations because their validity is not clearly defined or they are not valid where personal protective equipment (PPE) is worn. One of the simplest indices to both measure and assess the significance of the results obtained is the Wet Bulb Globe Temperature (WBGT) Index. This index was developed during World War II to ensure the safety of military personnel during training and was adopted by the American Conference of Government Industrial Hygienists (ACGIH) as the basis of their Threshold Limit Value (TLV) for heat stress and later in the standard BS EN 27243.

The WBGT is based on the environmental parameters: air temperature, measured using a dry bulb thermometer; water content of the air, measured using a natural, un-aspirated wet bulb thermometer; radiant heat measured using a globe thermometer; and air speed indirectly measured by both the wet bulb thermometer and the globe thermometer. All four important parameters are therefore measured using only three simple devices.

The standard is based on assessing four main factors:

- The thermal environment, expressed as WBGT;
- Work rates of the workers;
- The acclimatisation status of the individuals;
- The intermittency of the work.

The environmental WBGT, expressed in temperature units, is calculated from the following equations:

For indoor use, $\text{WBGT} = 0.7t'_n + 0.3t_g$

For outdoor use in sunlight, $\text{WBGT} = 0.7t'_n + 0.2t_g + 0.1t$

where t'_n is natural, un-aspirated, wet bulb temperature (°C); t_g is globe temperature (°C) and t is dry bulb temperature (°C).

The British Standard describes five bands of metabolic rates: 'resting', 'low' – equivalent activities such as sitting with light manual work or standing with light arm work; 'moderate' – sustained moderate hand and arm work or light pulling and pushing; 'heavy' – intense hand and trunk work, shovelling, manual sawing or pushing or pulling heavy loads and, 'very heavy' – very intense activities at a fast to maximum pace. The standard defines reference values for WBGT as shown in Table 15.1.

Note that sensible air movement is detectable by the individual.

The above-mentioned criteria should not be exceeded within any 1-h period of the working day. The standard provides a graph allowing adjustment of the WBGT reference values, depending on whether the workers are working continuously (as shown in Table 15.1), or working 75% and resting 25% in each hour, working and resting for equal amounts of time and working for 25% of the time and resting 75% of the time.

The standard does not contain any explicit adjustments for clothing worn by the workers. It is assumed that the clothing is normal work wear with a thermal insulation index of 0.6 clo (equivalent to 0.155 $m^2 \times K\ W^{-1}$, i.e. in metres squared $\times$ Kelvin per watt). The clothing adjustment factors shown in Table 15.2 can be used to adjust the environmental WBGT for some clothing ensembles.

All of the above-mentioned clothing ensembles are assumed to be worn over a light vest and underpants or shorts. Where multiple layers of clothing are worn, e.g. a vapour barrier garment worn over double-layered woven clothing: an ensemble widely used by fire fighters, the thermal consequence would be greater than given by the simple addition of the two individual correction factors above because of the additional insulation from the air layers trapped between the clothing. WBGT is not recommended as an exposure index in such extreme situations.

15.3 Measurement equipment

All thermal measurement equipment should be regularly calibrated against an appropriate standard instrument. This work can be carried out by you or others in a controlled thermal environment or by the equipment supplier.

Historically, dry bulb, wet bulb and globe temperatures were based on measurements made with mercury in glass thermometers. However, given the hazards associated with both mercury and glass in the workplace, most modern instruments are now based on electronic sensors, and mercury in glass thermometers are only used for calibration in the laboratory. However, in some situations it might be permissible to use the mercury in glass thermometers in a swing hygrometer for the dry bulb and wet bulb thermometers as they are mechanically protected. Note that for the WBGT Index the hygrometer is allowed to hang with the water reservoir at the bottom of the instrument rather than being swung around.

Table 15.1 WBGT reference values from BS EN 27243.

Metabolic rate class	Metabolic rate, M		WBGT Reference value			
	Related to a unit skin surface area (W m^{-2})	Total (for a mean skin surface area of 1.8 m^2) (W)	Person acclimatised to heat (°C)		Person not acclimatised to heat (°C)	
			No sensible air movement	Sensible air movement	No sensible air movement	Sensible air movement
0 (resting)	$M \leq 65$	$M \leq 117$	33		32	
1	$65 < M \leq 130$	$117 < M \leq 234$	30		29	
2	$130 < M \leq 200$	$234 < M \leq 360$	28		26	
3	$200 < M \leq 260$	$360 < M \leq 468$	25	26	22	23
4	$M > 260$	$M > 468$	23	25	18	20

177

Table 15.2 Clothing adjustment factors for WBGT.*

Clothing type	Addition to measured WBGT (°C)
Work clothes with long sleeved shirt and trousers	0
Cloth (woven material) overalls	0
SMS polypropylene overalls	0.5
Polyolefin overalls	1
Double-layered woven clothing	3
Limited use vapour barrier garments	11

*Based on guidance from the ACGIH

Apart from safety, a major benefit of electronic sensors is that the results from such devices can be read at a distance and can be electronically recorded.

15.3.1 Dry bulb thermometers

All dry bulb thermometer sensors should have a highly polished external surface to minimise the absorption or emission of radiant energy and should be shielded against the effects of air velocities greater than about 0.2 m s^{-1} over the surface of the sensor.

15.3.2 Wet bulb thermometers

These are simply dry bulb instruments as already described but with the sensor covered in a clean cotton wick wetted with distilled water. As the water evaporates from the wick, heat will be removed from the sensor, thus reducing the indicated temperature to below that of the dry bulb, unless the air is fully saturated with water vapour, in which case the wet and dry bulb temperature readings are identical. For measurement of WBGT, the monitor relies on natural air currents to remove evaporated water vapour from around the sensor. The wet bulb sensor must therefore not be shielded from environmental airflows. The result is referred to as the 'natural wet bulb temperature'. It is essential that the distilled water be permitted to reach the ambient dry bulb temperature at each measurement location before any measurement results are recorded.

15.3.3 Air speed

The measurement of air speed is quite difficult, although fortunately a direct measurement of air speed is not required for WBGT. There are very few low-cost instruments that can measure the relatively low air speeds that are often relevant to the thermal environment (i.e. less then 0.5 m s^{-1}) with the required accuracy and precision. The traditional instrument is in fact a special type of thermometer, the Kata thermometer, which is used to measure the cooling power of the air movement.

The Kata is an alcohol in glass thermometer with a large silvered bulb at its base and a small bulb at the top of the stem (Figure 15.1), which is inscribed with marks on the top and bottom corresponding to a temperature

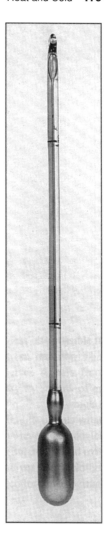

Figure 15.1 Kata thermometer. (© Casella Measurement Ltd. Reproduced with permission.)

difference of 3°C. Also inscribed on the stem is a number known as the Kata factor, which is specific to each instrument. The cooling power of the air is measured by timing the rate of fall of the liquid between the two marks having first heated the lower bulb to expand the liquid up the stem. From this the air velocity can be calculated or determined from a formula or chart supplied with the instrument. Kata thermometers with different temperature ranges can be used in different air temperatures to provide a suitable reading. There are now very few commercial suppliers of Kata thermometers. If you need to measure air movement then it may be easiest to use a sensitive anemometer (see Chapter 20).

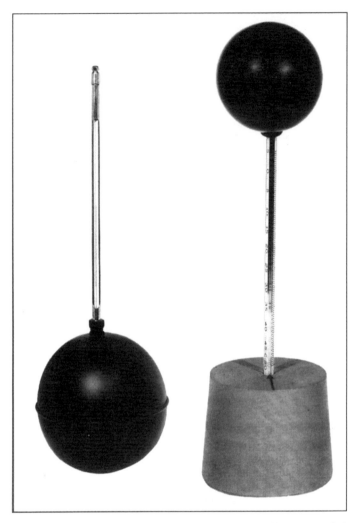

Figure 15.2 Globe thermometer with glass thermometer. (© Casella Measurement Ltd. Reproduced with permission.)

15.3.4 Globe thermometer

A dry bulb temperature sensor is placed at the centre of a matt black sphere or globe. Globes are usually available with 150 mm or 44 mm diameters. The larger globe takes up to 15–20 min to reach equilibrium with its surroundings but the smaller one is quicker. However, as the larger globe is more sensitive to airflow velocity than the small globe, and was used in most of the research on which the standard is based, use of the larger globe is recommended. Figure 15.2 shows a 150-mm diameter globe with glass thermometer, although we consider it is more appropriate to use a thermocouple or other electronic temperature sensor as an alternative to the mercury in glass thermometer.

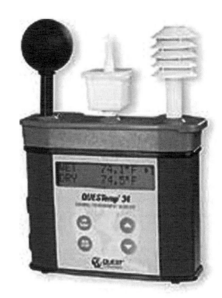

Figure 15.3 Integrating heat stress monitor.
(© Quest Technologies. Reproduced with
permission.)

15.3.5 Integrating instruments

Instruments are available that measure dry bulb, wet bulb, globe temperatures and air speed electrically and integrate the results into WBGT (Figure 15.3). As with any direct-reading instrument it must be regularly calibrated against accurate mercury in glass thermometers in an environmental chamber. Note that most integrating instruments use a small-diameter globe and they may not correctly adjust the globe thermometer readings to correct for the use of the smaller sensor. Before using any instruments with a globe thermometer less than 150 mm diameter, check with the supplier that the relevant correction for the globe sensor used has been incorporated into the instrument measurement results.

15.4 Personal monitoring

In addition to monitoring the working environment it is possible to monitor the worker by using a portable heat strain monitor or some other device to assess their physiological state. For example, the heat strain monitor consists of a miniature data logger that receives signals from various sensors attached to an employee's body by means of an elastic belt. Heart rate and temperature are sensed from which a 'strain index' is calculated and indicated with audible signals when the index reaches warning or action levels. The device can be set for three age ranges of worker (under 36, 36–50 and over 50 years) and for two levels of clothing: single layer (work clothes or cotton overalls) and multiple layers (double cotton or impermeable coveralls). The instrument is illustrated in Figure 15.4. Other instruments are also available to provide personal monitoring of heat strain.

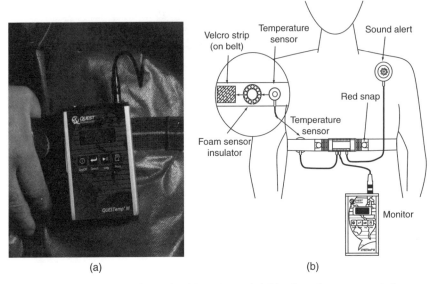

(a)   (b)

Figure 15.4 Portable heat strain monitor (a) monitor on belt (b) schematic arrangement of sensors. (© Quest Technologies. Reproduced with permission.)

European Standard EN ISO 9886 sets out methods available to measure and interpret the following:

- Body core temperature (estimated from rectal, oral, tympanic membrane and other temperature measurements);
- Skin temperature;
- Heart rate;
- Body-mass loss.

15.5 Measurement of the thermal environment

15.5.1 Aim

It is often necessary to examine the thermal stress imposed upon employees in hot or cold industries or in outdoor workplaces in hot or cold climates. By measuring three parameters – natural wet and dry bulb temperature plus globe temperature – the WBGT Index can be obtained and the thermal components making up the workplace environment evaluated.

15.5.2 Equipment required

A dry bulb thermometer, a wet bulb thermometer, a globe thermometer, distilled water, rubber bungs bored out to take one of the thermometers, aluminium foil, string, scissors and a tripod stand with clamps. Alternatively use an integrating direct-reading instrument as already described. The mercury thermometers in a swing hygrometer can be used for the dry bulb and wet bulb thermometers. However, the use of mercury in glass thermometers should be cleared with the site health and safety manger first.

15.5.3   Measurement methods

1. To prepare the dry bulb thermometer, when necessary, carefully attach a piece of aluminium to shield the sensor from radiation but not to restrict any air flow over it. The foil should be fitted shiny side out.
2. To prepare the natural wet bulb thermometer, attach the muslin wick over the sensor, covering it completely. Wet the wick with distilled water and allow the loose end of the wick to dip into the container of distilled water. Hang the container just below the sensor by means of string or sticky tape, ensuring that it is clear of the sensor in order to allow unrestricted airflow. Ensure that the distilled water reaches the ambient dry bulb temperature before any readings are taken. Where measurements have to be made at a number of locations with different dry bulb temperatures you may need to periodically top up the reservoir with distilled water.
3. To prepare the globe thermometer check that the sensor is in the centre of the globe and that there are no air gaps around the point where the thermometer or thermocouple wire enters the globe.
4. Arrange these three instruments on the tripod stand, as shown in Figure 15.5, and place it at the workplace to be measured. Ensure that the sensors are situated in the vicinity of the worker's chest or abdomen during normal operations and that the equipment does not impede the worker. (Note: BS EN 27243 recommends measurements be made at three heights – head, abdomen and ankles, although if only one height is to be used the chest/abdomen is recommended.) As noted above, a conventional swing hygrometer can be used to replace the wet and dry bulb thermometers. Ensure that the globe is not shadowed by the other thermometers, by the worker or by other equipment.
5. Allow about 20 min for the instruments to reach equilibrium and record the values of dry bulb, natural wet bulb and globe temperatures.

15.5.4   Observations

Where possible, take photographs of each subject monitored and his/her activities, preferably using a camcorder or the camcorder facility on a digital camera. The position of the worker in relation to radiant heat sources may be quite important in assessing their risk.

1. Make a careful record of all the sources that may impact on the thermal environment, e.g. radiant heaters or hot pipes, sources of water vapour, air vents.
2. Record each subject's activities so that his/her likely work rates can be estimated.
3. Record any intermittency in each subject's work pattern.

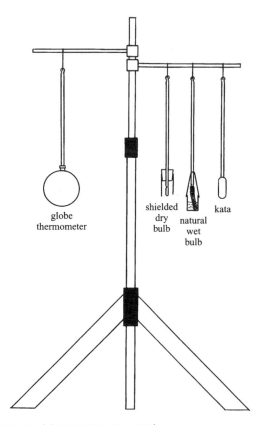

Figure 15.5 Arrangement of thermometers on a stand.

4. Record the type of clothing worn and the number and type of each layer of clothing for each subject.
5. Record whether any subject is wearing gloves or other personal protective equipment. If respiratory protective equipment is worn, record the type of equipment and note whether it is half-mask or full-mask, powered, air-fed or negative pressure.
6. Record whether any subject appears to be flushed or sweating. Note their fluid intake.
7. Once the measurements have been recorded ask each worker his/her opinion of the thermal nature of their work.

15.5.5 Results and calculations

The results from manual instruments should be recorded in a notebook or a pro forma recording form. It is strongly recommended that when direct reading heat stress or heart strain monitors are being used manual measurements should be also taken to check that the monitors are functioning correctly. To evaluate the WBGT Index, it is necessary to establish the work rate of the workers whose workplace is being measured – this can be done most simply by observation of the work and comparing these data with information tabulated in the standard, although there are more accurate instrumental methods available to measure workrate if required. By using Table 15.1, the recommended maximum WBGT can be established for different work rates, acclimatisation status and subjective airflow, and the measurements can be compared with the corresponding limits. Note that the WBGT reference values are fairly conservative and should ensure that most workers are unaffected by their thermal environment. Note also the WBGT reference values and limits for work-rest scheduling assume that the workers are resting in much the same conditions where they are working. If rest is possible in a cooler area this will result in a further reduction of any risk.

15.5.6   Possible problems

1. Dirty wicks or the use of non-distilled water on the wet bulb thermometer will result in a reduced evaporation rate, so giving an exaggeratedly high humidity.
2. When reading thermometers make sure that no other heat source such as human hands or breath comes into contact with them.
3. When undertaking an indoor survey it is useful to note the outdoor conditions with regard to air temperature, moisture content and wind speed as these factors can have an effect on indoor values.

15.6   Predicted Heat Strain Index

As we have noted the WBGT is a simple index that has several limitations. While it is easy to use for an initial assessment it may be overly conservative or may underestimate the risks when workers are wearing unusual protective clothing. The International Standards Organisation produced a standard based on the more sophisticated Predicted Heat Strain Index (BS EN 7933). The index is based on the physical and physiological process involved with heat exchange between the human body and the environment. The index requires measurement of air temperature, mean radiant temperature (calculated using the globe temperature), partial water vapour pressure and air speed. In addition, the mean metabolic rate and the clothing thermal characteristics are needed (there are separate standards that explain how to assess the latter two parameters – BS EN 28996 and BS EN 9920, respectively).

The measurements are used to calculate the required evaporative heat flow on the assumption that this is the mechanism by which the body will aim to achieve thermal equilibrium. This then determines the two key stress parameters: the skin wetness (as a fraction of the skin surface wet with sweat) and the required sweat rate (in grams per hour). The index also includes two predicted physiological stress parameters: the water loss (as a fraction of total body mass) and the rectal temperature (°C). The estimated maximum allowable exposure time (in minutes) is reached when either the estimated water loss or the rectal temperature reaches the limits set in the standard. The standard contains the limits for each of these along with a computer program to calculate the index values.

Although ISO7933 is nominally a more scientific assessment technique than WBGT and has been validated by extensive laboratory studies, the basis of the calculation of heat transfer from/to the body has a limited range of applicability, which has not been well defined. In addition, ISO7933 cannot be applied to clothing ensembles with a 'clo' value greater than 1 or which significantly affect the ability of sweat to evaporate.

Being less conservative than the WBGT Index, ISO7933 may permit people to work in situations that the WBGT Index would preclude. We consider that ISO7933 should only be used where heat strain is being measured or where medical supervision is present.

15.7   Risk assessment strategy

BS EN Standard 15265 provides a general strategy for the investigation of heat and cold stress problems. It is based around three strategies:

1. *Observation* of the work and work environment to identify the circumstances where there may be a risk, the simple steps that could be taken to eliminate or control the risk and whether further measurement of the thermal conditions is necessary.
2. *Analysis* of the work and the work environment at the time of day and year when the risk of heat stress is likely to be greatest.
3. Undertake a *detailed investigation* of the work and thermal environment by using sophisticated measurement methods.

In the observation phase the conditions should be assessed against a set of qualitative criteria for air temperature, humidity, thermal radiation, air movement, physical workload and clothing. The opinions of the workers should also be collected using a categorical scale. For air temperature the scale is shown in Table 15.3

Table 15.3   Examples of subjective environmental scoring scales in BS EN ISO 15265.

Score	Temperature condition
−3	Generally freezing
−2	Generally between 0 and 10°C
−1	Generally between 10 and 18°C
0	Generally between 18 and 15°C
1	Generally between 25 and 32°C
2	Generally between 32 and 40°C
3	Generally more than 40°C

Table 15.4   Summary table showing where the scores may deviate from the ideal.

	-3	-2	-1	0	1	2	3
Air temperature						X	
Humidity				X			
Thermal radiation						X	
Air movement				X			
Physical workload					X		
Clothing				X			

The results are marked on a grid with an "X". When the situation is judged as not ideal, i.e. outside +1 to −1, you should try to identify the reason. It is important to note it is not the score itself that is important but the analysis of why the score deviates from the ideal range. Note the shaded areas in the grid are outside the scoring range. An example of the scoring sheet is shown in Table 15.4.

In this example there is elevated air temperature and a high-radiant heat load; the worker is also working quite hard, but on its own this would not have provided any cause for concern.

Where there are undesirable conditions then one or more of the control approaches listed in the standard should be considered. These include the following strategies:

1. Air temperature
   - Eliminate the source of heat or cold.
   - Relocate the source of heat or cold away from the worker.
   - Insulate any hot surfaces.
   - Provide local ventilation, either exhausting or blowing
   - Use clothing that is more or less insulating depending on whether there is a heat or cold stress problem.
2. Humidity
   - Eliminate leaks of water vapour into the workroom.
   - Enclose cool surfaces to prevent condensation.
   - Use vapour-permeable waterproof clothing.
3. Thermal radiation
   - Reduce the number or size of radiating surfaces.
   - Use reflecting barriers.
   - Insulate radiating surfaces to reduce the surface temperature.
   - Move the worker further from the radiating surfaces.
   - Use special reflective suits to protect workers (normally only suitable for emergency workers such as firefighters).
4. Air movements
   - Eliminate hot air draughts in the workplace.
5. Physical workload
   - Minimise the speed and extent of movement of workers.
   - Provide mechanical aids to assist the worker.

6. Clothing
   • Use appropriately designed clothing for the thermal conditions.

Considering the example workplace with high-radiant heat and air temperature then the best solution might be to insulate the hot surfaces since this will tackle both problems, although it may take a little time to organise. In the short term, the manager could be advised to provide some localised cooling and some reflective barriers.

If it is unclear what the risks are or whether any of the control measures will work then the investigation should move on to Stage 2 – analysis, which will involve measurement of the key thermal parameters and an evaluation using either WBGT, the Predicted Heat Stress Index or some other appropriate index. In the unusual circumstance that this does not enable the selection of an appropriate control strategy then it may be necessary to call in an expert in heat stress assessment (Stage 3).

15.8 Cold

If the interaction of ambient thermal conditions, work rate and clothing type is such that the body can lose heat faster than it is generated, the body's deep core temperature can fall below the normal value of about 37°C and 'cold strain' can occur. In addition, workers may come into direct contact with cold surfaces and this may cause localised discomfort or injury.

BS EN ISO Standard 15743 – Ergonomics of the thermal environment – Cold workplaces – Risk assessment and management describes the methods for assessing and managing health and performance risks in cold workplaces. The standard describes the following:

• An approach to risk assessment in cold work;
• A strategy for occupational health professionals to identify workers with symptoms that increase their cold sensitivity, plus guidance and instructions for individual cold protection;
• Guidelines on different international thermal standards to help assess cold-related risks;
• An approach to cold risk management and
• Examples of working in cold conditions.

The first step outlined by this standard is to undertake a qualitative assessment of the work environment by using a pro forma scoring sheet. This focuses on assessments of the potential for problems from exposure to cold air, to excessive wind or localized air movements, contact with cold surfaces, contact with water or liquids on skin or clothing, the duration of the cold work, the work rate, the adequacy of protective clothing – both on the body and extremities – and the use of protective equipment such as hearing protection.

It may be necessary to augment the subjective assessment with simple measurements such as air temperature or wind speed. There is a simple

Table 15.5   Interpretation of the Wind Chill Index

t_{WC} (°C)	Interpretation
−10 to −24	Uncomfortably cold
−25 to −34	Very cold – risk of skin freezing
−34 to −59	Bitterly cold – exposed skin may freeze in 10 min
−60 and below	Extremely cold – exposed skin may freeze in 2 min

assessment of the required clothing insulation for cold conditions that can be made (the IREQ, described in BS EN ISO 11079), which is dependant on the air temperature, air speed, work rate and the air permeability of the outer clothing layer. For example, someone sedentary in 0°C with an air speed of 0.4 m s^{-1} would require clothing with an insulation of 3 clo (corresponding to heavy winter clothing with appropriate under clothes – BS EN ISO 7933 has some basic information about clothing insulation).

The effects of airflow over the body can enhance the heat lost by convection from the clothing surface and can result in a 'wind chill' effect. The Wind Chill Index (t_{WC}) is a useful way to assess clothing requirements in such conditions. The Wind Chill Index can be estimated using the following equation:

$$t_{WC} = 13.12 + 0.6215 \times t_a - 11.37.v^{0.16} + 0.3965 \times t_a.v^{0.16}$$

where t_a is the air temperature and v the air speed 10 m above the ground in km h^{-1} (you can find this out from a local weather station or estimate it by multiplying the wind speed at ground level by 1.5). This index is interpreted as shown in Table 15.5.

15.9   To calculate the wind chill factor

Wind chill is a function of the dry bulb air temperature and air speed only. That is it represents the worst case where there is no radiant heat gain component, and moisture content will be low because of the limited water-holding capacity of low temperature air, even if the air is saturated.

15.9.1   Procedure

1. Measure the dry bulb temperature and air velocity at the occupied site. Note that if measuring outdoor conditions, the wind direction is unlikely to be steady therefore a non-directional air speed meter should be used such as a hot wire anemometer. Adjust the wind speed to estimate the value 10 m above ground.
2. Use a calculator or a spreadsheet program to calculate t_{WC} using the formula provided above.

Example

Find the wind chill factor corresponding to a measured dry bulb temperature $-20°C$ at a speed of 15 km h^{-1}.

$$t_{wc} = 13.12 + (0.6215 \times (-20)) - (11.37 \times 15^{0.16}) + (3.965 \times (-20) \times 15^{0.16})$$

$$= -29°C$$

The calculated value is -29 °C, which corresponds to 'very cold'.

References and further reading

American Conference of Governmental Industrial Hygienists (2007). *Threshold Limit Values for Chemical Substances and Physical Agents and Biological Exposure Indices*. Cincinnati, OH: ACGIH.

American Conference of Governmental Industrial Hygienists (2007). *Documentation of the Threshold Limit Values for heat and cold stress*. Cincinnati, OH: ACGIH.

British Occupational Hygiene Society (1990). *The Thermal Environment*, Technical Guide No. 8. Leeds, UK: Science Reviews.

Aw TC, Gardiner K and Harrington JM. (2007). *Pocket Consultant in Occupational Health*, 5th edition. Oxford, UK: Blackwell Publishing.

Parsons KC. (2003). *Human Thermal Environments: The Effects of Hot, Moderate, and Cold Environments on Human Health, Comfort, and Performance*, 2nd edition. Lincoln, NE: CRC Press.

Parsons K. (2006). Heat stress standard ISO 7243 and its global application. *Industrial Health* 44: 368–379. Available at http://www.jniosh.go.jp/old/niih/en/indu_hel/2006/pdf/indhealth_44_3_368.pdf.

Youle A. (2005). The thermal environment. In: *Occupational Hygiene* (Gardiner K and Harrington, JM, eds), pp. 286-306. Oxford, UK: Blackwell Publishing.

Information from the HSE website. Available at http://www.hse.gov.uk/temperature/index.htm.

There is an extensive list of standards related to the thermal environment, which are available at www.bsi-global.com. Other standards are available on the International Standards Organisation website www.iso.org.

Some of the key standards are

BS EN 27243:1994: Hot environments – Estimation of the heat stress on working man, based on the WBGT-index (wet bulb globe temperature).

BS EN 7726:2001: Ergonomics of the thermal environment – Instruments for measuring physical quantities.

BS EN 7933: 2004: Ergonomics of the thermal environment – Analytical determination and interpretation of heat stress using calculation of the predicted heat strain.

16 Lighting

16.1 Introduction

Suitable and sufficient lighting is required for the purposes of safety, welfare and efficiency at work. Poor lighting does not cause disease, but it does increase fatigue and the risk of accidents. Poor lighting also reduces efficiency, hinders good housekeeping and increases worker dissatisfaction. This chapter briefly describes lighting, lighting standards and the methods available to measure illuminance.

For lighting to be considered to be both suitable and sufficient for the needs of individuals within the workplace it should:

- Provide sufficient light on the task to allow people to work safely and efficiently;
- Allow people to see movement and discriminate between colours and shapes accurately;
- Not produce glare, strong contrasts between adjacent areas, veiling reflections, flicker, or stroboscopic effects;
- Not contribute to making the conditions thermally uncomfortable; and
- Not introduce the risk of fire or explosion or produce a health and safety risk.

Lighting in the workplace usually comes from a mixture of natural and artificial light sources. Natural light comes from daylight entering through windows and skylights. Artificial lighting is produced by filament or discharge lamps to supplement natural day lighting and to maintain minimum levels of illumination throughout the workplace. Different types of lamp and lamp holders produce light with different characteristics; e.g. colours are not identifiable using low-pressure sodium discharge lamps.

The amount of light emitted by a source is known as luminance; this is measured in candela m^{-2} (Cd m^{-2}). The amount of light falling on a surface is known as illumination; this is measured in lumen m^{-2} (lux). As the eye does not react equally to light across the visible spectrum, measurement instruments need to be colour-corrected so that they match the human response to different frequencies of the visible light spectrum. Instruments also should be cosine-corrected to take into account the effects of light falling upon it from an oblique angle.

Glare is the visual sensation produced by bright areas within the field of view and may cause discomfort or interfere with our ability to see. Glare may also be caused by reflections from shiny surfaces usually known as veiling reflections. When there is direct interference with vision this is known as disability glare, e.g. from headlights from oncoming traffic. When vision is not directly impaired but there is discomfort, annoyance, irritability or distraction, the condition is known as discomfort glare, e.g. bright lights on ceiling on the edge of the field of view. People are particularly sensitive to discomfort glare at the edges of their field of view. Large differences in the levels of illumination between adjoining areas produce strong shadows, contrasts and reduce the ability to see detail. This can also cause discomfort glare.

Flicker is visible light modulation and we are particularly sensitive to it at 50 Hz at the edges of our field of view. It causes distraction, and may give rise to both discomfort and fatigue. In susceptible people flicker may also induce epileptic seizures. A stroboscopic effect occurs when a pulsating light from discharge lamps changes the perceived motion of rotating or reciprocating machinery. Stroboscopic effects can lead to major injuries by deceiving operators into believing that fast moving pieces of machinery are stationary or moving slowly.

Lamps and holders should be protected so that they do not produce a risk of fire or explosion. Lamps with large heat outputs should not touch or be close to combustible items, and must be 'ATEX' classified for use in flammable or explosive atmospheres where required – ATEX is the name given to the framework for controlling explosive atmospheres and the necessary standard of equipment and protective systems. Further information about ATEX requirements can be found on HSE's website. Lighting systems should be designed for ease of maintenance and cleaning.

16.2 Lighting Standards

There are no illumination standards laid down in health and safety regulations in Britain. Regulation 8 of the Workplace (Health, Safety and Welfare) regulations 1992 requires that every workplace must have suitable and sufficient lighting. The lighting in the workplace should as far as is possible, be natural. Guidance on minimum acceptable levels of lighting at work is given in the HSE publication 'Lighting at Work' (HSE, 2002). However, it does not explain how lighting can be used to maximise task performance or to enhance the appearance of the workplace. Standards for good lighting are given in British Standards and in Chartered Institute of Building Service Engineers (CIBSE) lighting guides.

The uniformity of the illuminance is the ratio of the minimum to the average value. The task area should be illuminated as uniformly as possible and within the workplace the illuminance should change gradually. The uniformity of

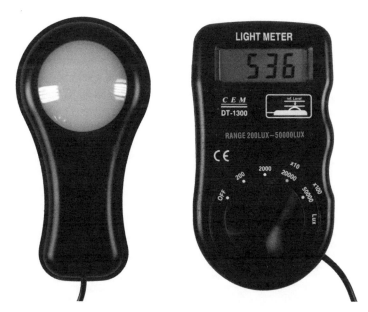

Figure 16.1 The light meter. (© Castle Group. Reproduced with permission.)

the task illuminance should not be less than 0.7 and the uniformity of the illuminance of the immediate surrounding areas should not be less than 0.5.

16.3   Equipment available

Light meters measure the electrical current produced by light falling on a photoelectric light cell. The best instruments for workplace measurements are illuminance meters that have a range of 0–5000 lux with the photocell connected to the meter by a length of cable to allow the meter to be read without the observer overshadowing the cell. Note that 2 lux is roughly equivalent to moonlight while 50,000 lux would be very bright sunlight. The photocell should be cosine-corrected to take into account the effects of light falling upon it from an oblique angle and colour-corrected to allow measurements to be taken over a wide range of lamps and in daylight. Figure 16.1 shows a light meter.

16.4   Calibration

Light meters should be calibrated against a primary standard at an accredited laboratory every 2 years to 'BS667: 2005 Specification for Portable Photoelectric Photometers.' If the instrument has been damaged or misused, it should be repaired and recalibrated before reuse. A battery check should also be carried out before you start to make any measurements. Cover the light cell with a soft cloth and check that the display reads '0' before using the instrument.

16.5 To measure lighting

16.5.1 Aim

To carry out a basic workplace lighting survey it is important to fully understand the distribution of light in a room and to determine whether workplace illumination levels are suitable and sufficient for the work to be undertaken. Two stages of assessment are required. The first is to complete a subjective examination of the general illumination and the second is to follow that up with some organised measurement of lighting levels.

16.5.2 Equipment required

In addition to a light meter the following equipment should be taken to site:

- Manufacturer's operating instructions;
- Clip board, squared paper, pencil, ruler and tape measure – plus a scale plan of the work site if possible;
- A visual assessment form;
- Camera;
- Screwdriver or Allen key for adjusting the instrument, if required;
- Spare batteries.

16.5.3 Method

Turn on the artificial lighting used on the site and allow it to stabilise before taking the first measurement. For filament lamps, the stabilisation period should be at least 10 min and for discharge lamps the stabilisation period should be at least 30 min. Draw a sketch plan of the room to show the principal working surfaces, windows, light fittings and other relevant features. This should be done to scale if possible. Draw separate floor and ceiling plans to avoid confusion between the furniture and the light fittings. Measure the major dimensions of the room and note them on the sketch plans. Record the positions and types of light fittings; the types and wattage of lamps; and the condition of the principal room surfaces.

Then note the following:

- The visual tasks being carried out;
- Your subjective impression of the natural and artificial lighting;
- Whether the light fittings, lamps and windows are clean or have accumulations of dirt or dust and
- The position of any light fittings or lamps that are damaged, missing or not working.

Survey the workplace; stop, look and listen! Walk around the area, stop frequently and observe what is going on; ask workers and supervisors about their work tasks and whether the lighting is satisfactory. If not, ask the reason why and in which parts of the room. Also ask what improvements they think can be made to the lighting arrangements. Determine whether there are any undesirable shadows or reflections on the work. Note whether the lighting fittings or windows cause discomfort or disability glare when seen separately or together and observe whether the windows are obstructed by internal furnishings or equipment and by outside trees, walls or other buildings, which may affect the illumination.

If the nature of the work requires the recognition of different colours, note whether the colour rendering of the lights is satisfactory. This may have to be done by removing some of the coloured material to the window or outside to observe it under natural daylight to see whether the colour changes.

Notice whether there is any flicker from discharge lamps including fluorescent tubes and if any stroboscopic effects on moving machinery are present.

To take measurements of lighting levels use the light meter to measure the illuminance readings at all work stations and on every work surface. This should be done with the normal workplace lighting switched on, that is, with general and local lamps on. Ensure you do not cast a shadow over the light meter. Natural lighting should be excluded as far as possible. If natural lighting cannot be excluded, measurements should be taken at night or on an overcast day unless simultaneous measurements can be taken of the natural and artificial lighting.

To measure average illuminance levels for comparison against BS ISO 8995 or CIBSE guides the workplace is divided into an equal number of areas and measurements are taken in the centre of each area. Measurements should be taken in a horizontal plane, ideally at 0.85 m above floor level. The minimum number of areas for measurements is calculated by producing a room index from the following equation:

$$k = \frac{L \times W}{Hm \times (L + W)}$$

where k is the room index, L is the room length, W is the room width, Hm is the height of lamps above working surface (0.85 m above floor level).

The minimum number of areas where measurement should be made are shown in Table 16.1.

Where the room is L-shaped or where the room is subdivided the room index should be calculated for each separate area.

Table 16.1 Minimum number of areas.

Room index	Minimum number of areas
Below 1	9
1 and below 2	16
2 and below 3	25
Above 3	36

Table 16.2 Recommended illuminance levels to prevent accidents and visual fatigue.

Activity or task	Typical workplace	Average illuminance (lux)	Minimum illuminance (lux)
General movement around the worksite	Corridors, circulation routes	20	5
Work involving limited perception of details	Factories assembling large components, kitchens	100	50
Work requiring perception of detail	Offices, metalworking plant	200	100
Tasks involving perception of fine detail	Electronics plants, textile factories	500	200

16.5.4 Possible problems

The main problems likely to be encountered are shadows and fluctuations due to the presence of natural lighting.

16.5.5 Results

Average illuminance is calculated by adding all measurements and dividing by the number of measurements. The uniformity ratio is calculated by dividing the lowest measurement by the average measurement. Use CIBSE or HSE guidance to judge whether the illuminance is adequate for the tasks being carried out in the workplace. Table 16.2 shows the recommendations based on guidance from HSE.

Note that the recommended illuminance levels given in the CIBSE guidance are generally higher than those shown above, for example for offices they recommend 300–500 lux.

16.5.6 Reporting

The monitoring report should provide the following information:

- General information about the purpose of the measurements, the date of evaluation and who has carried out the measurements and evaluation;
- Measurement instrumentation, including instrumentation details, calibration traceability and the calibration checks;
- Environmental conditions at the workplace, with the location of measurements (e.g. indoor, outdoor, factory area), air temperature, and how daylight was excluded or compensated for during the survey;
- Sketch plans, with dimensions, showing principal working surfaces and furniture, windows, light fittings and any other relevant features.
- Describe the visual tasks being carried out, the positions and types of light fittings, the types and wattage of lamps and the condition of the principal room surfaces;

Table 16.3 Possible solutions to poor lighting

Problem	Possible solutions
Tasks are difficult to see	Replace failed lamps and clean luminaires
	Remove obstructions
	Increase the reflectance of surfaces
	Move the working area
	Provide local or task lighting
	Provide magnification or vision aids
	Increase number of luminaires to provide more illuminance
Uneven lighting or strong shadows on the task	Replace failed lamps and clean luminaires
	Remove obstructions
	Increase/decrease the reflectances of the room surfaces which are too dim or too bright
	Increase number of luminaires, or change the type of luminaires or change their spacings to provide a more even illuminance
Glare	Move any bright sources
	Increase/decrease the reflectances of surfaces which are too dim or too bright
	Use luminaires that prevent direct sight of lamps.
	Change the orientation of linear luminaires to provide an end-on view
	Raise height of luminaire or move lamp outside field of vision.
Flicker	Change lamps near the end of their life
	Check electrical circuit for any faults in the supply
	Use high frequency control gear
	Supply adjacent rows of luminaires from different phases of the electricity supply

- Your subjective impression of the natural and artificial lighting;
- Describe whether the light fittings, lamps and windows are clean or dirty, and the position of any light fittings or lamps that are damaged, missing or not working;
- Show results of illuminance measurement on the sketch plan;
- Calculate the average illuminances and uniformity ratios;
- Comment on the results in relation to the relevant standards;
- Clearly set out your recommendations, making sure that they are realistic and practicable.

16.6 Control

Where there is poor lighting the following actions should be considered to resolve the problem (Table 16.3).

References and further reading

Smith, NA. (2005). Light and lighting. In: *Occupational Hygiene*, 3rd edition (Gardiner K, Harrington JM, eds). Oxford, UK: Blackwell Publishing.

Smith, NA. (2000). *Lighting for Health and Safety*. Oxford, UK: Butterworth Heineman.

Relevant British Standards:

BS 667: 2005: Specification for Portable Photoelectric Photometers.

BS ISO 8995:2002: Lighting of indoor work places.

The Chartered Institute of Building Services Engineers (CIBSE) publishes codes for different environments, including

- Code for Lighting 2006.
- Lighting Guide 1: Industrial Lighting.
- Lighting Guide 7: Offices.
- Lighting Guide 12: Emergency Lighting Design.

HSE (2002). *Lighting at Work*. HSG38. Sudbury, UK: HSE Books.

ATEX requirements and information about the Dangerous Substances and Explosive Atmospheres Regulations 2002 (DSEAR) are described at http://www.hse.gov.uk/fireandexplosion/atex.htm.

17 Ionising Radiation

17.1 Introduction

Radiation hazards can occur in many workplaces, but this area of monitoring hazards is sufficiently specialised to remain outside the jurisdiction of most health and safety personnel unless they have undergone special training. When a radiation hazard is present in a workplace it is normally an integral part of the work process, with the full knowledge of all concerned. Unlike many chemical hazards, a radiation hazard cannot be immediately perceived; therefore no warning signs are noticed if exposures are too high. Because of its specialised nature, the reader is strongly advised to consult a radiation expert whenever a problem is suspected or further information is required. In Britain, under the Ionising Radiation regulations 1999, a Radiation Protection Advisor (RPA) needs to be appointed for certain conditions.

There are two types of radiation: ionising and non-ionising. The main difference between these is in the way they interact with matter, including human tissue, and whether they cause ionisation of constituent atoms. The ionisation creates chemical species known as free radicals that can cause damage to the complex biological molecules that form chromosomes. These processes can result in severe acute effects in humans, if the radiation dose is high enough then it may cause cancer or hereditary effects in their offspring.

All matter consists of atoms that comprise a nucleus-containing protons and neutrons, surrounded by a 'cloud' of electrons. The number of protons in the nucleus, also known as the atomic number, determines the chemical properties of the atom; atoms with atomic number 1 are all hydrogen, those with atomic number 2 are helium, and so on. Atoms of a specific chemical can have a range of neutrons in the nucleus, and so phosphorus, which has atomic number 15, can have between 13 and 19 neutrons. Atoms with the same number of protons and different numbers of neutrons are known as isotopes. The total number of protons and neutrons in an atom is known as the mass number. Ionising radiation often results from an unstable isotope changing to a more stable form. Note that all the isotopes of a given element are chemically identical, since the chemical properties are determined by the atomic number of the element.

Examples of radiation encountered in work areas are given in Table 17.1 and the frequencies and wavelengths of the various forms of electromagnetic radiation are shown in Figure 17.1.

Table 17.1   Examples of ionising and non-ionising radiation.

Ionising radiation	Non-ionising radiation
Alpha (α)	Radiowaves
Beta (β)	Microwaves
Gamma (γ)	Visible light (e.g. lasers)
X-rays	Ultraviolet
Neutrons	Infrared

In this chapter we describe the physics of ionising radiation and the methods available for measurement of exposure and associated dose limits. In the following chapter we discuss non-ionising radiation.

17.2   Ionising radiation

Ionising radiation, which may be produced during radioactive decay, interacts with body tissue and loses energy by ionising surrounding molecules. This type of radiation can be hazardous to health because, if it penetrates living tissue, the resulting ionisation can cause chemical changes in the body that lead to harmful effects.

The damage to health caused by radiation exposure can result in two types of effect:

Non-stochastic effects (for example, cataract of the lens of the eye, skin ulceration and impaired fertility), which are assumed to vary in severity with the level of radiation dose received, but are not detectable until a threshold dose has been received.

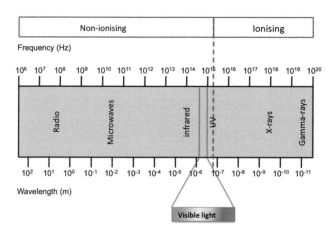

Figure 17.1   The electromagnetic spectrum. (Reproduced with permission from *Occupational Hygiene*, 3rd edition, edited by Kerry Gardiner and J. Malcolm Harrington, Blackwell Publishing Ltd., 2005, p. 308.)

Stochastic effects (for example, induction of carcinogenesis or genetic damage) are such that the chance of the disease occurring increases progressively with the dose received. It is assumed that there is no detectable threshold for stochastic effects and the severity of the effect, if it occurs at all, is independent of the dose responsible for it. The hazard from radiation can arise either from the uniform irradiation of the whole body or part of a body (external radiation) or from irradiation due to ingested, inhaled or absorbed radioactive material concentrating in particular organs and tissues of the body (internal radiation).

17.3 Background radiation

Artificial ionising radiation has been used for several decades in the development and understanding of the sciences including medicine, and in industry. Naturally occurring radioactivity, on the other hand, has always existed and pervades the whole environment. Background radiation varies from place to place and is made up of radiation from the sun and outer space, from naturally occurring radioactive materials on earth, and radioactive aerosols and gases in the atmosphere. Added to this, recently, are artificial sources of radiation such as escapes from nuclear installations, fall-out from nuclear explosions, radioactive waste and occupational exposure. Natural and artificial radiations are the same in kind and effect.

In common with other hazards encountered in work environments, radiation carries a risk of causing harm, and employees must be protected from unnecessary or excessive exposure to it. Although for most people radiation of natural origin causes the highest exposure, much of it is unavoidable – although in some circumstances (e.g. radon in buildings) control can and should be put in place. Exposure to artificial radiation is more readily controlled by a system of radiological protection procedures, some of which are mentioned briefly later in this chapter.

17.4 Basic concepts and quantities

The notation used to describe isotopes is as follows:

$$^{A}_{Z}X$$

where X is the chemical symbol of the element, A, the number of neutrons and protons (known as the mass number) and Z, the atomic number (or number of protons).

For hydrogen the classification for its three isotopes is

$$^{1}_{1}H \qquad ^{2}_{1}H \qquad ^{3}_{1}H$$

hydrogen   deuterium   tritium

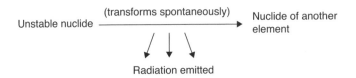

Figure 17.2 Decay of an unstable nuclide to a stable one. (Reproduced with permission *Monitoring for Health Hazards at Work*, 3rd edition, by Indira Ashton and Frank S. Gill, Blackwell Publishers Ltd., 2000. pp. 165.)

Often the chemical symbol of the element is written with the mass number only since the atomic number is always the same. For example: ^{14}C or carbon-14 for $^{14}_{6}C$.

Some atoms are unstable. The stability of a nucleus is determined by the numbers of neutrons and protons, their configuration and the forces they exert on each other. To attain stability, changes take place within the atom that result in the emission of radiation. The process of spontaneous transformation of an unstable atom into an atom of another element while emitting radiation is called radioactivity (Figure 17.2).

An atom whose nucleus is unstable is known as a radioactive isotope or radionuclide. The transformation is termed decay and the radiation emitted is called ionising radiation. For example, carbon-14 is a radionuclide that decays by emitting β radiation to nitrogen-14, a stable nuclide (Figure 17.3).

Radioactive decay can take place in stages with a succession of transformations with the last decay product being a stable isotope (Figure 17.4). Of the 1700 or so known nuclides, about 280 are stable. The behaviour of stable and unstable nuclei and the characteristic of any nucleus can be found in a *nuclide chart* linked to that radionuclide.

17.5 Types of radiation

The main forms of radiation that result from radioactive decay are either particulate (α and β particles) or electromagnetic (γ rays and X-rays).

Alpha (α) particles are streams of positively charged helium nuclei, which comprise two protons plus two neutrons. The particles are relatively heavy and their range in air is 2–5 cm; paper, thin foil or the skin easily stop them. Their range in body tissue is less than 1 mm and they are only hazardous if α-emitting materials are taken into the body. Examples of the use

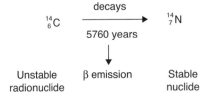

Figure 17.3 Decay of carbon 14. (Reproduced with permission *Monitoring for Health Hazards at Work*, 3rd edition, by Indira Ashton and Frank S. Gill, Blackwell Publishers Ltd., 2000. pp. 165.)

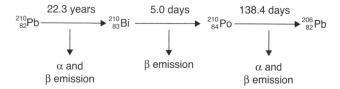

Figure 17.4 An example of decay in stages: lead to bismuth to polonium to lead. (Reproduced with permission *Monitoring for Health Hazards at Work*, 3rd edition, by Indira Ashton and Frank S. Gill, Blackwell Publishing Ltd., 2000. pp. 166.)

of alpha sources are in static eliminators, smoke detectors and thickness gauges.

Beta (β) particles have mass and charge equal to an electron, although this can be either positive or negative, i.e. β^+ or β^-. Their range in air is 4–5 m and they can be stopped by thin layers of water, glass, perspex or aluminium. Their range of penetration depends on their energy. They have greater penetrating power in body tissue, approximately 2 cm and so may present an external radiation hazard. Beta emitters are also hazardous if taken into the body. Examples of applications of β-emitting sources are in static eliminators, thickness gauges, luminescent materials and selected radioactive materials used in research and diagnostics.

Gamma (γ) rays are discrete quantities of energy without mass or charge and are propagated as waves. Gamma rays are electromagnetic radiations similar to light and radiowaves but with shorter wavelengths and higher energies. Their range in air can be greater than 100 m. They are highly penetrating to body tissue and are hazardous when external to the body. Only heavy shielding materials such as lead or concrete can attenuate them. Gamma radiation is used in medical diagnosis and therapy, thickness gauges, level gauges, and pipeline flow rate measurement. Gamma rays and X-rays are indistinguishable from each other and only differ in how they are produced.

X-rays are also electromagnetic rays with approximately 60 m range in air. Bombarding a metal target with electrons in an evacuated tube produces them. X-rays are less penetrating to body tissue than γ rays but are equally hazardous when external to the body. High-density materials like lead or concrete are required to attenuate them. X-rays are used in radiography and fluoroscopy.

Neutrons are electrically neutral particles. Their range in air is greater than 100 m and they are highly penetrating to body tissues. When neutrons are first produced in a nuclear reactor or in a particle accelerator such as a cyclotron, they are known as fast neutrons. Thick shields of materials containing light atoms such as water, wax or graphite are effective in slowing them. Shields of cadmium or boron can then efficiently absorb slow (thermal) neutrons. Neutron-emitting radioactive sources are used for activation analysis in a variety of medical and industrial applications, in prospecting for oil and gas, for measuring the moisture content of soils and cements and for testing reactor instrumentation.

17.6 Energy

The energy with which radiations are produced is expressed in *electron volts* (eV). This is equivalent to the energy gained by an electron in passing through an electrical potential difference of 1 V. Multiples of this unit are commonly used, mainly the kiloelectron volt (keV) and mega electron volt (MeV).

1 keV = 1000 eV

1 MeV = 1000 keV = 1,000,000 eV

For non-β radiation, the electron volt is used as the unit energy from the relationship,

$$E_k = 0.5 \, mv^2$$

where E_k is kinetic energy, m is the mass of the particle and v is the velocity.

17.7 Activity

A radioactive material comprising millions of individual atoms does not emit radiation indefinitely. The activity or source strength of a radionuclide is the rate at which spontaneous decay occurs in it. As soon as a radionuclide is formed, its activity decays with time and this process cannot be changed.

The time taken for a radionuclide to decay to half of its original value is known as the half-life. Each radioactive substance has a unique and unalterable half-life. Half-lives range from millions of years to fractions of seconds. In successive half-lives, the activity of a radionuclide is reduced by decay to one-half, one-quarter, one-eighth, one-sixteenth and so on, of the initial value. It is therefore possible to predict the activity remaining at any time. A stable nuclide is a radionuclide with an infinite half-life.

The rate of decay depends on the type of radioactive substance. *Activity* is expressed in *becquerels* (Bq) or disintegrations per second. Examples of the half-life and radioactive emission are given for a selection of radionuclides in Table 17.2.

Full details about radioactive decay from unstable isotopes are available at http://en.wikipedia.org/wiki/Index_to_isotope_pages.

Table 17.2 Example of types of radiation emitted by a selection of radionuclides.

Isotope	Half-life	Radioactive emission
Vanadium-52	3.8 min	β^-
Radon-222	3.8 days	α
Chromium-51	27.7 days	γ
Hydrogen-3	12.3 years	β^-
Caesium-137	30 years	β^-
Carbon-14	5760 years	β^-

Table 17.3 Types of radiation and quality factor

Types of radiation	Quality factors
X-rays, γ rays and electrons	1
Thermal or slow neutrons	2.3
Fast neutrons and proton particles	10
α-particles	20

17.8   Radiation dose units

17.8.1   Absorbed dose and dose equivalent

Absorbed dose is a measure of energy deposition in any medium by all types of ionising radiation and expressed as the energy absorbed per unit mass of materials. The unit of absorbed dose is called the *gray* (Gy) and is defined as an energy deposition of 1 joule per kilogram (J kg^{-1}).

In biological systems the same absorbed dose of different types of radiation gives rise to different degrees of biological damage. To take this into account the absorbed dose of each type of radiation is multiplied by a *quality factor (Q)*, which reflects the ability of the particular radiation to cause damage, to give the dose equivalent.

The *sievert* (Sv) is the unit of dose equivalent, which is related to the Gray as follows:

Dose equivalent (Sv) = absorbed dose $\times Q \times N$

where N is a further modifying factor, which accounts for other factors such as absorbed dose rate and fractionation, although N is normally assigned the value 1.

The values of the quality factor depends on the density of ionisation caused by the radiation. They are given in Table 17.3.

The sievert is too large a unit for ordinary use, so millisievert (mSv) and microsievert (μSv) are generally used.

17.8.2   To calculate dose equivalent

An employee can be exposed to different types of radiation during a period of work. An indication of the exposure is required. For example, during an experiment an employee received the following amounts of radiation:

0.03 Gy of γ dose
0.07 Gy of X-ray dose
0.001 Gy of fast neutron dose.

To calculate the total dose equivalent we use the relationship:

Dose equivalent = absorbed dose $\times$ quality factor, summed over the different doses.
Gamma dose equivalent = 0.03 Gy $\times$ 1 = 0.03 Sv

X-ray dose equivalent $= 0.07 \, \text{Gy} \times 1 = 0.07 \, \text{Sv}$
Fast neutron dose equivalent $= 0.001 \, \text{Gy} \times 10 = 0.01 \, \text{Sv}$
Therefore the total dose equivalent $= 0.11 \, \text{Sv}$.

17.8.3 Dose rate

The dose rate is the rate at which a dose is received. The accumulation of dose received by an employee is equal to the dose rate multiplied by the exposure time; the shorter the time the smaller the dose. The rate is usually expressed per hour. Therefore

Total dose = dose rate × time

where the dose rate is in Sv h^{-1}, and the time in hours.

Here is an example of how dose rate can be used. A classified worker is allowed to receive a dose equivalent of 1 mSv in a week (Note: 1 mSv equals 1000 μSv). How long can he work in an area in which the dose equivalent rate is 50 μSv h^{-1}?
Rearranging the relationship, we have

Allowable time = total dose/dose rate

$$= 1000/50$$

$$= 20 \, \text{h}$$

17.9 Dose limits

Radiation dose limits are set so that non-stochastic effects are prevented completely and stochastic effects are kept within acceptable limits. The principle of ALARA (As Low As Reasonably Achievable) is encouraged. Employers are required to restrict the dose received by employees and other persons. This is achieved by (1) the use of engineering controls and design features, including shielding, containment of radioactive substances, ventilation, the provision of safety features and warning signs; (2) by administrative procedures, such as local rules and (3) by designating categories to work areas (e.g. controlled and supervised) and personnel (e.g. classified).

Where possible, work with unsealed sources should be carried out in fume cupboards behind appropriate shielding. In addition, safe systems of work in the form of site and departmental local rules covering procedures should be established. Facilities for personal hygiene, decontamination and waste disposal procedures and appropriate protective equipment should be provided. Compliance with these features should be monitored.

Safe dose limits are recommended by the International Commission on Radiation Protection (ICRP) and have been adopted in the Britain by the Health and Safety Executive (HSE) as published in the Ionising Radiation Regulations. The current dose limits for the Britain are given in Table 17.4.

For women of reproductive capacity the equivalent dose limit for the abdomen is 13 mSv in any consecutive period of 3 months. Once a pregnancy

Table 17.4 Dose limits, which must not be exceeded in a calendar year.

	Employees aged 18 years or over	Trainees aged under 18 years	Members of the public
Whole body	20 mSv	6 mSv	1 mSv
Individual organs and tissues (skin, hands, forearms, feet and ankles)	500 mSv	150 mSv	50 mSv
Lens of the eye	150 mSv	45 mSv	15 mSv

has been confirmed and the employer notified, the equivalent dose to the foetus should not exceed 1 mSv during the remainder of the pregnancy.

It is interesting to note that for someone living and working in Cornwall, where there is exposure to γ radiation from naturally occurring radon emissions from the granite rocks, the contribution to their absorbed dose from background radiation could be about 0.6 mSv year^{-1}. Cosmic radiation adds about another 0.3 mSv, which brings the total absorbed dose close to the limit for a member of the general public (i.e. 1 mSv year^{-1}).

17.10 Derived limits

Derived limits (DLs) can be used to control the radiation dose from specific sources to ensure the annual dose limit is not exceeded. Limiting the airborne concentration and level of surface contamination will generally control the internal radiation dose. DLs for surface contamination can vary, depending on the type and toxicity of radioactive material and the classification of the area in which it can be handled safely. Derived limits for air contamination that can be inhaled are often referred to as Derived Air Concentrations (DACs) and these vary for the different radioactive substances.

The Annual Limits of Intake (ALI) is the limit placed on the amount of a radionuclide ingested or inhaled in becquerels, which would give a harm commitment to the organs it irradiates; the committed dose equivalent is equal to that resulting from whole-body irradiation of 20 mSv in a year. These are estimated by the International Commission for Radiological Protection (ICRP) and take into account chemical forms and translocation of radionuclides by using three models; the models use the respiratory system, gastrointestinal tract, and skeletal system. They relate the intake of radionuclides to organ dose and therefore to risk.

The derived air concentration is therefore the concentration that, breathed each week for 40 h, leads to the absorption of ALI. ALIs and DACs for selected radionuclides are listed in the relevant ICRP publication.

17.11 Procedures to minimise occupational dose

Occupational exposure comprises all dose equivalents and committed dose equivalents received at work. The nature and magnitude of occupational radiation exposure varies over a very wide range. Hence, the type and extent of individual monitoring required is dependent on the work environment. For example, a person working in a nuclear processing plant or in radioisotope manufacturing will require different levels of monitoring from someone working with low levels of radiation such as in a university laboratory, using unsealed radionuclides.

The Ionising Radiation regulations and the recommendations of the ICRP control the handling, use and disposal of radioactive materials and apply to all premises where ionising radiations are handled.

To ensure control of exposure received, it is recommended that all persons using ionising radiation should register with a central body within an organisation so that the health and safety services in that organisation are aware of the location and type of work being undertaken. All registered employees must undergo formal training in radiation protection principles and safe working procedures.

Working areas are classified in the regulations according to the potential level of exposure. These are the following:

- *Uncontrolled areas.* The annual dose is less than 1 mSV.
- *Supervised areas.* The annual dose is likely to exceed 1 mSv or an equivalent dose greater than 1/10 of any relevant dose limit. Employees are subject to routine personal monitoring.
- *Controlled areas.* The annual dose is likely to exceed 6 mSv or an equivalent dose greater than three-tenths of any relevant dose limit. Employees are subject to medical surveillance and routine personal monitoring if they work regularly in these areas. Other employees can only enter under a written system of work.

An external radiation hazard can arise from sources of radiation outside the body. It can arise from a sealed or unsealed (sometimes called closed) source. A sealed source is where the radioactive material is enclosed in a strong container and cannot be removed by normal means. An unsealed source is a source such as a phial containing a liquid or powder; or radioactive particles that are made to accelerate in machines and reactors. The hazard from external radiation may be due to β, X, γ and neutron radiations. Alpha radiation is not normally regarded as an external hazard as α-particles cannot penetrate the outer layers of skin.

There are four basic methods of protection against external radiation. These are shielding the worker from the radiation, arranging that the distance from the source to the worker is as long as possible, reducing the handling time to a minimum, and restricting the strength of the source to the minimum necessary for the task. A combination of these methods will give the protection necessary to ensure that doses are kept below the relevant dose limits. It may be necessary to consult an expert to get the balance right. For example, it may be more dangerous if the source is shielded too much, making handling cumbersome and thereby increasing the exposure time.

Generally, shielding is the preferred method as it results in intrinsically safe working conditions. Reliance on distance or time of exposure involves continuous administrative control over employees. The different types of radiation have different powers of penetration, although some form of shielding materials can stop all of them. Advice may be obtained from manufacturers or a RPA on the type and thickness of shielding necessary. The half-thickness or *half-value layer* (HVL) for a particular shielding material is the thickness required to reduce the intensity to one half of its incident value. Charts for various isotopes are available in the literature.

The intensity of a point source radiation decreases with increasing distance, obeying the Inverse Square Law. Simply, this means that by doubling the distance the radiation level is reduced to one-quarter, by trebling the distance the radiation level is reduced to one-ninth, and so on. This works in reverse as well, so the nearer a worker is located to a source the higher the radiation exposure. The radiation dose close to a low activity source can be very high so it should never be touched with the bare hands; tongs or tweezers should always be used.

17.12   Personal dosimetry and medical surveillance

The UK regulations require the monitoring of the doses received by classified persons and certain other employees and the maintenance of dose records for 50 years by a dosimetry service approved by the HSE.

On registration each worker is categorised for personal dosimetry based on the type and quantities of radioactive sources to be used and the nature of the work. If an employee is likely to exceed three-tenths of a set dose limit he or she is designated as a classified person and has to undergo more rigorous dosimetry and medical surveillance.

Film badges, body and extremity thermoluminescent dosimeters (TLD) can be used to monitor dose. These are supplied and analysed by an approved dosimetry service, such as the Health Protection Agency (a full list of providers is available on the HSE website). Dosimeters are usually changed every 4 weeks. Small pocket monitors, with pre-set alarms, are used for the daily monitoring of operators of large sealed sources or X-rays. Quarterly and annual doses are calculated and the records archived for the statutory period. Termination records are prepared by the approved dosimetry service when an employee leaves. A copy is given to the employer and another is forwarded to the HSE.

Health surveillance of registered employees is carried out by an appointed doctor (approved by the HSE). When an employer has an occupational health service, one of their occupational physicians is normally the appointed doctor. The health record of classified persons, which must be kept for 50 years, is updated every 12 months, although a medical examination of the individual is not normally carried out unless personal dosimetry or other factors suggest that it would be advisable.

17.12.1 Monitoring of ionising radiation in work areas

Monitoring the levels of radiation in each 'controlled' or 'supervised' area is required, with records being kept for at least 2 years.

The local rules should require that working areas and adjacent areas be monitored routinely. Hand-held monitors are used or wipe tests where there are unsealed sources. More comprehensive monthly monitoring should be carried out in all working areas, with the emphasis placed on those most likely to be contaminated. All areas external to radiation working areas (e.g. offices and corridors) should be monitored on a 3-monthly basis to ensure that contamination is not spreading.

All monitoring equipment must be tested and calibrated annually by a competent person as defined in the regulations.

There is a plethora of radiation monitoring instruments on the market. Instruments that measure external radiation rely on detection devices based on the physical or chemical effects of radiation such as ionisation in gases, ionisation and excitation in certain solids, changes in chemical systems and activation of neutrons. They therefore vary in their sensitivity to radiation, the type of radiation to which they respond, their response to radiations of the same type but of different energies, the volume of the detector, the time taken to obtain a reading and the type of detector. Advice must be sought from an RPA on suitability and selection of appropriate instruments.

Radiation intensity is measured most commonly by an ionisation chamber, a proportional counter, Geiger–Muller counter (Figure 17.5) or a scintillation detector (Figure 17.6). Most provide a numerical value known as a 'count' but to relate that count to true radiation intensity it is necessary to calibrate the instrument against a known value of intensity.

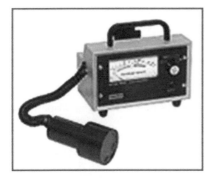

Figure 17.5 A Geiger–Muller counter.
(© Thermo Fisher Scientific. Reproduced with permission.)

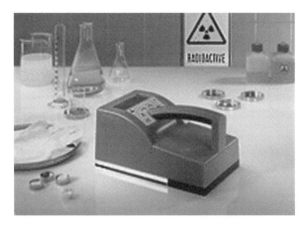

Figure 17.6 A scintillation detector. (© Berthold Technologies (UK) Ltd. Reproduced with permission.)

17.12.2 Personal monitoring for external dose

There are three commonly used devices for monitoring external dose received by the individual. They are the following:

1. Thermoluminescent dosimeters (TLD, shown in Figure 17.7).
2. Film badge dosimeters (Figure 17.8).
3. A direct-reading device such as a pocket ionisation dosimeter or quartz-fibre electroscope.

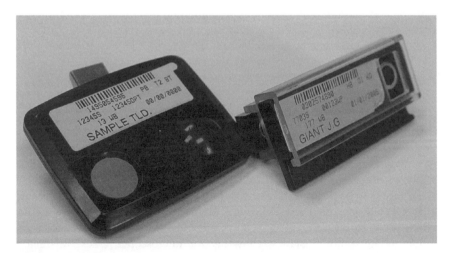

Figure 17.7 Two thermoluminescent detectors (TLDs). (© Mirion Technologies, Inc. Reproduced with permission.)

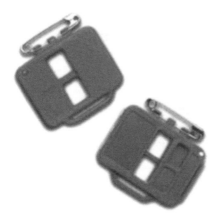

Figure 17.8 Two film badges. (© Loxford Equipment Company Ltd. Reproduced with permission.)

Personal monitoring with a film badge or TLD is usually undertaken by an approved dosimetry service. Each dosimeter is numbered and is for use by one person only. The length of each monitoring period depends on the dose likely to be received during the period. Normally, a dosimeter is worn for 4 weeks, but this can vary from 1 day to 3 months, depending on type of dosimeter used and circumstances of work and nuclides handled.

The dosimeter is normally worn on the trunk at chest or waist height. The main concern is with the whole-body dose from external radiation. Film badges and body TLDs are worn with the label (open window) facing away from the body. For finger or wrist doses, the extremity TLD must be turned toward the area of highest potential dose. If there is any reason to suspect that doses to other parts of the body such as fingers or eyes may be received, extremity TLDs may be required as well as whole-body dosimeters. If protective clothing such as an apron is worn, the dosimeter is usually worn on the trunk under the apron. A dosimeter is also worn on the unprotected parts of the body if there is likely to be an exposure.

17.12.3 Film badge dosimeter

Where exposure is from external sources such as X-rays, γ rays (e.g. from caesium-137) or high-energy β emitters (e.g. phosphorus-32), personal monitoring is widely carried out by means of a film badge. The film is sensitive to radiation and is housed in a specially designed plastic casing containing windows of various materials that shield certain kinds of radiation but which allow others to pass through. The dosimeter must be worn all the time when working with ionising radiation as it is monitoring an integrated dose to the whole body. However, work close to small sources or with narrow beams of radiation (e.g. X-ray crystallography, electron microscopes, cracks in shielding) involves exposure to many non-uniform fields. In such cases there is no simple method of obtaining a more accurate estimate of the whole-body dose.

17.12.3.1   Advantages of the film badge dosimeter
1. Inexpensive and easily available.
2. Capable of integrating doses over a wide range.
3. Able to measure different radiation types and energies.
4. The developed film can be stored to provide a permanent record that can be read again if required.

17.12.3.2   Disadvantages
1. It has an energy dependent response especially for low energy radiation.
2. Response varies with angle relative to incident radiation.
3. There is a latent image fading of the film, which limits the monitoring period (4 weeks is best).
4. When the dosimeter is not being worn, care should be taken to prevent it from being exposed inadvertently to ionising radiation.
5. It is sensitive to heat and humidity so, if subjected to these conditions, the assessment of doses may be affected.

17.12.4   Thermoluminescent dosimeter
Some materials such as lithium fluoride can change to an 'excited' state when bombarded with ionising radiation. When the device is heated the crystals return to normal and emit a measurable emission of light. Thus a small badge containing these crystals can be used as a dosimeter as the degree of irradiation can be related to the amount of light produced on heating. An advantage with this type of dosimeter is that it is small and its analysis can be quickly and automatically performed.

They are sometimes used in combination with the film badge – a film badge for whole-body dose monitoring and an extremity TLD strap for finger dose monitoring.

17.12.4.1   Advantages thermoluminescent dosimeter
1. A wide-dose integration range.
2. A more energy-independent response than film badges.
3. No appreciable latent image fading or angular response variation.
4. Not as sensitive to the effects of heat and humidity as film badges.

17.12.4.2   Disadvantages
1. More expensive than film badges.
2. Dose information is destroyed at read-out, which eliminates the possibility of a re-check of the dose at a later date.
3. The thermoluminescent crystals or powder can give erroneous readings if damaged or if they become dirty through careless handling.

Film badges or TLDs will not detect low energy β emitters emission (e.g. tritium, carbon-14, sulphur-35) as they will not penetrate the outer casing of the monitor.

17.12.5 Direct-reading monitors

In situations where an immediate indication of X or γ dose rate is desirable, then a direct reading monitor is commonly employed. They are normally self-indicating on a calibrated scale or a digital read-out so that the dose can be assessed at any stage of an operation involving potentially high exposures. For example, a self-indicating pocket dosimeter, about the size of a pen, is useful for measuring doses in situations where the dose rate is high since they allow a continuous indication of the rate of accumulation of dose. Devices in this group include miniature quartz-fibre ionisation dosimeters, charged with a small battery unit and the dose received since it was switched on can be read at any time.

The direct-reading instruments are normally used in conjunction with a film badge or TLD, which provide the permanent record of radiation dose received by the individual.

17.12.5.1 Disadvantages of direct-reading monitors

1. Must be calibrated with known dose levels.
2. Fairly expensive.
3. Insensitive to low energy radiation.
4. Can lose sensitivity due to leakage.
5. Fragile, so are easily damaged.

17.12.6 Air monitoring

Airborne radioactive dust from unsealed sources can be sampled on a filter by using a high-volume air sampler. A known volume of air is drawn through a filter, which is removed at the end of the sampling period and scanned for its radioactivity using a counter. This technique is similar to that used for harmful dusts described in Chapter 9.

Radon is a radioactive gas that is one of the decay products from uranium that is found in some rocks and soil. Radon is found in all parts of the Britain, although the levels are higher in the North East of Scotland, the South West of England and several other parts of the country. The gas disperses outdoors but if radon permeates inside poorly ventilated buildings then it can give rise to elevated levels. Radon levels may also be elevated in underground mines and in caves.

There are a number of passive monitors that are available to measure radon levels, but the commonest method used in the Britain is the 'etched track' monitor. These monitors are based on small pieces of sensitive plastic with a hemispherical diffusive cover through which radon can permeate. When the plastic is struck by an α-particle from radon or from its decay products, the plastic structure is damaged. When the strip is returned to the laboratory it can be etched to reveal the damage. The number of tracks is proportional to the total exposure to radon decay products.

If the measurement level is above 400 Bq m^{-3} the employer needs to take immediate action to manage the exposures and plan for some remediation of the building to reduce the levels. This may include providing a barrier to stop the ingress of radon into the building or installing additional ventilation in basements or other underground areas.

References and further reading

Clayton RF. (2005). Ionizing radiation: physics, measurement, biological effects and control. In: *Occupational Hygiene*, 3rd edition (Gardiner G, Harrington JM, eds). Oxford, UK: Blackwell Publishing.

Martin A, Harbison S. (2006). *An Introduction to Radiation Protection*, 5th edition. London: Hodder and Arnold.

HSE (2000). *Work with Ionising Radiation. Ionising Radiations Regulations 1999 Approved Code of Practice and Guidance*. L121. Sudbury, UK: HSE Books.

HSEs ionising radiation website has useful information. Available at http://www.hse.gov.uk/radiation/ionising/.

Information about ionising radiation from the Health Protection Agency (HPA). Available at www.hpa.org.uk/radiation/.

Details of the risks form radon exposure and the possible means of controlling exposure are available at http://www.hse.gov.uk/radiation/ionising/radon.htm.

Details of the International Commission for Radiological Protection (ICRP) website is http://www.icrp.org.

The history of recommendations from the ICRP can be downloaded at: http://www.icrp.org/docs/Histpol.pdf.

18 Non-Ionising Radiation

18.1 Introduction

Non-ionising radiations make up most of the low energy or longer wavelength of the electromagnetic spectrum as shown in Figure 17.1. These electromagnetic fields (EMF) include radiowaves, microwaves, static magnetic fields, ultraviolet radiation (UV), visible light and infrared (IR) radiation. Both the frequency of the radiation and its intensity are important in determining the potential risks for employees. Lasers are a particular type of device, which emit a high-intensity beam of electromagnetic radiation and for this reason they are particularly hazardous. This chapter discusses the measurement of each of these non-ionising radiations and associated standards.

Table 18.1 lists some common sources of non-ionising radiation.

It is helpful to know that the frequency and the wavelength of EMF are related to each other so that knowing one you can calculate the other. The equation relating wavelength and frequency is

$$f = \frac{v}{\lambda}$$

where f is the frequency in hertz (Hz), λ the wavelength (m) and v the speed of light (about 3×10^8 m s^{-1}).

So a wave with a frequency of 300 MHz (300×10^6 Hz) has a wavelength of 1 m; i.e.

$$\lambda = \frac{v}{f} = \frac{3 \times 10^8}{3 \times 10^8} = 1 \text{ m}$$

Ultraviolet radiation can affect the skin and eyes. After high-intensity exposure the eyes can suffer from serious damage to the cornea (photokeratitis), sometimes called 'arc eye' or 'welder's flash' or 'snow blindness'. The symptoms are pain as if having grit in the eye and an aversion to bright lights. The symptoms do not cause permanent damage and usually disappear after about 36 h of rest. Chronic exposure to the eye can cause cataracts and welders are at risk of melanoma of the eye.

Acute skin exposure to UV radiation can cause erythema (which is reddening of the skin, i.e. sunburn). Chronic exposure of the skin can cause aging and skin cancer (both melanoma and non-melanoma skin cancer), although the available evidence suggests that the risk of melanoma is generally not

Table 18.1 Common sources of non-ionising radiation.

UV	IR	Microwaves	Other EMF	Static magnetic fields
Sunshine	Furnaces and	Ovens	Mobile phones	Magnetic
Welding equipment	other hot sources	Radar	and	resonance
Carbon arcs	in the glass, steel,	Communica-	base-stations	imaging (MRI)
Sterilising equipment	and aluminum	tion systems	Radio	Strong magnets,
Cadmium or	industries	Scientific	transmitters	e.g. in aluminium
mercury lamps	IR lamps in	equipment	Electrical power	production
Fly-killing tubes	medical treatment	WiFi systems	lines	
(Insectocutors)	Lasers			
Lasers				

increased amongst outdoor workers who might be considered to have the greatest potential for UV exposure. Small amounts of UV exposure are essential for the production of vitamin D in humans; i.e. there are also health benefits from UV exposure.

Infrared exposure may result in heating of the body and so may add to the problems of heat stress in hot environments. Acute exposure to very high-intensity IR radiation can cause local burns on the skin; repeated sub-acute exposure may cause erythema and discolouration of the skin. Repeated exposure of the eye to high-intensity IR radiation can cause cataracts, as for example amongst glass blowers.

Microwaves are used for heating and cooking and are emitted from radio and radar transmitters. Absorption of microwave energy causes rapid local heating particularly if the material contains a high proportion of water, because the resonant frequency of water molecules is within the microwave range. Since human tissue is mostly made up of water it is particularly sensitive to heating from microwave exposure.

There have been a number of epidemiological studies of workers exposed to radiowaves and more recently to radio transmissions from mobile telephones, particularly in relation to brain tumours. The evidence of adverse health effects from radiowaves is equivocal.

It has been suggested that there may be a range of adverse health effects associated with extremely low frequency (ELF) electric and magnetic fields, for example from power lines, but there is no consistent scientific evidence to support most of these suggestions. There is limited scientific evidence that ELF can cause childhood leukaemia but there is inadequate evidence for all other types of cancer.

Exposure to very high static magnetic fields produces unpleasant transient sensations, e.g. vertigo, although there is no evidence of long-term health effects. People with cardiac pacemakers or persons with metallic clips and other metallic implants must be particularly careful about being exposed to high-magnetic fields.

18.2 Ultraviolet radiation

The ultraviolet radiation spectrum is conventionally subdivided into three regions: ultraviolet A (UVA) covering wavelengths 400–315 nm; ultraviolet B (UVB) for wavelengths 315–280 nm and ultraviolet C (UVC) for wavelengths 280–100 nm. The longer wavelength rays (i.e. UVA) are considered to be less hazardous than the shorter wavelength radiation. UV radiation between about 100 and 200 nm wavelength is not transmitted in air and so is not relevant to human health. Occupational exposure limits for UV radiation are recommended by the International Commission for Non-Ionising Radiation Protection (ICNIRP). These limits are dependent on the wavelength of the radiation and are intended to provide guidance to protect people from both the long-term and acute effects of exposure.

The radiant power in watts (W) describes the rate of energy output of an optical source. Two quantities are used to quantify human exposure to UV radiation: irradiance, which is the rate of surface exposure in watts per metre squared (W m^{-2}) and radiant exposure, which is the radiant energy per unit area accumulated over a time interval in joules per metre squared (J m^{-2}).

The ICNIRP guidelines for human exposure of the eye and skin to UV radiation is 30 J m^{-2} over an 8-h day. The radiant exposure must be mathematically weighted using the hazard sensitivity spectrum 180–400 nm, which has a peak response at 280 nm. Figure 18.1 shows the weighting and the response of a broad spectrum UV monitor along with the monitor. An additional requirement of the ICNIRP is that the un-weighted UVA exposure should not exceed a daily limit value of 10^4 J m^{-2}.

There are also a number of monitors with detectors specific to UVA, UVB and UVC, although these need to be used with care as they will give a biased result if they are used in situations where the UV radiation is spread across a wide range of wavelengths.

There are a number of personal UV monitors, but these have mostly been used in research projects rather than in routine surveillance.

Before undertaking a survey to measure UV exposure from artificial sources, it is important to obtain details of the spectral emission from the lamp from the manufacturer's data. In making the measurements the probe should be located at critical points in relation to exposure, e.g. the eye and exposed skin. You should also consider the potential for UV radiation to be reflected from surfaces within the workroom when making measurements.

The main engineering controls used for artificial UV sources are the use of 'light-tight' cabinets and UV-absorbing glass or plastic shielding. Care should be taken in the use of shiny reflecting surfaces inside equipment as these will also reflect UV radiation. Access to enclosures should be interlocked so that it is not possible to breach the containment while the lamp is on. For some jobs, such as welding, personal protection must be used to protect against UV radiation and other non-ionising radiation. For outdoor workers exposed to

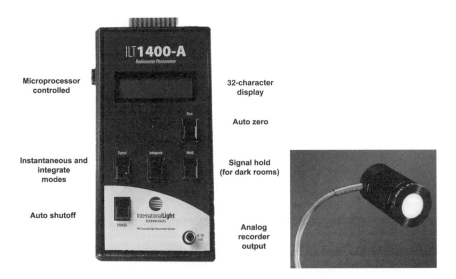

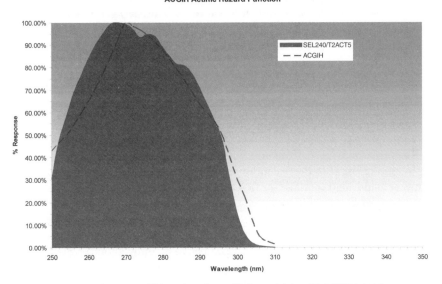

SEL240/T2ACT5 Relative Response Compared to ACGIH Actinic Hazard Function

Figure 18.1 A broad-spectrum UV monitor along with the weighting. (© LOT-Oriel Ltd. Reproduced with permission.)

UV radiation the control strategies can include the following:

- Avoiding direct sunlight exposure or seek shade around noon in spring and summer;
- Wearing clothing and eyewear that provide protection from UV radiation;
- Use of topical sunscreens with a sun protection factor (SPF) greater than 30.

18.3 Infrared radiation

Electromagnetic radiation with wavelengths between 780 nm to 1 mm is known as infrared (IR) radiation. The infrared region is subdivided into IRA (wavelengths 0.78–1.4 μm), IRB (wavelengths 1.4–3 μm) and IRC (wavelengths 3 μm to 1 mm). IRA radiation penetrates several millimeters into human issue whereas IRB penetrates less than 1 mm. IRC does not penetrate beyond the outer layers of the dead skin cells known as the *stratum corneum*.

Most high-intensity broadband IR sources such as arc or incandescent lamps produce negligible levels of IRC compared with the emissions at shorter wavelengths. Only lasers present a potential hazard in this region of the IR spectrum. The ICNIRP guidelines for IRA and IRB to protect the cornea is that exposure should be less than 100 W m^{-2} for lengthy exposure periods (>1000 s) or steadily increasing levels for shorter exposure periods given by the equation:

$$E_{IR} = 18,000 \times t^{-0.75} \text{ W m}^{-2}$$

where t is the time in seconds.

However, in cold conditions where the IR radiation is used for heating, the limit can be increased, so at 10°C it is 300 W m^{-2} and at 0°C it is 400 W m^{-2}.

For skin the limit is given as the energy deposited per square metre by the following equation depending on the duration of exposure less than 10 s:

$$H = 20000 \times t^{0.25} \text{ J m}^{-2}$$

No limit is specified for longer durations as it is assumed that the normal response to the discomfort or pain of the IR radiation will cause the person to remove their skin from the exposure.

Limits are also provided to protect against retinal damage from IRA.

The measurement instrumentation is identical to that used for visible light or UV radiation, with the exception that a different sensor is used. Figure 18.2 shows a hand-held monitor for IRA and part of IRB.

The approach to engineering controls for IR radiation is similar to that for UV, i.e. total enclosure of the source and all reflective pathways. Where it is not possible to control the risk with engineering measures, eye protection by using suitable visors or goggles and protective clothing should be used. Administrative controls may be necessary, e.g. controlling access to certain areas, training and appropriate supervision.

18.4 Microwaves and radiowaves

Microwaves have wavelengths from about 1 m (frequency 300 MHz) down to 1 mm (300 GHz) and radio waves cover wavelengths from about 1m up to 30 km (10 kHz), although the frequency of the waves are most often cited. The safety levels are based on the heating effect or other acute effects such as induced electrical currents in the body. Organs such as the eye, the gall bladder

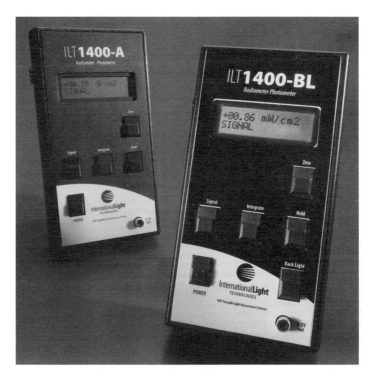

Figure 18.2 A hand-held monitor for IRA and part of IRB. (© LOT-Oriel Ltd. Reproduced with permission.)

and parts of the gastrointestinal system are particularly at risk from localised heating since relatively little blood circulates in these tissues to provide the required cooling effect. The limit on occupational exposure recommended by ICNIRP expressed as power density to EMF between 10 kHz and 300 GHz is 50 W m^{-2}. Separate limits are placed on the electric and magnetic field strengths, measured as the root mean square value, as shown in Table 18.2. Note that '*f*' is the frequency of the radiation.

In the cases of pulsed sources or intermittent exposure, higher levels are acceptable as the energy is absorbed for a shorter period of time. It is the total energy that can safely be received in a given time that should be controlled. This is covered by the appropriate averaging time for the measurement, i.e. 6 min. Measurements should generally be made over a 20 cm^2 area.

When microwave ovens are used it is appropriate to test for leakage by using a simple monitor designed for this purpose (Figure 18.3). It is considered reasonably practicable to control radiation leakage to below 50 W m^{-2}. Leakage above this should be considered an indicator that maintenance is required.

The most effective controls for EMF are engineering controls. Sources of EMF should be properly shielded to minimize stray radiation. Any devices

Table 18.2 Exposure limits for EMF.

Frequency range	E field strength (V m^{-2})	H field strength (A m^{-2})	Magnetic field (μT)	Power density (W m^{-2})
<1 Hz	–	1.63×10^5	2×10^5	–
1–8 Hz	20,000	$1.63 \times 10^5/f^2$	$2 \times 10^5/f^2$	–
8–25 Hz	20,000	$2 \times 10^4/f$	$2.5 \times 10^4/f$	–
25–820 Hz	500/f	20/f	25/f	–
820 Hz – 65 kHz	610	24.4	30.7	–
65 kHz to 1 MHz	610	1.6/f	2/f	–
1–10 MHz	610/f	1.6/f	2/f	–
10–400 MHz	61	0.16	0.2	10
400–2000 MHz	$3f^{0.5}$	$0.008f^{0.5}$	$0.01f^{0.5}$	$f/40$
2–300 GHz	137	0.36	0.45	50

that can produce acute thermal injuries, such as industrial microwave ovens, should have interlocked doors. Devices that produce high levels of stray radio frequency radiation (e.g., induction heaters) should, whenever possible, be operated remotely. Administrative control measures should include restricted access to areas of potential exposure, limitation of exposure times plus appropriate training and supervision. When exposures cannot be reduced to acceptable levels by other measures it may be necessary to consider specialized personal protective equipment, e.g. radio frequency or microwave protective suits.

18.5 Lasers

Lasers cause damage because the energy is concentrated into a very small area and can burn the skin or parts of the eyes. Where the eye transmits the frequency, the dangers are especially high as the energy can be focused to very high-power densities and damage the retina. There is generally no need to measure the intensity of emission as it is often known or can be calculated from the manufacturer's data. Special attention must be paid to pulsed lasers as their average power can be low but the peak power can be extremely high.

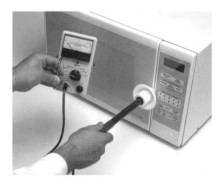

Figure 18.3 A leak monitor for microwave ovens. (© ETS-Lindgren. Reproduced with permission.)

The exposure from a continuous wave laser is measured in power surface density (W m^{-2}) and from pulsed lasers in energy surface density per pulse (J m^{-2}).

Exposure limits are imposed at the following:

Constant power levels are applied at long exposure and very short exposure times.

Constant energy levels are applied at short exposure times for wavelengths greater than 400 nm. In the ultraviolet and visible it applies at longer exposure times of greater than 10 seconds.

The safety standards are complex to interpret. The conditions are given for laser exposure for ultraviolet, visible and infrared radiation and for the exposure times from less than 1 nano-second (1 ns) up to 8 h. The limits also cover skin and eye exposure to continuous, pulsed and multi-pulsed conditions.

Lasers are categorised into the following classes:

Class 1 are lasers are devices where the irradiance of the accessible beam does not exceed the exposure limit and their use does not require any special precautions provided they are used as the manufacturer specifies.

Class 1M lasers produce either a highly divergent beam or a large diameter beam. Lasers in this class can only be harmful if viewed using magnifying optical devices.

Class 2 lasers have a maximum output power of 1 mW and wavelength between 400 nm and 700 nm. Anyone accidentally exposed to the beam will be protected by her or his natural involuntary aversion response.

Class 2M lasers produce either a highly divergent beam or a large diameter beam, again with wavelength between 400 and 700 nm. Avoid viewing with a magnifying device.

Class 3R lasers can have a maximum output power of 5 mW. Accidental viewing may damage the eye, but the risk of injury from a short exposure is small.

Class 3B lasers may have an output power of up to 500 mW. These lasers can cause an eye injury from viewing the direct beam and from reflections. Class 3B lasers are considered hazardous to the eye and should be used with particular care.

Class 4 lasers have an output power more than 500 mW. These lasers can cause serious injury to the eye and skin and will also present a fire hazard if sufficiently high-output powers are used. They may be used for laser displays, laser surgery or cutting metals, and should only be used with great care.

It is good practice to take advice from a qualified laser protection advisor when using Class 3B or 4 lasers.

References and further reading

Chadwick P. (2005). Non-ionizing radiation: electromagnetic fields and optical radiation. In: *Occupational Hygiene*, 3rd edition (Gardiner K, Harrington JM, eds). Oxford, UK: Blackwell Publishing.

ICNIRP (1998). Guidelines for limiting exposure to time-varying electric, magnetic and electromagnetic fields (up to 300GHz). *Health Physics* 74(4): 494–522.

ICNIRP (1997). Guidelines on limits of exposure to broad-band incoherent optical radiation (0.38–3μm). *Health Physics* 73(3): 539–554.

ICNIRP (2006). ICNIRP statement on far infrared radiation exposure. *Health Physics* 91(6): 630–645.

ICNIRP (2000). Revision of guidelines on limits of exposure to laser radiation for wavelengths between 400 nm and 1.4 μm. *Health Physics* 79(4): 431–440.

ICNIRP (2004). Guidelines on limits of exposure to ultraviolet radiation of wavelengths between 180 nm and 400 nm (incoherent radiation). *Health Physics* 87(2): 171–186.

Vecchia P, Hietanen M, Stuck BE, van Deventer E, Niu S. (2007). *Protecting Workers from Ultraviolet Radiation*. ICNIRP 14/2007. Oberschleißheim, Germany: ICNIRP.

Ahlbom A, Green A, Kheifets L, Savitz D, Swerdlow A. (2004). Epidemiology of Health Effects of Radiofrequency Exposure. *Environmental Health Perspectives* 112(17): 1741–1754.

Independent Advisory Group on Non-Ionising Radiation (2008). *Static Magnetic Fields. RCE-6*. Didcot: Health Protection Agency.

HSEs non-ionising radiation website: http://www.hse.gov.uk/radiation/nonionising/.

US NIOSH electric and magnetic field's website: http://www.cdc.gov/niosh/topics/EMF/.

ICNIRP guidelines and other useful information are available at http://www.icnirp.de/documents/downloads.htm.

5 Assessing the Effectiveness of Control

19   Introduction to Control

19.1   Introduction

The basis for control of health hazards at work is based on the concepts of prevention and control; where possible risks should be prevented and where this is not possible, the risks should be reduced to some level that is considered acceptable. In Britain, a set of principles for good control practice is used as the basis for judging whether control is adequate for hazardous substances. We have generalized these principles to apply to all hazardous agents:

- Design and operate processes and activities to minimize emission and the spread of agents;
- Take into account all relevant routes of exposure when developing control measures;
- Control exposure by measures that are proportionate to the health risk;
- Choose the most effective and reliable control options that minimize the emission and spread of health hazards;
- Provide suitable personal protective equipment, in combination with other control measures, in situations where adequate control cannot be achieved by other means;
- Check and review regularly all aspects of control measures for their continuing effectiveness;
- Inform and train all employees about the hazards and risks from the agents with which they work and the use of control measures developed to minimize the risks;
- Ensure that the introduction of any control measures does not increase the overall risk to health and safety.

Where it is not possible to achieve adequate control of exposure through the use of engineering controls or by changing the work then suitable personal protective equipment (PPE) must be provided in addition to the other control measures. It is often said that this implies that PPE is the 'last resort' and should only be used when all other forms of control are impracticable. However, in many situations, such as in maintenance or other transitory work, the pragmatic approach is to rely on PPE to protect the workers.

This chapter focuses on control of hazardous substances and other hazardous agents, and the specific approaches that can be used for risk management.

19.2 Specific control measures

The above-mentioned principles are sometimes expressed in the form of a 'control hierarchy', with the implication that those measures near the top of the list are more effective or reliable in controlling exposure. In fact, as the principles of 'good control practice' recognize it is often not so simple and control measures may vary in their effectiveness and suitability, plus different control approaches may be used in combination rather than as alternatives. For example, local ventilation systems can vary in their effectiveness in reducing exposure from virtually no effect to a reduction in exposure to less than one-thousandth of the original figure.

The following is a list of specific control options:

- Elimination;
- Substitution;
- Total enclosure;
- Technological solutions;
- Segregation;
- Partial enclosure;
- Local ventilation;
- General ventilation;
- Personal protection equipment.

Elimination and substitution are removing or reducing the hazard or risk. Total enclosure should provide a barrier to prevent release of the hazard into the work environment. The other controls all attempt to mitigate the effects of the hazardous agent once it has been emitted into the workplace.

19.2.1 Elimination

Elimination of risk by changing the processes or substances, e.g. eliminating a painting process by replacing painted materials with corrosion resistant materials or replacing a noisy riveting process with the use of a high-performance adhesive. However, note that such elimination in one workplace might just shift the risk to another workplace; e.g. the manufacture of corrosion-resistant materials might involve hazardous metal-plating processes. Alternatively, the elimination of one hazard might result in another hazard arising in the same workplace, e.g. in the riveting to gluing example above the replacement of a physical hazard, noise, might result in a chemical hazard from the adhesive. It is therefore essential to ensure that the elimination of one hazard does not introduce another hazard, with possibly greater risk to the workers.

19.2.2 Substitution

Replacing a hazardous substance by lower hazard substance or the same substance in a form that reduces the exposure, e.g. in shot blasting replacing sand containing silica by silica-free substances such as olivine or plastic pellets, producing enzymes as granules rather than powders, replacing a hazardous solvent, such as toluene, with a less hazardous ketone or by replacing a solvent-based paint with a water-based paint. However, it is again essential to ensure that the replacement of one hazard does not introduce another hazard; e.g. although ketones are generally less chemically hazardous than toluene, it is important that the replacement substance does not have a lower flash point than toluene and although water-based paints may be inherently less hazardous than solvent-based paints, water-based paints generally contain fungicides and/or antifoaming agents, some of which cause respiratory effects, or substances that can cause respiratory sensitisation. In any substitution it is therefore essential to fully assess the relative hazards and risks associated with the original and replacement substances and processes.

19.2.3 Total enclosure

Fully contained processes, such as in ventilated glove boxes for unsealed radioactive materials or an enclosed chemical process can provide a very high level of containment. However, no system is completely enclosed and it may be necessary to break the enclosure to collect quality assurance samples or for maintenance. In addition, during normal use there may be slight leaks from flange joints, pumps and other process equipment. However, in situations where this may be critical it is possible to design 'layers of protection', for example in the pharmaceutical industry where you may have an enclosed powder material transfer point inside an enclosure, e.g. split butterfly valve inside a glove box.

19.2.4 Technological solutions

Such control solutions include the use of water sprays to prevent the emission of dust from cutting blades or discs, 'squeeze' piling to very substantially reduce the noise and vibration generated by piling processes, the use of chemical feedstocks in pre-reacted form, e.g. as in the replacement of highly volatile isocyanate monomers by substantially less volatile homopolymers in polyurethane paints and lacquers. The application of 'anti-noise' materials can very substantially reduce the noise levels generated by large slow-moving equipment where a significant proportion of the noise energy released is at frequencies below about 500 Hz.

19.2.5 Segregation

Segregation involves separating the worker from the process. Such segregation can involve total enclosure of the process or the worker. In many work situations it is difficult to totally enclose the process, so suitable work havens are provided for the operator. For example, 'noise havens' are widely used to minimise the noise exposure of workers involved in the use of equipment to which it would be difficult to apply effective noise control at source. Such havens can also be provided with clean filtered air to minimise exposures to airborne hazardous substances.

19.2.6 Partial enclosure

Partially contained processes, such as in a conventional fume cupboard or a down-draught booth, can provide high levels of control, but correct operating

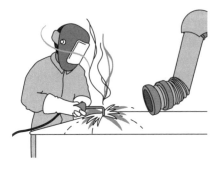

Figure 19.1 Diagram showing the incorrect placement of a hood while welding, i.e. too far from the source.

procedures must be adhered to in order to ensure good control. The correct use of partial enclosure therefore involves the stringent training and supervision of users.

19.2.7 Local ventilation

This is very widely used to capture dust, fumes, gases and vapours from processes such as cutting and welding. Sometimes known as 'local exhaust ventilation' or LEV because it is often the case that air is extracted or exhausted from the workroom. However, it is also possible to provide local ventilation by using supplied air or supplied air in combination with exhausted air. There is also increasing use of re-circulation of filtered air back into the workroom to save on energy costs. Unless correctly used local ventilation can be ineffective. For example, Figure 19.1 illustrates the incorrect placement of a flexible LEV hood during the welding of stainless steel and Figure 19.2 illustrates operators placing their heads between the emission source and extraction inlet and hence being unnecessarily exposed. The correct use of LEV therefore involves training and supervision of users.

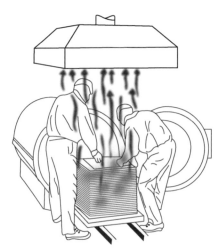

Figure 19.2 Operators placing their head between the emission source and the extraction hood.

19.2.8 General ventilation

General ventilation is often regarded as being a low effectiveness form of control as it acts to simply dilute substances that have already become airborne. However, in small rooms, e.g. less than about 100 m^3, adequate general ventilation is one of the best ways to ensure that contaminant air concentrations are controlled to a safe level; without sufficient ventilation in these rooms high levels of vapours or fumes could arise. If high levels of general ventilation are used to control hazardous substances the air flows may cause thermal discomfort in cool conditions and if the replacement air has to be heated to maintain safe and comfortable working conditions, the cost of such heating can be substantial. General ventilation should be designed to provide some minimal level of control in a workroom. It is sometimes recommended that general ventilation is only used to control exposure to contaminants when:

- There is low and uniform contaminant release rate;
- The substances are of relatively low toxicity;
- The sources are in the far-field of the workers.

However, these are quite restrictive and used in combination with other control measures general ventilation has an important role in all work situations.

19.2.9 Personal protective equipment

PPE, which includes ear defenders, respirators, gloves, protective clothing, boots and many other items, is generally regarded as the 'last resort', e.g. see Regulation 7 of the Control of Substances Hazardous to Health regulations. In most work situations, PPE should be regarded as a temporary measure while other, more effective, control measures are being implemented or as back-up in high-risk situations in case other control measures, such as total enclosure, were to fail. If one enters a workplace and finds workers wearing PPE for routine operations the immediate question should be 'Where are the other, effective, controls?' However, in emergency situations, such as firefighting, rescue or incident situations, PPE might be the only or primary form of control available. The effectiveness of PPE is critically dependent on its correct use by each individual employee. All form of PPE therefore involve the selection of equipment adequate to provide the required protection, the stringent selection of equipment to match each individual wearer, the training and supervision of wearers and, where relevant, the cleaning and maintenance of the PPE.

19.3 The effectiveness of control measures

The effectiveness of the above control measures may vary considerably. If elimination or substitution work well they can virtually eliminate the risk, but there are several reports of cases where the changes made have been unsuccessful and exposures have only reduced slightly or in some cases increased. The effectiveness of other types of localized control will depend on the background levels in the workplace, and it will not be possible to reduce exposure below the general ambient levels.

Complete enclosure of a process emitting a hazardous substance in a workplace where there are no other sources might be expected to give more than a 90% reduction in exposure; i.e. the level will be less than one tenth of those without the controls in place. A well-designed local ventilation system with partial enclosure (e.g. fume cupboard in a laboratory) might give about a 99% reduction in exposure whereas a poorly designed system might only give 50% reduction in exposure. Local ventilation systems fixed at appropriate points on a machine or process should give about 90% reduction in exposure, but mobile ventilation, for example a mobile hood used to capture welding fume, poorly maintained or badly designed systems may only give about a 30% reduction or less. Partial enclosures without any extraction are likely to give fairly limited control, e.g. 10–35% reduction in exposure.

In laboratory and field tests, PPE is perhaps surprisingly effective. For respiratory protection the average protection offered may reduce exposure by 90–99.9% or better. However, once we take account of the variability in effectiveness between individual workers, the reduction in exposure is more modest. The British Standards Institute recommends assuming effectiveness between 75 and 95% for half-mask devices and between 75 and 97.5% for full-face devices.

The impact of introducing control measures can be estimated using the figures on the likely effectiveness. For example, in a powder-handling operation putting the workstation inside a carefully designed local ventilation booth might reduce exposure by 90%. If the average exposure measured before the hood was installed was 15 mg m^{-3} then it might be expected that the average exposure after introducing the hood would be 1.5 mg m^{-3}, i.e. 90% lower.

All control measures require routine evaluation and testing of their effectiveness. This must be augmented with regular maintenance procedures. The testing is designed to check that the system is functioning as it was originally designed and installed. Any measurements should be compared with the corresponding data obtained at the time of commissioning to show any changes in performance are not likely to compromise effectiveness.

One last piece of general advice about control measures – careful observation of their use or otherwise will generally show any limitations and help pinpoint what steps may need to be taken to improve effectiveness.

References and further reading

Gardiner K. (2005). Control philosophy. In: *Occupational Hygiene*, 3rd edition (Gardiner K, Harrington JM, eds). Oxford, UK: Blackwell Publishing.

Health and Safety Executive (2005). *Control of Substances Hazardous to Health, 5th edition. Approved Code of Practice*. L5. Sudbury, UK: HSE Books.

Fransman W, Schinkel J, Meijster T, Van Hemmen J, Tielemans E, Goede H. (2008). Development and evaluation of an exposure control efficacy library (ECEL). *Annals of Occupational Hygiene* 52(7): 567–575.

20 Ventilation

20.1 Introduction

In many workplaces, local ventilation systems are provided to supply or extract air locally. Such systems incorporate an air mover, generally in the form of a fan; an inlet hood or hoods; ducting; and a filter or other air cleaner to prevent atmospheric pollution from the discharge of dirty air. Where air is supplied into a workplace the system may additionally include heaters, coolers, humidifiers or a combination of these items. Entry hoods may be in the form of flexible or fixed inlets, booths, fume cupboards or other enclosures. Ductwork may be of considerable length containing bends, changes of cross-section, branch pieces and other fittings. This chapter deals with measurements made to test local ventilation systems to ensure they are functioning as designed and in a way that will ensure effective control. We do not describe how to design a local ventilation system, which is discussed in other texts.

The performance of local ventilation systems needs to be regularly examined to ensure their satisfactory operation. Current British legislation, such as the Control of Substances Hazardous to Health (COSHH) regulations, impose the duty to ensure that engineering controls are maintained 'in an efficient state, in efficient working order, in good repair and in a clean condition', with tests of their effectiveness carried out at least once every 14 months and to maintain records of examination and tests carried out for at least 5 years from the date of the tests. These assessments would generally include visual examination of the system to ensure its integrity and measurement of air volume flow rates, air velocities and pressures at extraction points and inside ducts and other points, e.g. across filters and fans. These measurements can be supplemented by the tracing of airflow patterns around ventilation terminals such as extraction hoods, slots, enclosures and fume cupboards.

As local ventilation systems are provided to protect workers' health, a surprising omission from the various regulations is the duty to monitor exposure levels for workers on the process to demonstrate that the ventilation systems do adequately reduce workers' exposures. However, we recommend that exposure measurements are made when a new system is commissioned and when any major modifications are made to a system.

20.2 Air pressure

Air pressures are usually quoted as gauge pressures, i.e. the pressure difference between inside the system and atmospheric pressure or that of the room in which the equipment is installed. The unit of pressure is the pascal (Pa). However, as pressure gauges may be simple U tubes containing a liquid such as water or paraffin, tradition has it that pressures are sometimes quoted as the length or height of a column of liquid, for example, millimetres of water (mm H_2O). In general, 1 mm water gauge can be considered to be a pressure of 10 Pa. If a fluid other than water is used the following equation is employed the pressure 'p' (Pa):

$$p = \rho_L \times g \times h$$

where ρ_L is the density of the liquid in the gauge in kg m^{-3}; h is the height of the column in metres and g is the acceleration due to gravity (9.81 m s^{-2}).

Note that given the accuracy and repeatability of such measurements it is adequate to record and report pressures to two significant figures.

It is necessary to differentiate between three different types of pressure in ventilation systems: static pressure, velocity pressure and total pressure.

20.2.1 Static pressure (p_s)

Static pressure (p_s) is the pressure exerted in all directions by a stationary fluid or gas. If the fluid is in motion, it is the pressure exerted at right angles to the direction of flow. Static pressure can be either positive or negative in relation to atmospheric pressure. For example, on the suction side of a fan it would be negative but on the delivery side it would be positive.

20.2.2 Velocity pressure (p_v)

Velocity pressure (p_v) is defined as the pressure equivalent of the kinetic energy of a fluid in motion although it is perhaps best illustrated as that pressure which is exerted on a surface placed across an airstream as in the force imposed on the palm of your hand if you blow against it. It is calculated from the expression

$$p_v = 0.5 \times \rho \times v^2$$

where ρ is the density of the air in kg m^{-3} (1.2 kg m^{-3} at normal room temperature) and v is the velocity of the air in m s^{-1}.

Note that in physics velocity is taken to be a vector quantity having both direction and magnitude. The magnitude of an air velocity is termed the air speed. For simplicity, in the text we use the term velocity rather than switch between speed and velocity. Velocity pressure is always positive.

20.2.3 Total pressure (p_t)

Total pressure (p_t) is the algebraic sum of the static and velocity pressures at a point in an airstream and can be either positive or negative in relation to atmospheric pressure. For example, in a duct downstream of the fan the static

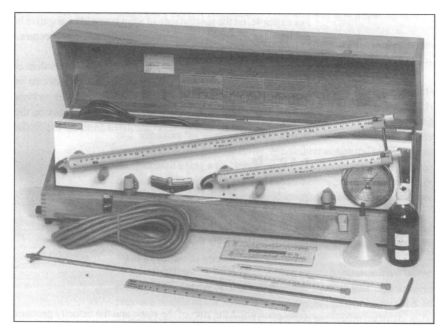

Figure 20.1 Portable inclined manometer. (© Airflow Developments Ltd. Reproduced with permission.)

pressure is −30 Pa and the velocity pressure is 50 Pa, giving a total pressure of −30 + 50 = 20 Pa.

20.3 Measurement equipment

20.3.1 Pressure-measuring instruments

It is possible to make a simple pressure gauge by taking a glass or plastic tube bent in a U shape and filling it half full with water. With one limb connected to the inside of the ventilation duct by means of rubber or plastic tubing at the point where the pressure measurement is required, and the other limb open to the atmosphere, the water will take up different levels in each limb of the tube. The difference in vertical height between the two liquid levels represents the pressure in the duct (in mm H_2O). By using the formula given earlier, this pressure in pascals can be calculated. For pressures below about 50 Pa, this instrument will be imprecise because it will be difficult to measure the difference in height of the two columns. If more precision is required then it is necessary to incline one limb of the U tube as in the manometer in Figure 20.1.

There is a range of commercially available manometers from simple vertical U tubes to instruments whose angle of inclination can be varied in known fixed positions and whose scales are calibrated in various units of pressure. The liquids used in the more sophisticated instruments are usually of a lower specific gravity than water thus providing a more extended scale than

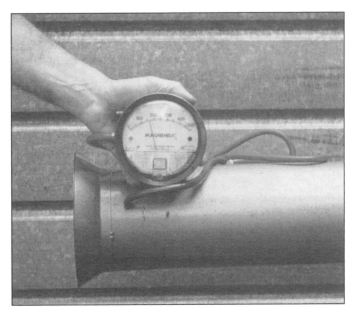

Figure 20.2 Magnehelic diaphragm pressure gauge. (Reproduced with permission *Monitoring for Health Hazards at Work*, 3rd edition, by Indira Ashton and Frank S. Gill, Blackwell Publishing Ltd., 2000. p. 89.)

would be obtained with water for the same pressure. It is important to ensure that such gauges are filled with the correct liquid or the scales will give the incorrect value. Also with gauges having variable inclinations, it is important to multiply the reading obtained by a scale factor appropriate to the angle of inclination as provided by the manufacturer.

Liquid-filled gauges have the disadvantage that they can be difficult to transport without losing the liquid, and the liquid must be free of bubbles when being used. Overloading the gauge can result in bubbles being formed or the liquid being blown out of the tubes. Also, vertical U tubes must be held vertically when in use and inclined manometers must be carefully levelled and zeroed before use and kept level whilst being read.

Diaphragm pressure gauges do not have these disadvantages as a reading is obtained on a dial by a pointer actuated by the movement of a diaphragm, one side of which is exposed to the pressure to be measured. A mechanical or magnetic linkage moves the pointer. Such gauges are much easier to use in industrial situations but they need to be regularly calibrated against an accurate inclined manometer set up under suitable laboratory conditions. They must also be zeroed before taking a set of readings, which can be done by joining the two pressure tappings by a tube and making the appropriate adjustment. Gauges of this type can be read by placing either in a vertical or horizontal position but they must be zeroed in the plane in which they are to be used. An example of a diaphragm pressure gauge is shown in Figure 20.2.

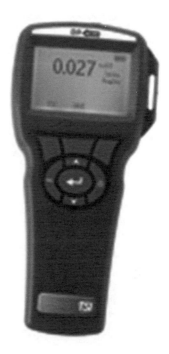

Figure 20.3 Digital micromanometer. (© TSI Instruments Ltd. Reproduced with permission.)

A wide range of pressures can be measured using a battery-powered micromanometer, as illustrated in Figures 20.3. Displays can be digital or analogue and some have the facility to display an air velocity corresponding to a measured velocity pressure when coupled to a pitot-static tube (see Section 2.3.2.3), assuming standard air density.

20.3.2 Air velocity measuring instruments

The magnitude of air velocity is measured in metres per second (m s^{-1}). A wide variety of air velocity measurement instruments are available and they can be classified into three main groups: vane anemometers, heated sensor anemometers and velocity pressure devices.

20.3.2.1 Vane anemometers

Modern instruments are small rotating windmills electrically or optically coupled to a meter or a digital indicator to give a direct reading in units of air velocity. Modern instruments are available in diameters from 20 to 100 mm, as for example shown in Figure 20.4. As the rotating vanes are extremely light and are suspended on jewelled bearings it is important to ensure that they are handled carefully, that nothing is allowed to touch the vanes and the instruments are not used in air velocities above the specified limit. This

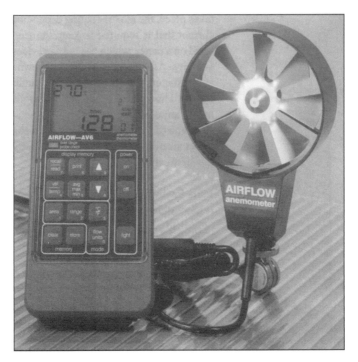

Figure 20.4 Electronic vane anemometer. (© Airflow Developments Ltd. Reproduced with permission.)

type of instrument requires regular calibration if reliable results are to be obtained. Electrically powered instruments should not be used in flammable atmospheres unless they are certified as being intrinsically safe.

It must be appreciated that vane anemometers are sensitive to 'yaw', i.e. the angle of the instrument to the air movement direction. The vane axis must be parallel to the airstream lines during the measurement. If you are uncertain of the direction of the airflow use a smoke indicator tube to make the flow direction visible (see Section 20.3.2.4 on smoke tubes).

20.3.2.2 Heated sensor anemometers

These devices rely upon the cooling power of air movement, affecting a small sensor made from a thin wire, a metal film or a thermistor bead (i.e. a material whose electrical resistance changes with the temperature). As air blows over the sensor cooling takes place, the rate of cooling depending upon the air velocity. The electrical current that is required to keep the sensor temperature constant is registered on a meter, which has been previously calibrated in units of air velocity. An example of this type of instrument is shown in Figure 20.5. As with vane anemometers they require careful handling and regular calibration against known air velocities. Also, they should not be used in

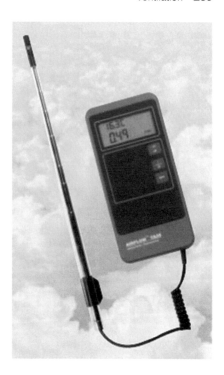

Figure 20.5 Heated sensor anemometer.
(© TSI Instruments Ltd. Reproduced with
permission.)

flammable atmospheres unless certified as being intrinsically safe. Some such
instruments may be damaged by corrosive atmospheres or if exposed to
'sticky' dusts or grit.

Some of these instruments have a cowl over the sensing head to direct
air over it, which means that they must be carefully placed in the airstream
aligned with the airflow direction.

20.3.2.3   Velocity pressure devices

It is possible to measure velocity pressure by using a pressure gauge as already described in conjunction with a probe known as a 'pitot-static' tube
(Figure 20.6). This device consists of two tubes, one concentrically placed inside the other. The inner tube is positioned facing into the airstream with its
axis parallel to the streamlines – sensing the total pressure. The outer tube is
sealed at the end and around the outer part of the tube there is a ring of holes
that are at right angles to the airstream – sensing static pressure. At the opposite end to the pitot, the tubes are each fitted with a tapping to connect to
the pressure gauge via flexible tubing. To facilitate insertion into the side of
ducting the whole device is bent at a right angle. The principle of operation is
as follows: as the static pressure inside the duct is acting upon both tubes it is
also acting upon each side of the pressure gauge and therefore cancels itself

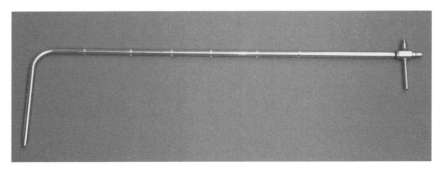

Figure 20.6 Pitot-static tube. (© JS Holdings. Reproduced with permission.)

out leaving only the velocity pressure to provide the reading on the gauge. This is illustrated diagrammatically in Figure 20.7. Rearranging the velocity pressure formula mentioned earlier the air velocity (v) can be calculated from the measured pressure as follows:

$$v = \sqrt{\frac{2p_v}{\rho}}$$

Example: a velocity pressure p_v of 100 Pa is measured using a pitot-static tube, assuming air density ρ is 1.2 kg m^{-3} the air velocity is

$$v = \sqrt{\frac{2 \times 100}{1.2}} = 12.9 \text{ m s}^{-1}$$

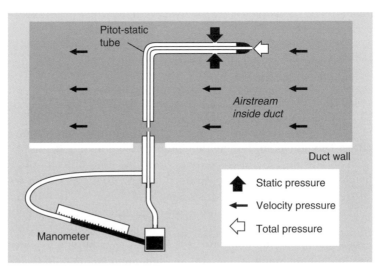

Figure 20.7 Principle of operation of pitot-static tube. (Reproduced with permission from *Occupational Hygiene*, 3rd edition, edited by Kerry Gardiner and J. Malcolm Harrington, Blackwell Publishing Ltd., 2005, p. 443.)

It is important to note that most such instruments are unsuitable for air velocities below about 3 m s^{-3}, as precision is low. If air velocities are likely to be below 3 m s^{-3} an alternative airflow meter should be used. Also, with pitot-static tubes, it is important to ensure that the tube points directly into the airstream since any deviation will result in errors. To this end, some makes of pitot-static tube have a pointer at the lower end to indicate the direction in which the head is pointing. A pitot-static tube should only be used for measuring duct air velocity. It is unsuitable for measuring the air velocity at the face of hoods or booths.

20.3.2.4   Smoke tube kit

A smoke tracer can be used to visualise the patterns of airflow outside ducts, to spot leaks of air from ventilation systems, to identify sources of draught, and to visualise turbulence, for example, at the edges of fume cupboards or booths. White smoke can be produced in a variety of ways but the most convenient method is a smoke tube kit, which consists of a rubber bulb fitted with one-way valves and a small sealed glass tube containing a chemical that, when exposed to air, gives off a stream of white 'smoke'. To activate the chemical it is necessary to break the sealed ends of the glass tube and attach one end to the bulb. By squeezing the bulb air is passed through the tube producing a stream of dense white particulate. Rubber end seals can be fitted to the tube to conserve the chemical for later use. The tube may seal itself with a deposit of white powder before all of the chemical is exhausted but this can be cleared with a thin spike.

A useful feature of smoke produced this way is that it is at the same temperature as the surrounding air. It is not recommended that smoke from a combustion source such as a match is used as it is hotter than the surrounding air and will tend to rise, giving a false picture of the airflow patterns.

It should be noted that the smoke produced by such tubes can be toxic and corrosive, and they should not be used unless authorised by the health and safety manger of the premises being assessed. Such tubes must not be used in food, drink or drug manufacturing premises. Care should also be taken to ensure that the sharp glass edges on the broken tube do not injure anyone.

It is sometimes necessary to generate larger clouds of smoke than can be produced from a tube kit. For example, to trace the emissions from the stack of a chemical fume cupboard amongst many in a laboratory block or to observe the behaviour of a plume leaving the stack. Larger, more stable and continuous streams of smoke can be produced using an ignitable chemical smoke producer similar to fireworks and supplied by firework manufacturers. Theatrical smoke machines may also be useful in these circumstances where the 'smoke' is blown out by a fan integral to the machine. This device is a standard method of visually testing the containment of a chemical fume cupboard in some countries.

These 'smoke' aerosols may also be toxic and the firework type sources may constitute a fire hazard. Sources that emit large quantities of smoke can cause fire alarms to go off and they should therefore not be used unless authorised by the health and safety manger of the premises being assessed.

20.3.2.5   Calibration

It is necessary to regularly check the performance of air velocity measurement instruments against accurately known air velocities. Calibration of anemometers is best done in a wind tunnel but such devices are large, expensive and are limited in location to the larger research establishments and universities, and may not be easily accessible. As an alternative, it is possible to use a small, relatively inexpensive wind tunnel known as an 'open jet' wind tunnel, which can guarantee air velocities to within $\pm 2\%$ of the true value. This is sufficiently precise for most field measurements. However, most equipment manufacturers also offer a calibration service at a modest cost.

20.3.2.6   Tyndall beam

The Tyndall beam (described in Chapter 9) is a useful device for assessing the effectiveness of local ventilation hoods in capturing aerosols. The light can be positioned to one side of an exhaust hood to observe the path of the dust cloud.

20.3.3   Barometric pressure instruments

Barometric pressure can be measured by a variety of devices. The absolute instrument is the Fortin barometer, which is a column of mercury contained in an inverted sealed tube standing in a trough of mercury. The column is held up by air pressure whose value is expressed by the height of the column supported in millimetres. For example, standard atmospheric pressure is 760 mm of mercury (mm Hg). This value can be converted into pascal and hence into bar or millibar (1 mbar = 100 Pa). Note in the European Union the sale of mercury is now restricted.

The barometric pressure can also be measured by an aneroid barometer, which is essentially a sealed bellows-type chamber that expands and contracts with changes in pressure and moves a needle on a suitably calibrated dial. Modern devices use pressure transducers, which can provide a signal to a digital display. Aneroid and digital barometers require regular calibration.

Alternatively, figures for local atmospheric pressures can be obtained from the Met Office website.

20.4   Ventilation measurement records

Two types of measurement are generally made on local ventilation systems: routine checks by supervisors or workers using the system and a statutory thorough examination and test carried out by an expert. In Britain, statutory measurements and records of those measurements are required to be kept for at least 5 years. For routine measurements to be of any value the current performance figures need to be compared with the previous ones to obtain a trend. In this way the capability of the system to control can be judged.

The employer should have two documents for each local ventilation system: the user manual, which should contain information about how to use the system and how to maintain it, and the logbook, containing schedules for daily/weekly/monthly checks and maintenance, records of maintenance, the basis of performance of the system and compliance with the correct way of working with the system. These documents constitute a statement of the design specification of the ventilation system and should include a sketch or photograph of its layout. The routine checks could include a variety of observation data, such as the integrity of hoods and ducts, the static pressure measured just behind the hoods and the static pressure difference over the filter or air cleaner.

If the system is used to control large quantities of hazardous materials the performance of the system may deteriorate due to heavy deposits on certain parts such as dampers and fan blades. In addition, some substances may react with the materials making up the control system and damage them. For example, acid vapour mists could corrode the ducting if it is made of certain metals. This emphasises the importance of including health and safety professionals at the design stage of the control system so that appropriate systems are selected and installed.

The following information should be available in the system documentation:

Identification details – the name and number of the plant; its location; the type of plant; and the hazardous substances that are being controlled. It is useful to take photographs of each component of the system and to refer to the relevant photograph(s) for each measurement made. Such photographs can also allow any changes to the system between examinations to be identified and defined.

Enclosures and hoods – maximum number to be in use at any time; location or position; static pressure behind each hood or extraction point; face velocity. Each individual hood or extraction point should be tested.

Details of the inlet design should be recorded, namely a glove box or total enclosure, a booth or fume cupboard, a canopy hood, a side hood, a flexible arm moveable hood, or a slot. Note the face dimensions, duct diameter, area, face velocity, duct velocity, volume flow rate and static pressure. With regard to total enclosures such as glove boxes, air velocities and volume flow rates are not relevant and in any case may not be measurable. However, static pressure is important as is the negative static pressure that prevents the pollutant being controlled from escaping.

Ducting – dimensions; transport air velocity (i.e. the minimum design velocity to transport the contaminant through the system); actual duct air velocity and the volume flow. The ductwork can be described in the sketch with the duct dimension written by each length. The dimensions of the ducts leading from the hoods etc. can be inserted in a table summarising the data for each of the extract points.

Filter/collector – specification; volume flow; static pressure at inlet, outlet and across filter. There are many types of filter to be found in industry, all variations of basic types: dry centrifugal (cyclones); electrostatic; fabric (bag or cartridge filters); wet scrubbers; absorbers; thermal oxidisers and catalytic cleaners. All that needs to be recorded is one of these descriptions. The make and serial number can be obtained from the identification plate on the device. If it is a fabric filter the total surface area of the filtration medium is useful to have as a filter air velocity can be calculated from the volume flow rate.

The static pressure across the device, particularly if it is a fabric filter, will indicate the condition of the fabric, therefore it is useful to know what it should be when in good condition. If it is higher than normal it indicates blocked or partially blocked fabric; if it is below normal it will indicate either a hole in the fabric or a reduced flow rate for some other reason. By subtracting the static pressure at the filter outlet from that at the inlet the pressure across the filter can be calculated. Static pressure at the inlet will indicate the condition of the ductwork system: if it is higher than normal it may indicate a blockage in the ductwork and if lower, it may indicate a reduced flow rate of the fan or a hole in the system. Some systems have a secondary filter or a combination of two filters in series.

Fan or air mover – specification; volume flow; static pressure at inlet; direction and speed of rotation.

Identify the fan maker and the serial number. This is usually found on a plate riveted to the fan casing. In some instances this may be missing or the plate is so corroded that it cannot be read, in which case 'information not available' should be entered. The type of fan is usually obvious by inspection. The most common fans are either axial flow or centrifugal, the former normally being cylindrical in shape with a propeller type of impeller rotating inside and an electrical cable attached to a junction box on the casing. The centrifugal fan has a casing that is scroll-shaped with the inlet duct entering at the centre and the outlet duct connected to the periphery, i.e. the inlet flow direction is at right angles to the outlet flow. Very occasionally, a mixed-flow configuration is found, where a centrifugal impeller rotates within what appears to be an axial-flow casing. If there is any doubt, and the fan identification plate is readable, a telephone call to the maker will confirm the type.

The type of drive describes the way the fan impeller is connected to the drive motor: either direct, where the impeller shaft is the same as that of the motor, or V-belt driven, where a pulley is attached to the fan shaft and another to the motor and V-shaped belts connect the two like a chain on a bicycle. The pulleys should always be covered with a guard, which may make counting the number of belts difficult. The fan diameter means the outside diameter of the rotating impeller and will be almost the same as the inlet duct diameter in the case of the axial flow fan and slightly larger than inlet duct diameter on the centrifugal type. Many of the centrifugal impellers are designed to be withdrawn through an opening in the casing of the inlet duct side, and an estimate of the diameter of that opening will indicate the diameter of the impeller.

The fan rotational speed will be the same as the motor speed with direct-driven fans, and that can be read either from the identification plate of the motor or the fan casing. With V-belt driven fans, it will be necessary to measure the speed by placing a portable tachometer on the end of the fan shaft and this may involve removing the guard: an operation that must be done with the fan stationary. The fan must then be started up and the shaft speed carefully measured, making sure that no part of the measurer's body or clothing can come into contact with the belts or pulleys. Ideally, arrangements should be made to have a small opening cut into the casing opposite the end of the fan shaft sufficiently large to allow the tip of the tachometer to be pushed into the shaft.

The direction of rotation is extremely important to note, particularly with fans driven by three-phase electric motors. If the wiring to the motor has been connected incorrectly, the motor will run in reverse. With axial-flow fans this results in the air flowing in the opposite direction, and is usually quickly noticed and rectified, but with centrifugal fans the air continues to flow in the correct direction but at a greatly reduced flow rate. The direction of rotation needs to be described in relation to one side or the other of the fan. It is recommended that the fan be viewed from the side of the electric motor and described as 'clockwise' or 'anti-clockwise'. Some fans have the correct direction marked on the casing, but if not the correct direction of a centrifugal fan can be deduced by observing the scroll shape of the fan casing. The impeller should rotate towards the expansion of the scroll. Any other relevant information about the fan can usually be obtained from the label either on the motor or the fan casing.

Systems that return exhaust air to the workplace – filter efficiency; concentration of contamination in return air. Note that care must be taken where air is returned to a workplace after it has been filtered to remove contaminants. There must be some form of sensor in the return airflow to detect a failure of the filter, e.g. in the case of an activated charcoal filter becoming overloaded, to automatically shut down the recirculation pathway.

The thorough examination and test should be carried out by a competent person. The assessment must be made at intervals not greater than 14 months, but this is generally done at least annually and for many systems more frequent examination and monitoring may be required. The assessor will rely on the existing records, such as the logbook, user manual and maintenance records. In addition, they will undertake their own investigation in three stages:

- A thorough visual examination to check the local ventilation is in efficient working order, in good repair and is clean;
- Measurement of key system parameters to check the system still conforms with commissioning data;
- An assessment that the control of worker exposure is adequate.

The measurements made at stage 2 might include:

- Measuring the air velocities in ducts and at the face of some hoods;
- Measuring static pressure at suitable test points, for example behind hoods, in ducting, across air cleaners;
- Checking the fan speed, plus the motor speed and the electrical power consumption;
- Measuring the quantity of the replacement air supplied into the workroom;
- Testing system alarms;
- Measuring air temperatures throughout the system;
- Assessing performance of the air cleaner, particularly if the air is re-circulated back into the workroom.

20.5 Measurement of air flow in ducts

20.5.1 Aim

Ducted ventilation systems require to be checked at regular intervals to ensure that the designed air-flow rate is being maintained. Deterioration occurs gradually due to a variety of factors, but mainly because of a build-up of deposits on the fan blades, duct walls and other parts of the system. If a record of the results is routinely made, then trends can be spotted and remedial action taken.

20.5.2 Equipment required

An air velocity measuring device – which can be either a vane anemometer, a heated head air velocity meter or a pitot-static tube and pressure gauge – a tape measure and a marker pen are needed. It should be borne in mind that whatever instrument is chosen, an access hole or holes are required in the duct wall to allow the instrument to be inserted, thus the smaller the instrument the smaller the hole. It will therefore be necessary to have a drill and suitable drill bits at hand. In this respect, the pitot-static tube is the most suitable, requiring a hole no larger than about 12 mm in diameter, although some of the smaller heated head instruments will also fit that size hole. Vane anemometers are less suitable for this purpose.

Note that if the ducting handles air containing radioactive, pathogenic material or toxic chemicals, then drilling holes may lead to contamination of the drill, the measuring instruments and escape of the pollutant into an occupied area. After the measurements are made the hole must be sealed with a grommet or industrial adhesive tape, although this is good practice regardless of the type of contaminant being handled by the system.

20.5.3 Method

1. Select a suitable length of duct in the airstream to be measured. Ideally, the measuring station should be in an airstream that is free from turbulence, which means the ducting should be straight and there should be

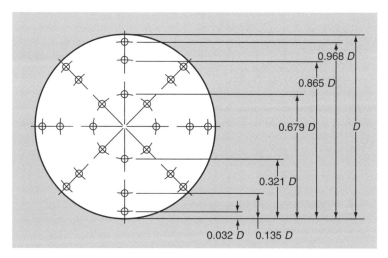

Figure 20.8 Measuring positions for placing pitot-static tubes in circular ducting.

no obstruction or changes of direction in the duct for at least 10 diameters upstream of it and none should appear downstream for 5 diameters. In many installations it is not possible to find such a place, therefore the longest length of straight ducting should be chosen and the measuring station taken as far downstream as possible from the last cause of turbulence. The reliability of the results will be affected by the degree of turbulence in the airstream.

2. Having chosen a measuring station it is necessary to place the instrument's sensing head in representative places over the cross-section of the duct to obtain an average air velocity. This is because the air moves at a higher velocity towards the centre than it does close to the walls of the duct. British Standard 848 recommends positions for the instrument as set out in Figures 20.8 and 20.9 for circular and rectangular cross-sections. Circular ducts are divided according to a log-linear rule and the rectangular according to a log-Tchebycheff rule (these are simple sets of rules for deriving where in the duct measurements should be made to give a representative measurement of average airflow). Thus it may be necessary to drill various holes in the duct walls to suit the size of the measuring station. Plugs of rubber or other suitable material should be available to cover the holes after use.

3. To assist in placing the sensing head of the instrument in the correct position inside the duct, the stem or carrying arm should be marked so that when the mark is aligned with the side of the duct the head is in one of the positions indicated by Figures 20.9 or 20.10. For example, if the duct is circular in cross-section and of 300 mm diameter, the stem should be

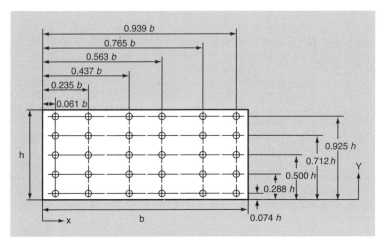

Figure 20.9 Log-Tchebycheff rule for traverse points in a rectangular duct.

marked at the following six distances from the head:

$300 \times 0.032 = 9.6$ mm	$300 \times 0.679 = 203.7$ mm
$300 \times 0.135 = 40.5$ mm	$300 \times 0.865 = 259.5$ mm
$300 \times 0.321 = 96.3$ mm	$300 \times 0.968 = 290.4$ mm

Note: With some pitot-static tubes the stem has rings of spring steel that can be adjusted to mark the appropriate position.

4. With battery-driven instruments, check the battery as indicated by the maker and turn on the meter and, where necessary, zero the scale in still air. This can be done by placing the head in a small closed container such as a tube sealed at one end.

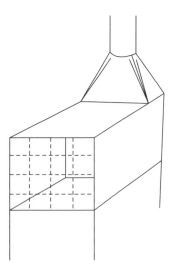

Figure 20.10 Face of booth showing measurement positions. (Reproduced with permission *Monitoring for Health Hazards at Work*, 3rd edition, by Indira Ashton and Frank S. Gill, Blackwell Publishing Ltd., 2000. p. 106.)

5. With pitot-static tubes it is necessary to set up the pressure gauge. Inclined manometers require to be levelled and zeroed, but this is best done after the connecting tubes have been attached so as not to disturb the setting by so doing. The high-pressure side of the gauge must be connected to the central tube of the pitot-static tube and the low-pressure side to the outside tube. Diaphragm gauges must be zeroed in the position in which they are to be read, i.e. either flat or vertical, but the position must not be changed after that. Electronic manometers have less restricted-use conditions.

6. Remove any protective cover from the sensing head and insert it through the hole in the duct. It can be helpful to first do a 'quick traverse' to check whether there is a lot of turbulence and/or an even flow across the duct. Also a centre-point measurement can give a 'quick and dirty' estimate of average air velocity in the duct, assuming the approximation that velocity is 0.9 times the centre-point velocity.

7. To make an accurate measurement of duct velocity, position the pitot tube so that the first mark is against the duct wall. If the duct is circular, then the stem of the instrument must be held along the line of the diameter, but if it is a rectangular cross-section then the stem must be at right angles to the duct wall. Ensure that the sensing head is exactly facing into the airstream. This is important with instruments that have a directional shield around the head and with pitot-static tubes, which often have a pointer at the lower end to indicate the position in which the head is facing. Some heated head instruments have no directional characteristics so this is not important. When using pitot-static tubes and liquid filled manometers it is a wise precaution to bend and squeeze both flexible connecting tubes to cut off the pressure in the gauge, releasing them simultaneously only when the pitot-static tube is in the correct position. Alternatively, use a simultaneous switching device available with some liquid-filled manometers. This can prevent an excessively high static pressure from blowing the fluid out of the gauge. If the air temperature and barometric pressure are very different from standard conditions (i.e. 20°C and 1013 mbar), then these parameters should also be measured.

8. Note the reading of the meter or the gauge and if necessary convert it to pascals according to the scale factor or the conversion factor.

9. Move the head to the next position and repeat step 7 and so on until all positions in the diagram have been measured.

10. It is wise to repeat the complete set of readings at least once more.

11. Where necessary measure duct temperature and obtain barometric pressure close to the measuring station.

12. Obtain the internal dimensions of the measuring station either by direct measurement, manufacturer's data or, in the case of a thick-walled duct, by measuring the outside dimensions and subtracting the thickness of the walls.

20.5.4 Calculation

Where air velocity meters have been used, it may be necessary to correct each reading from the latest calibration chart for the instrument concerned. The corrected velocities in each set of results should then be averaged to obtain the average air velocity at the measuring station.

The pitot-static tube and gauge method has obtained a set of velocity pressure readings, which must be converted to a air velocity before calculating an average. *Do not average the pressure readings.*

Calculate the air velocity as follows:

$$v = \sqrt{\frac{2p_v}{\rho}} \ \text{m s}^{-1}$$

where p_v = the reading of the velocity pressure in Pa, and

ρ is the air density in kg m^{-3}, which can be taken as 1.2 kg m^{-3}, unless the air temperature or barometric pressure is very different from 20°C or 1013 mbar (standard conditions).

To correct for temperature and pressure:

$$\text{new density } \rho_1 = \frac{1.2 \times P_{at} \times 293}{1013 \times (273 + t)} \ \text{kg m}^{-3}$$

Use ρ_1 in place of ρ in the above formula, where

P_{at} is barometric pressure in millibars (mbar), t is duct air temperature in °C.

The volume of air flowing (Q) is calculated from the formula: $Q = v \times A$ m^3 s^{-1}, where v is the average air velocity at the measuring station in m s^{-1}, that is, the arithmetic mean of the air velocities measured at that measuring station, which could be the mean of 30 readings in a rectangular duct, or 20 or 24 in a circular duct, and A is the cross-sectional area of the duct at the measuring station in m^2.

With circular cross-section:

$$A = \frac{\pi \times d^2}{4} \ \text{m}^2$$

where d is diameter of duct in metres; and with rectangular cross-section, A is $a \times b$ m^2 where a and b are the dimensions of the two sides of the rectangular duct at the measuring station.

20.5.5 Example

To measure the volume flow rate in a circular duct whose diameter is 200 mm, a six-point traverse was undertaken using a pitot-static tube and manometer. The following velocity pressures were obtained:

210, 213, 224, 230, 219, 214 (Pa).

Air temperature in the duct was 25°C and the barometric pressure was measured to be 982 mbar, which are non-standard conditions.

Calculation of volume flow rate:

To calculate the new non-standard air density:

$$\rho = \frac{1.2 \times 293 \times P_{at}}{1013 \times (273 + t)}$$

$$= \frac{1.2 \times 293 \times 982}{1013 \times (273 + 25)}$$

$$= 1.14 \text{ kg m}^{-3}$$

$$v = \sqrt{\frac{2p_v}{\rho}} \text{ m s}^{-1}$$

$$= \sqrt{\frac{2 \times 210}{1.14}} = 19.2 \text{ m s}^{-1} \text{ at the first traverse point}$$

Similarly $v_2 = 19.3 \text{ m s}^{-1}$

$v_3 = 19.8 \text{ m s}^{-1}$

$v_4 = 20.1 \text{ m s}^{-1}$

$v_5 = 19.6 \text{ m s}^{-1}$

$v_6 = 19.4 \text{ m s}^{-1}$

$$\bar{v} = \frac{19.2 + 19.3 + 19.8 + 20.1 + 19.6 + 19.4}{6} = 19.6 \text{ m s}^{-1}$$

$$A = \frac{(0.2)^2 \pi}{4}$$
$$= 0.031 \text{ m}^2$$
$$Q = vA \text{ m}^3 \text{ s}^{-1}$$

$$= 19.6 \times 0.031 = 0.62 \text{ m}^3 \text{ s}^{-1}$$

Note: The calculations are only to three significant figures as the precision of ventilation measurements of this nature is unlikely to be greater that ±2%.

20.5.6 Possible problems

1. Ventilation flow rates fluctuate for a variety of reasons:
   - some fans have a fluctuating output;
   - external influences such as wind and weather can affect flow rates; and
   - internal influences such as the movement of large loads across the entrance or exit of a ventilation system can affect flow rates. Therefore, it is important to take more than one set of readings.
2. Some flow rates pulsate, so, when reading meters, some estimate of the mid-point of the pulse should be taken.

3. Due to deposits of dust or sticky particles on the insides of ducting, the cross-sectional area may not be as expected. This is particularly prevalent in the ducting on paint spray booths. Adjustments can only be made by inspection.

20.6 Measurement of pressure in ventilation systems

20.6.1 Aim

In order that air should flow in ventilation systems it is necessary to create a pressure difference between the inside of the duct and the atmosphere. This is usually achieved by means of a fan. If the ducting is connected to the suction side of the fan the pressure inside is negative, thus drawing air into the system. A positive pressure is found on the discharge side, thus ducting on that side will deliver air under the influence of that pressure. Pressure is absorbed by the ducting, fittings and obstructions such as dampers and filters. With some ventilation systems dirt can build up inside, which can restrict the flow and increase the pressure absorbed. Also, fabric filters will gradually increase in resistance as dust is collected, resulting in an increase in pressure absorbed. It is, therefore, useful to measure pressures at various places in the system and, if done routinely, the trend can provide an indication of any deterioration in performance.

20.6.2 Equipment required

A manometer or diaphragm gauge, flexible plastic tubing of sufficient length to suit the siting of the gauge in relation to the measuring point (if pressure is to be measured on either side of an item, then it is useful to have tubing of two different colours), some moulding clay or plasticine to act as a sealant, a hand or electric drill capable of drilling holes the same diameter as the outside diameter of the flexible tubing, some rubber plugs or tape to seal up the hole after measuring.

20.6.3 Method

1. Select places to insert the tubing to suit the requirements of the system. For example, on either side of a filter, on either side of the fan, and/or at chosen places along the ducting. Drill a hole into the duct at each place. If the site is to be measured regularly then it may be advantageous and labour saving if a permanent nozzle is soldered or fixed to the duct wall to take the flexible tubing. The inner edge of the nozzle must be flush with the inside of the duct so that none protrudes into the airstream, and a cap should be fitted to prevent leakage after use.
   Note: If the ducting handles air containing radioactive, pathogenic material or toxic chemicals, then drilling holes may lead to contamination of the drill, the measuring instruments and escape of the pollutant into an occupied area.
2. Connect a length of flexible plastic tubing to each side of the gauge.

3. Level and zero the gauge as necessary.
4. By using the highest pressure range available, connect the other ends of the tubing to the places to be measured. With liquid filled manometers it is necessary to think carefully about the pressures to be measured before connecting the tubing into the system, as liquid can be easily removed by the ventilation pressure. The following points should be borne in mind:
   - Positive pressure will depress and negative pressure will elevate the liquid in the limb to which it is connected;
   - If a gauge pressure is to be measured, that is, with one side of the gauge open to atmosphere, then all parts of the ventilation system on the suction side of the fan will be at a negative pressure, whilst those on the delivery side will be at a positive pressure;
   - If a pressure difference is to be measured between two parts of the system – that is, both tubes are connected into the ducting – then, with the exception of the fans themselves, the air flows from the high to the low pressure, which means that the upstream side will be at the higher pressure;
   - With fans, the higher pressure will be on the delivery side.
     Note that electronic manometers are now widely used and they avoid most of these difficulties.
5. Having selected the highest range, if the pressure reading is low then a lower range can be used.
6. Note the reading, remove the tubing and seal the hole.
7. The recorded value may need to be multiplied by the scale factor of the range used.

20.6.4 Results
Little information can be gained from the results unless the design values of the system are known, against which the measurements can be compared. However, if routine measurements are taken, say once every month, and a continuous record kept then the condition of the ventilation system can be observed regularly, and if any deterioration is noted then corrective action can be taken. It is suggested that for each measuring station, a record sheet be kept containing the information.

20.6.5 Possible problems
1. Ventilation pressures may fluctuate due to external influences. If this is the case, then the cause should be removed if possible and the readings repeated.
2. If the pressure continues to fluctuate or pulsate then a mean or mid-point of the pulsation must be taken.
3. If the ventilation pressure has been misjudged when using a liquid filled gauge and the liquid has bubbled or blown out, then it is important to ensure that the flexible tubing is cleared of fluid and the liquid replenished in the gauge and all bubbles removed. It may be necessary to hang the tubing

in a vertical position to drain for some time or to blow it through with a jet of compressed air. Bubbles may be removed by gently rocking the fluid in the gauge from side to side by using a blowing action through a short length of clean tubing.

20.7 To measure the face velocity on a booth or hood

20.7.1 Aim

Fume cupboards, paint spray booths and other ventilated enclosures control the emission of substances by providing an enclosure on five of the six sides around the source, and on the sixth, maintaining an inward velocity of air such that the pollutants released in the enclosure should not escape. The velocity maintained on the open face is known as the 'face velocity' and for most situations should be kept within the range 0.5–2.5 m s^{-1}. Note that the face velocity of interest is the face of the booth and not the face of any air duct inlet within the hood, e.g. in a 'walk-in' booth with a open face 2 m × 2 m and an internal air inlet duct 0.5 m × 0.5 m the 'face' of interest is the 2 m × 2 m face. The aperture height could be critical when highly toxic materials are handled. An indication of the average velocity plus a profile of the range of velocities at different points across the face is required. Remember, record the direction of the airflow as well as the air velocity.

20.7.2 Equipment required

A rotating vane anemometer or heated head instrument, tape measure and marker pen are required.

20.7.3 Method

By using a tape measure and marker pen, the face of the enclosure should be divided into imaginary rectangles as shown in Figure 20.10. The air velocity measuring instrument should be held in the centre of each imaginary rectangle and allowed to remain there for a few seconds to adjust to a steady velocity (the larger the diameter of the vane anemometer the longer it will take to reach this velocity). The reading should be noted on a sketch of the face with the positions and distances labelled. When the measurement is noted, move to the next rectangle and so on until the whole face is measured. Measurements should also be made at the position of the operator's breathing zone and the position and distance from the inlet face recorded.

It is advisable to repeat all readings at least three times or until consistent results readings are obtained.

20.7.4 Results

If necessary, use the calibration chart of the air velocity instrument used to correct all the readings taken to provide the true velocity. Examine the individual spot readings to ascertain if any parts of the face have an inconsistent reading, such as too low or too high, and try to establish the reason. The air velocity at the face should be between about 0.5 m s^{-1} to about 0.8 m s^{-1}. It is useful to calculate the arithmetic mean of the velocities across the face, and then check each reading to see whether it is within ±20% of that mean. If any is outside this range, then the reason should be sought; e.g. the inlet duct may not be fitted with a means of ensuring uniform flow over the whole of the face area, and the condition remedied. If the velocity profile looks reasonably even, calculate the arithmetic mean of the spot air velocity readings to present as the average face air velocity and note it.

20.7.5 Possible problems

1. With a hand-held instrument it is possible to affect the readings by having an arm or other part of the body too close to the face, thus creating air currents that are not typical of normal conditions. Care should be taken to ensure that the minimum of obstruction is caused by the measurer and the instrument.
2. If the profile of air velocity is very uneven such that at some places the velocity is virtually zero then an unsatisfactory situation is indicated, which should be noted and rectified as soon as possible. Furthermore, the average air velocities obtained would be imprecise and of little value.

20.8 To measure the face velocity on a fume cupboard

20.8.1 Aim

Chemical fume cupboards are a special type of enclosure having a sliding front cover or sash. This serves two purposes: it protects the eyes and face of the operator from splashing of chemicals released inside, and it improves the enclosure by partially enclosing the sixth side, i.e. the front. The position of the sash may affect the velocity of the entering air as the area of opening will vary. The aim is to ensure that the face velocity is within an appropriate range. Low air velocities, e.g. less than 0.3 m s^{-1} may be particularly susceptible to loss of control from cross-droughts. High face velocities, e.g. more than 0.8 m s^{-1}, may produce re-circulating wakes in front of the user, which can draw contamination out of the cabinet.

Note that in some workplaces, such as semiconductor or drug manufacturing or testing sites, such fume cupboards are intended to protect the items inside the cupboard rather than the operator and that the fan blows filtered air *into* the cupboard. It is therefore important to measure the relative pressure between the inside and outside of the fume cupboard to ensure that the cupboard is protecting the operator.

Any measurements taken should be combined with inspections of the condition of the structure and services provided in the fume cupboard and the free movement of the sash. All defects should be reported.

20.8.2 Equipment required

A rotating vane anemometer, heated head anemometer or pitot probe, tape measure and marker pen are required.

20.8.3 Method

Set the sash to the normal operating position. In well-regulated laboratories this will normally be indicated by an arrow on the side of the frame.

By using the tape measure and marker pen, divide the face into imaginary rectangles similar to those shown in Figure 20.10. As a general guide, the rectangles should have the long side between 200 and 300 mm and the short side between 100 and 200 mm, depending upon the area of opening.

Hold the air velocity meter in the centre of each marked rectangle and allow it to remain there for a few seconds before noting the reading. Write down the results on a sketch of the face with the positions and dimensions labelled. Include a diagram showing the direction of the airflow.

Having noted the reading, move to the next rectangle and repeat until all the rectangles have been measured.

20.8.4 Results

If necessary, use the calibration chart of the air velocity instrument to correct all readings to obtain the true velocities. Calculate the arithmetic mean of the face velocities and check against the recommended face velocity. If the mean is below the recommended value it may be necessary to lower the sash to achieve the correct velocity. In this case, the arrow marking the normal operating position must be moved to indicate the new sash position. Also, check each reading to see whether it is within $\pm 20\%$ of that mean. If any is outside this range then the reason should be sought and the condition remedied.

20.8.5 Possible problems

The position of the user or equipment inside the fume cupboard may influence individual readings. This is particularly so if the equipment is too close to the air inlet. Ask the operator whether the equipment can be placed further inside the cupboard and if possible, move it. Not only will this improve the distribution of air velocities on the face, but it will probably also reduce any risk of pollutants escaping. It is prudent to use smoke tubes to check that with the operator and any equipment in place that there is no escape of air from the fume cupboard, e.g. from re-circulating air wakes in front of the operator. Release some smoke at the source of hazardous substance inside the cupboard and observe if smoke is drawn out of the cabinet because of turbulent wakes (see 'To measure the performance of a suction inlet' section for further details of how to systematically investigate the effectiveness of fume cupboards and other inlets).

Note: Most modern fume cupboards have a device to ensure a reasonably constant face velocity whatever the position of the sash and to prevent excessively high velocities when the sash is nearly fully closed. This may take the form of a by-pass grille or duct or by means of a variable speed fan. Do not estimate the volume flow rate of the fan by using the face velocity unless the sash is in the fully opened position as some air may be flowing through the by-pass.

Face velocity measurements may be combined with fan inlet flow rate, static pressure measurements and, where possible, discharge stack velocity.

20.9   To measure the performance of a suction inlet

20.9.1   Aim

Extract hoods, slots and enclosures are intended to capture air pollutants to prevent them from being released into the general room atmosphere. Unfortunately, many have insufficient air flowing or have their suction inlet too far away from the point of release of the pollutant, or they have inadequate enclosure around the source. Thus, some means of checking the airflow patterns and air velocity in and around the inlet is useful so that the full extent of the zone of influence of the device can be ascertained.

20.9.2   Equipment required

A smoke tube kit, a tape measure and an air velocity indicator such as a thermistor bead flowmeter are required.

20.9.3   Method

It should be pointed out that this method is intended to trace airflow patterns and measure air velocities around the inlet and not to check on the absolute efficiency of the suction device. To achieve the latter, it would be necessary to release a tracer gas whose decay of airborne concentration with distance from the source could be measured using some direct reading analysis instrument. This last technique is considered to be a specialist task and is not discussed further in this book.

1. Ensure that cross-draughts and local air turbulence are minimised during the test. For example, close doors or windows and restrict the movement of people in the vicinity. In particularly busy workplaces, it may be necessary to undertake this work outside working hours.
2. Break the ends of the smoke tube and insert it in the rubber bulb, puff smoke around the suction inlet gradually moving further away from the mouth until the full extent of the zone of influence (*'capture bubble'*) can be observed. The locations where the smoke is no longer being drawn in mark the edge of the zone of influence of this inlet.
3. Make a sketch drawing of the inlet and the work equipment that lies within the zone of influence.
4. Plot on the sketch an imaginary grid of squares across the face of the inlet and in the area in front to cover the whole zone of influence in the horizontal plane containing the source of pollutant. Other planes, both vertical and horizontal, can be chosen if a full picture is required. The dimensions of the

grid squares should be 100–150 mm depending upon the size of the inlet, the smaller ones using the smaller squares.

5. By using the tape measure as a guide to the measuring positions place the sensing head at the corner of each grid square taking care to ensure that the instrument is, as far as possible, axial to the airstreams' lines. This may be difficult as the airstreams around suction inlets are curved as air enters from all sides. Also the sensing head should be carried on a long probe so that the position of the observer's arms and body does not interfere with the flow patterns. Note the air velocity at each place by writing it on the sketch at the appropriate position.

6. Measure the air velocity on the face of the inlet along the centre line at the intersection with each of the grid lines. Note the results on the sketch. If there is a flat surface in front of the hood, such as a workbench, do not allow the instrument head to touch the surface but lift it clear of the surface, level with the centreline of the hood. Also record the airflow direction.

7. Repeat item 5 mentioned above for as many planes that have been chosen.

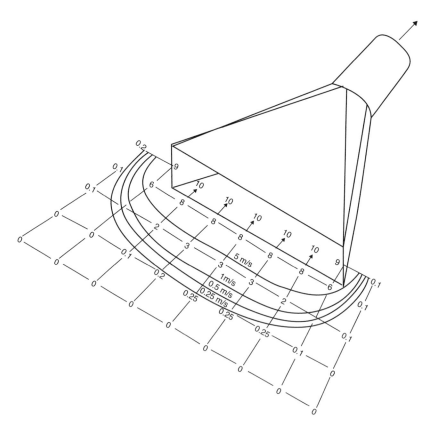

Figure 20.11 Extract slot showing measured air speed results and plotted contours. (Reproduced with permission *Monitoring for Health Hazards at Work*, 3rd edition, by Indira Ashton and Frank S. Gill, Blackwell Publishers Ltd., 2000. p. 110.)

20.9.4 Results

If necessary, correct each reading by using the appropriate calibration chart. Calculate the average of the velocities across the face of the inlet and note the range of the readings in relation to the average. If there is a wide variation then the airflow distribution is uneven and may require some means of equalisation by using face slots or airflow splitters or guides.

Inspect the results on any chosen plane of grids and try to estimate the position of points of equal velocity. For example, draw a cross or spot at the points, where in your opinion, the 5, 1, 0.5 and 0.25 m s^{-1} velocities occur. Join up the spots of equal velocity to produce a velocity contour of that air velocity as shown in Figure 20.11. The lowest contour should be 0.25 m s^{-1}. Any pollutant released outside this contour is unlikely to be captured or drawn into the inlet even if released into an undisturbed airstream, and if turbulence is caused by cross-draughts due to the presence of external influences such as open windows, doors or the movement of people or vehicles then pollutant will escape the zone of influence and be released into the general air.

References and further reading

Gill FS. (2005). Ventilation. In: *Occupational Hygiene*, 3rd edition (Gardiner K, Harrington JM, eds). Oxford, UK: Blackwell Publishing.

American Conference of Government Industrial Hygienists (2007). Testing of ventilation systems. In: *Industrial Ventilation: A Manual of Recommended Practice for Design*, 26th edition. Lansing, MI: ACGIH.

Burgess WA, Ellenbecker MJ, Treitman RD. (2004). *Ventilation for Control of the Work Environment*. Hoboken, NJ: Wiley-Interscience.

Daly BB. (1992). *Woods Practical Guide to Fan Engineering*, 3rd edition. Colchester, UK: Woods of Colchester. Available at http://www.flaktwoods.com/169/0/1/34bd869d-e1da-4f17-9209-8bb33b2ffa8a.

Nicholson GP, Clark RP, Grover F, de Calcina-Goff ML. (2000). A simple method for fume cupboard performance assessment. *Annals of Occupational Hygiene* 44(4): 291–300. Available at http://annhyg.oxfordjournals.org/cgi/content/abstract/44/4/291.

HSE (2000). *General Ventilation in the Workplace*. HSG 202. Sudbury, UK: HSE Books.

HSE (2005). *Control of substances hazardous to health (Fifth edition) and Approved Code of Practice to Control of Substances Hazardous to Health Regulations 2002 (as amended)*. L5. Sudbury, UK: HSE Books.

HSE (2008). *Controlling Airborne Contaminants at Work. A Guide to Local Exhaust Ventilation (LEV)*. Sudbury, UK: HSE Books.

British Standards relevant to local ventilation include
BS 848-1:1997: Fans for General Purpose. Methods of testing performance.
BS EN 14175-2:2003: Fume cupboards. Safety and performance requirements.

There is information for employers, employees and designers/installers/testers of LEV on the HSE's LEV home page. The site includes videos of common processes and sources. Available at http://www.hse.gov.uk/lev/index.htm.

21 | Personal Protective Equipment

21.1 Introduction

In assessing the effectiveness of a personal protective equipment (PPE) programme it is necessary for the assessor to be aware of the components of an effective programme. The overall effectiveness of any PPE is only partly determined by the quality and appropriateness of the equipment selected and so understanding what component systems should be in place is essential. This chapter describes the key elements of a successful PPE programme and the methods that can be used to measure the effectiveness of the PPE.

21.2 Components of an effective PPE programme

An effective PPE programme involves at least the following:

- Assess risks and identify where control is required;
- Implement all feasible controls other than PPE;
- Identify who needs residual protection;
- Select PPE adequate to control residual exposure;
- Involve wearers in the PPE selection process;
- Match PPE to each individual wearer;
- Carry out objective fit tests for respiratory protective equipment (RPE);
- Ensure that PPE does not exacerbate or create risk;
- Ensure that different items of PPE selected are mutually compatible;
- Train wearers in the correct use of their PPE;
- Supervise wearers to ensure correct use of PPE;
- Maintain PPE in efficient and hygienic condition;
- Inspect PPE to ensure it is correctly maintained;
- Provide suitable storage facilities for PPE;
- Monitor the PPE programme to ensure its continuing effectiveness.

The above-mentioned points are described in greater detail later as is the information to be gathered to assess the effectiveness of each step of the programme.

21.2.1 Assessment of risks and identification of where control is required

Identify any likely hazards and quantify any risks. The assessment should identify and quantify all unacceptable risks during both routine operation, planned maintenance activities and in foreseeable situations where the controls may fail, and provide the information needed for selecting adequate PPE.

You should ensure that an adequate risk assessment has been carried out. The assessment should identify likely chemical, biological and physical hazards. It should evaluate the likely level and duration of exposure in routine operations and in cases where there may be accidental exposure. These items of information will be required to help select the most appropriate PPE. The risk assessment should be based on all practicable control requirements being in place and operating. It should also contain the information necessary to select adequate PPE for both routine and foreseeable failure situations.

21.2.2 Implement all feasible controls

If hazardous substances or processes must be used, all feasible means of reduction of risk must be considered before adopting PPE, e.g. to substitute the hazardous agent with a hazard-free or lower hazard material, enclose any process involving hazardous substances or to apply local ventilation to such processes etc. If there are additional controls that could be installed then these should be introduced and the risk assessment updated accordingly. The selection of PPE should be based on controlling the residual risk once feasible controls have been introduced. PPE may also have a role in controlling risk in the interim until other controls have been commissioned.

21.2.3 Identify who needs residual protection

From the assessment of likely risks and of the effectiveness of any procedures applied to reduce these risks, all persons still potentially at risk should be identified. Make sure you consider all people who may have unacceptable exposure, including maintenance staff, cleaners and others involved in irregular tasks.

21.2.4 Inform wearers of the consequences of exposure

To ensure that all workers fully utilise their PPE, they should be fully aware of the risks to their health in the workplace and the potential consequences if these risks are not adequately controlled. If the correct use of PPE involves inconvenience or discomfort it is important to ensure that all PPE wearers have a perception of the risks to which they are exposed and of the level of protection the PPE can reliably achieve when properly worn. It is important to ensure that the information provided complies with the requirements of Regulation 12 of the Control of Substances Hazardous to Health (COSHH) regulations or other appropriate legislation.

21.2.5 Select PPE adequate to control residual exposure

PPE should be selected to reduce any risks to acceptable levels; e.g. in the case of airborne hazardous substances, exposure levels inside the respirator facepiece should be reduced to below any occupational exposure limit (e.g. the WEL in Britain). For any substances classified as a carcinogen, mutagen or asthmagen then it is prudent to ensure that the ultimate exposure is well below the limit value; e.g. a tenth or less is a good target. If manufacturers cannot supply workplace data or written assurance as to the level of performance that can realistically be achieved in real workplaces, their PPE should not be used.

The effectiveness of respiratory protection is indicated by the assigned protection factor (APF), which is an indication of the minimum level of relative protection that might be expected by workers properly wearing the device. Figure 21.1 shows a range of respiratory protection and Table 21.1 shows the APF for the various types of RPE. For example, a respirator with an APF of 4 should reduce a worker's exposure by at least a factor of 4, i.e. to one-quarter of the exposure level outside the mask. There are four levels of APF that are generally used in the Britain: 4, 10, 20 and 40. Positive demand breathing apparatus providing fresh air has a much higher APF, but this type of PPE is much specialised in its application. Therefore the maximum exposure that someone should be allowed to experience while wearing respiratory protection should be 40 times the occupational exposure limit.

Someone asked to clean a duct containing vanadium pentoxide (WEL 8 h TWA = 0.05 mg m^{-3}) has an estimated maximum exposure level of 0.4 mg m^{-3}, averaged over a whole work shift, will require a respirator or breathing apparatus to complete their tasks. The required protection factor (PF) is estimated:

$$PF = \frac{E}{OEL}$$

where E is the exposure averaged over either 8 h or 15 min, and OEL is the limit value over the same averaging period.

$$PF = \frac{0.4}{0.05} = 80$$

None of the available devices is suitable and meets this requirement, and it is inappropriate to recommend self-contained positive demand breathing apparatus. It is therefore necessary to review the proposed work methods to improve the controls. Introducing local ventilation to extract air through the duct away from the worker and providing a high-efficiency vacuum cleaner rather than a brush might reduce exposure by about a factor of 10, which would mean that a the required protection factor would be 8. Because of the toxicity of vanadium pentoxide, we would still recommend using equipment with a higher AFP than the minimum, e.g. using a powered helmet respirator with an APF of 40, along with other carefully planned controls including impervious protective clothing, gloves. The work should also be done at times when there is minimal opportunity for others to be exposed.

21.2.6 Involve wearers in the PPE selection process

As many types of PPE impose some discomfort on the wearer to achieve adequate fit, wearers should be fully involved in the PPE selection process to

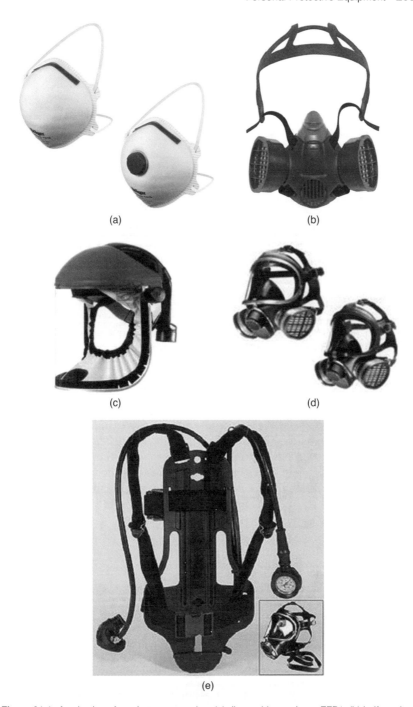

Figure 21.1 A selection of respiratory protection: (a) disposable respirator FFP1; (b) half-mask respirator; (c) powered hood TH2; (d) full facepiece respirator; (e) full mask breathing apparatus. (© Draeger Safety UK Ltd. Reproduced with permission.)

Table 21.1 Assigned protection factors for a selection of RPE

RPE type	APF
Filtering facepiece respirator (FFP1)	
Rubber half-mask with P1 filter	4
Filtering facepiece respirator (FFP2)	
Half or full-facepiece respirators with P2 filters	10
Powered hoods (TH1)	
Filtering facepiece respirator (FFP3)	
Half or full-facepiece respirators with P3 filters)	20
Powered hoods (TH2)	
Full-facepiece respirator with P3 filter	
Powered hoods or blouses (TH3)	
Constant flow airline hoods, blasting helmets, or full masks breathing apparatus)	40
Self-contained negative pressure demand valve breathing apparatus	

Note: Assigned protection factors in the United States and other parts of the world are different from those shown in the table. Make sure that the APF quoted by the supplier is relevant to your circumstances.

ensure that the equipment does not impose unacceptable discomfort and to help give the wearers 'ownership' of the PPE programme. It is not necessary to consult every individual in the selection process but rather that the workforce has been adequately consulted.

21.2.7 Match PPE to each individual wearer

Even in a small workforce there may be large differences in the physical characteristics of PPE wearers. Because PPE that fits one person may not fit another: e.g. a respirator that correctly fits a large male might not correctly fit a petite female, it is essential that each individual is provided with equipment that suits them. Although no one would consider it sensible to buy safety shoes in only one size, many employers appear to consider that one size of respirator, earmuff or gloves can correctly fit all wearers.

Given the range of differences in body sizes in a typical workforce, employers should ensure that the equipment provided adequately fits all those required to wear them. It might be necessary to provide a range of equipment of different shapes and sizes to ensure that all potential wearers can be adequately protected. Suppliers should be consulted for guidance on selection and to provide test data demonstrating that the PPE provides wearers with adequate protection. Note that most items of PPE are required to be either CE certified or to meet National Standards and that the tests involved in such certification or testing are generally defined or interpreted to involve mainly test subjects with a limited range of body sizes.

For PPE that imposes significant stress on the wearer, e.g. heavy chemical protective suits that can cause heat strain, or breathing apparatus that may weigh up to 18 kg or which requires the wearer to breathe pure oxygen, it may be necessary to ensure that only medically fit and suitable persons will be required to wear the equipment. In such cases you must consult an occupational physician for guidance.

21.2.8 Carry out objective fit tests of RPE

Current British guidance requires that all persons provided with RPE as a means of the employer complying with their legal duties undergo suitable fit tests with their RPE. Fit testing can range from qualitative tests using for example substances with a bitter or sweet taste, or quantitative tests using measurements of the difference in particle concentrations inside and outside the mask (Figure 21.2). Qualitative tests will only identify gross misfits between the RPE and the wearer. The results from any fit test should not be taken as evidence that the RPE fits the wearer or as any indication of likely protection in the workplace. Some RPE suppliers provide fit tests as part of a 'package', although you may wish to ensure that fit tests are carried out by an independent agency or by your own organisation.

21.2.9 Ensure that PPE does not exacerbate or create risks

Some types of PPE can exacerbate or create risks. For example, eye protectors or full-facepiece respirators can affect the field of vision, hearing defenders can reduce the ability to hear warning signals or the approach of vehicles, chemical-protective clothing can reduce the body's ability to lose metabolic heat. If the required PPE encloses a significant proportion of the body, for example torso, head and face, the possibility of the wearer being at risk due to thermal strain should be addressed and action taken if harmful levels of thermal strain are likely.

If wearers perceive that the consequences of such potential risks are more severe than the risks that the PPE is intended to protect against then they may refuse to wear the PPE. For example, coalminers traditionally refused to wear hearing defenders because they needed to hear the 'strata creak' to warn of potential roof collapse. The risk from an accidental roof fall was perceived to be more serious than the hearing loss risk from noise.

Care should be taken to ensure that any risks likely to be created by PPE are fully investigated and reduced to acceptable levels. Where some residual risk remains, action should be taken to minimize the risk created by the PPE at source. For example, if hearing defenders are used where moving vehicles may be present, the vehicles should be fitted with warning lights so that realization of the approach of the vehicles does not rely on aural warning.

For PPE intended to prevent eye or skin exposure the manufacturer should be able to provide guidance on maximum wear periods for foreseeable conditions of use and the supplier should be consulted to provide the relevant information. Equipment should only be purchased from manufacturers who are able to supply such information. In some cases, the PPE has caused its own unintended health problems, for example in the past some disposable respirators were identified that released fine glass fibres from the filter material

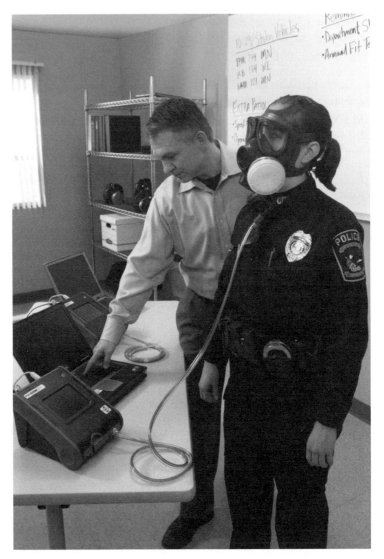

Figure 21.2 Face-fit testing kit – PortaCount. (© TSI Instruments Ltd. Reproduced with permission.)

into the wearer's breathing zone and in some cases disposable latex rubber gloves containing powder-released proteins that caused skin sensitisation in the wearers. Generally when such problems are identified the equipment is withdrawn from the market.

21.2.10 Ensure PPE are mutually compatible
Where two or more types of PPE are to be worn simultaneously, the different types of PPE can interact to reduce the protection provided by one or both

items. For example, for safety helmets worn with full-facepiece respirators, the facepiece can force the safety helmet to tip backwards. Other examples of potentially adverse interactions are respirators worn together with eye protectors where the respirator can prevent the correct fitting of the eye protectors and lead to misting up of inside surfaces, or eye protectors worn with earmuffs where the legs of the eye protectors can prevent a good seal between the head and the muff. In such situations it is essential that each item of PPE provides the required level of protection without affecting the effectiveness of any other PPE. Care must therefore be taken when selecting PPE for such situations to ensure that all equipment that may have to be worn together are mutually compatible.

While it is important to select PPE that do not individually cause unacceptable discomfort, it should be appreciated that wearing two or more items of PPE together can result in previously 'comfortable' equipment being considered 'uncomfortable'. Care must therefore be taken to ensure that the overall ensemble is acceptable to the wearers. The user should seek guidance from the supplier about equipment compatibility, e.g. ask what type of safety helmet can be worn together with his respirator. While it may be difficult for individual users to ensure mutual compatibility where different companies manufacture various items of PPE, it may be simpler to buy equipment made by the same manufacturer since they are required to be able to supply information regarding their mutual equipment compatibility.

21.2.11 Train wearers in the correct use of their PPE

Wearers and their supervisors should be thoroughly trained in how to fit the PPE correctly, how to assess whether the equipment is correctly fitted, how to inspect the PPE to ensure that it has been correctly manufactured and assembled, and, for reusable equipment, whether it has been adequately cleaned and maintained.

The potential consequences of PPE failure should be reflected in the thoroughness of the training, i.e. the greater the risk, the more thorough the training needs to be. One aspect of training is to convince wearers that the equipment provided would protect them. Generating such conviction is generally most easily achieved by practical training that allows the wearer to assess how well the PPE can perform when fitted and worn correctly. Where possible the training should involve practical sessions by using suitable training tools, e.g. where the wearers carry out representative tasks for appropriate time periods. Videos can be a useful 'second best'.

Training should cover the correct use of PPE ensembles, e.g. for RPE and protective clothing ensembles, to fit the RPE first, not to wear the RPE facepiece or head harness over the hood of protective clothing and to remove RPE last after completing all required decontamination procedures. Wearers of RPE should be aware that correct fit may depend on there being no facial hair which can lie between the facepiece and their face and that stubble can be more detrimental to good fit than a beard. Employees should therefore be aware that being 'clean-shaven' means having shaved immediately before the start of each shift during which RPE might have to be worn and possibly shaving again during the shift if they have heavy beard growth.

For highly complex PPE that may be used in situations of acute risk, e.g. breathing apparatus, manufacturers often offer training courses for wearers and for maintenance and inspection staff.

21.2.12 Supervise wearers to ensure correct use of PPE

Supervision should be provided to ensure that PPE is correctly worn at all times when wearers may potentially be at risk, that wearers are correctly prepared for wearing their PPE and that the correct personal decontamination procedures are followed where necessary. The overall effectiveness of any PPE programme can be critically dependent on the actions of workplace supervisors who are close enough to the wearers to actively enforce correct usage of PPE.

Supervisors should be trained in how to ensure that wearers are likely to be able to fit their PPE correctly, e.g. to ensure that RPE wearers are clean-shaven or that wearers of hearing protectors do not have hairstyles that might prevent earmuffs sealing adequately to the sides of the head. Maintenance and inspection staff should be trained in the relevant procedures with particular emphasis being given to ensuring that they are able to carry out such tasks without placing themselves at risk from contamination on the PPE, e.g. when cleaning PPE that may be contaminated with asbestos or isocyanates.

The responsibilities and authority of supervisors within the PPE programme should be specified in the supervisors' job descriptions so that they are fully aware of their role and that their health and safety duties take precedence over production. Leading by example is important – supervisors and other management staff should wear PPE properly whenever in the controlled area, even if only for a short visit.

21.2.13 Maintain PPE in efficient and hygienic condition

Reusable PPE will need to be cleaned, serviced and maintained, both to ensure the ongoing efficiency of the equipment and to ensure that the wearer is not exposed to contamination caused by poorly cleaned equipment. Many wearers will understandably be unwilling to fit into obviously dirty or faulty equipment. In setting up a PPE programme, the persons responsible should ask themselves, 'would I be prepared to wear the equipment provided?'

The legal duty to maintain equipment is imposed on the employer. The employer cannot delegate such a responsibility unless the person to whom the responsibility is delegated is 'competent'. Even where competent persons are available, the employer still has the responsibility to ensure that they carry out their duties in a competent manner.

Personnel carrying out maintenance should be trained in the tasks they are to undertake, in the identification of any risks that may arise during such work and in the use of any PPE necessary to protect themselves during such work.

21.2.14 Inspect PPE to ensure it is correctly maintained

Regular inspection and testing of serviced PPE enables the employer to ensure that the equipment is complete and is in good condition. For example, the COSHH regulations requires that, for other than disposable RPE, the employer shall ensure that thorough examination and, where appropriate, testing of the equipment shall be carried out at suitable intervals.

21.2.15 Provide suitable storage facilities for PPE

Legislation requires that PPE should generally be properly stored in a well-defined place. This is not an aspect that an employer should overlook and it is part of ensuring that the equipment that is provided is clean and serviceable. Separate segregated storage of clean and contaminated equipment is important.

21.2.16 Record maintenance and inspection data

Although there is no legal duty to record maintenance data, there is a legal duty to record inspections. Maintenance data provide the employer with a means of checking if all those who should wear PPE actually do so and to ensure that those who do not wear PPE are identified so that corrective action can be taken. The maintenance and inspection records can also provide employers with 'proof' that their legal duties to maintain and inspect relevant equipment have been met.

21.2.17 Monitor programme to ensure its continuing effectiveness

As with any intervention programme, it is generally inadequate to put a system into operation and assume that it will continue to function adequately without any further action. It is therefore prudent to routinely check the operation of the programme, to retrain and 're-indoctrinate' all personnel involved at suitable intervals and to take any remedial action that may be required.

A senior named individual with the necessary authority to ensure compliance should be appointed to manage the continuing effectiveness of the PPE programme.

21.3 Face-fit testing using a particle counter

21.3.1 Aim

The aim of this measurement is to fit-test workers wearing respiratory protective equipment with an APF of 10 or more by using a particle counting device. The method does not work with equipment with low APF because it relies on the difference in the concentration of ambient particles inside and outside the mask and the assumption that the particles inside the mask arrived there through a leak between the face and the mask. For equipment with a low level of protection this assumption does not hold since a proportion of particles (perhaps 5% of the outside aerosol) will have passed through the respirator filter. There is really just one company (TSI Inc) marketing equipment to undertake these tests and they provide guidance on the procedure on their website (www.tsi.com).

21.3.2 Equipment required

A TSI PortaCount Plus and N95-companion, which supplements the ambient particles and is essential for devices with an APF of 10 (Figure 21.1) is required. A suitable personal computer to run the provided software program is also required. Tests should be carried out in a quiet room with a table and chairs – the room volume should be less than about 100 m^3 to ensure there is sufficient ambient airborne particulate.

21.3.3 Method

1. Ensure that respirator wearers are trained and know how to properly fit the respirator they have been assigned. It is not necessary to check the training records – a few simple questions and observation of their ability to don the device is sufficient. Make an assessment of whether the mask is likely to fit the wearer – either by observation or using a qualitative fit test.
2. Arrange the equipment on the table and connect all of the tubing. Start the particle generator to boost the particle concentration for the test – it should have been running for about 15 min before the first test.
3. Perform the recommended start-up checks using the TSI FitPlus software package – zero check, particle check and max fit factor check.
4. Fit the sampling probe into the mask to enable the instrument to obtain a sample from the inside of the mask.
5. Ask the wearer to put on the N95-Companion sampling pendant and attach the tube to the mask.
6. Start the test sequence by using the FitPlus software – this also records the results, along with details of the wearer and respirator make and model. Wearers have to undertake a sequence of activities, e.g. normal breathing, touch toes, grimace, each lasting about 90 s.
7. Once the test is complete the results can be printed out and discussed with the wearer. If the test failed to meet the criteria then the tester should attempt to investigate the reason, e.g. poor fitting procedure, inappropriate size mask, and then retest if appropriate.

21.3.4 Possible problems

1. Wearers should not smoke for at least 1 h prior to the test – particles may continue to be exhaled throughout this time and these will bias the result.
2. Excessive moisture in the respirator facepiece or tubes to the monitor can cause water droplets to be measured, resulting in an erroneously low result.
3. In some environments, there may be insufficient ambient aerosol for the test – try using a smaller room if this is a problem.
4. Note that like all direct reading aerosol monitors the PortaCount requires regular (annual) maintenance and calibration checks.

References and further reading

Howie RM. (2005). Personal protective equipment. In: *Occupational Hygiene*, 3rd edition (Gardiner K, Harrington JM, eds). Oxford, UK: Blackwell Publishing.

BSI (2005). *Respiratory Protective Devices Recommendations for Selection, Use, Care and Maintenance Guidance Document-Supersedes BS 4275: 1997*. BS 529. London: British Standards Institution.

BSI (2001). *Selection, Use and Maintenance of Chemical Protective Clothing*. BS 7184. London: British Standards Institution.

HSE (2005). *Respiratory Protective Equipment at Work – A Practical Guide (HSG 53)*. Sudbury, UK: HSE Books.

HSE (2003). *Selection of Personal Protective Equipment: Chemicals Causing Harm Via Skin or Eye Contact (Control Guidance Sheet S101)*. Sudbury, UK: HSE Books. Available at http://www.hse.gov.uk/pubns/guidance/s101.pdf.

HSE (2003). *Selection of Personal Protective Equipment: Control Approach S Supplementary Advice (Control Guidance Sheet S102)*. Sudbury, UK: HSE Books. Available at http://www.hse.gov.uk/pubns/guidance/s102.pdf.

HSE (2006). *COSHH Essential: Respiratory Protective Equipment (RPE): UK Standard Assigned Protection Factor 4*. Sudbury, UK: HSE Books. Available at http://www.hse.gov.uk/pubns/guidance/rpe1.pdf.

HSE (2006). *COSHH Essential: Respiratory Protective Equipment (RPE): UK Standard Assigned Protection Factor 10*. Sudbury, UK: HSE Books. Available at http://www.hse.gov.uk/pubns/guidance/rpe2.pdf.

HSE (2006). *COSHH Essential: Respiratory Protective Equipment (RPE): UK Standard Assigned Protection Factor 20*. Sudbury, UK: HSE Books. Available at http://www.hse.gov.uk/pubns/guidance/rpe3.pdf.

HSE (2006). *COSHH Essential: Respiratory Protective Equipment (RPE): UK Standard Assigned Protection Factor 40*. Sudbury, UK: HSE Books. Available at http://www.hse.gov.uk/pubns/guidance/rpe4.pdf.

HSE (2006). *COSHH Essential: Respiratory Protective Equipment (RPE): Breathing Apparatus with UK Standard Assigned Protection Factor 40*. Sudbury, UK: HSE Books. Available at http://www.hse.gov.uk/pubns/guidance/rpe5.pdf.

HSE (2003). *Fit Testing of Respiratory Protective Equipment Facepieces. (OC 282/28)*. Sudbury, UK: HSE Books. Available at http://www.hse.gov.uk/foi/internalops/fod/oc/200-299/282_28.pdf.

Clayton MP, Bancroft B, Rajan B. (2002). A review of assigned protection factors of various types and classes of respiratory protective equipment with reference to their measured breathing resistances. *Annals of Occupational Hygiene* 46(6): 537–547. Available at http://annhyg.oxfordjournals.org/cgi/content/full/46/6/537.

Howie RM. (2005). Respiratory protective equipment. *Occupational and Environmental Medicine* 62: 423–428. Available at http://www.pubmedcentral.nih.gov/picrender.fcgi?artid=1741040&blobtype=pdf.

6 Risk Assessment and Risk Communication

22 Risk Assessment

22.1 Introduction

The need for risk assessment is central to many of the regulations in the Britain, including the Control of Substance Hazardous to Health (COSHH) regulations through to legislation covering noise, asbestos, lead, and the use of personal protective equipment.

The Management of Health and Safety at Work regulations state that all employers shall make a suitable and sufficient assessment of the following:

- Risks to the health and safety of their employees;
- Risks to the health and safety of persons not in their employment.

This assessment should:

- Be a systematic general examination;
- Identify and record the significant risks;
- Identify and prioritise the measures to comply with relevant legislation.

A competent risk assessment involves a number of discrete steps and the HSE guidance on the five steps to risk assessment available at http://www.hse.gov.uk/risk/fivesteps.htm provides an excellent overview of how to carry out a risk assessment. For hazardous substances it is recommended that risk assessments be completed for tasks or processes rather than by substance.

In performing a risk assessment for hazardous substances, it is useful to consider the following points:

- Identify all hazardous substances or agents likely to be used or generated in the task;
- Assess the likely levels of exposure to hazardous substances for the task;
- Identify all persons likely to be exposed to the hazardous substances;
- Assess whether the exposures are likely to cause harm to those exposed;
- If the exposures are likely to cause harm, assess whether the use or generation of these materials can be eliminated or if they can be replaced by less hazardous substances;
- If elimination or replacement cannot be used to reduce the risks then define the control measures necessary to reduce the harm to socially acceptable levels;

- Define the maintenance programme necessary to ensure that the control measures are maintained to provide effective performance;
- Define the information and instruction required to ensure that all relevant personnel are fully aware of the hazards and risks associated with the task;
- Define the training and supervision necessary to ensure that the control measures are fully implemented;
- Define the monitoring and health surveillance programmes necessary to ensure that the control measures are and continue to successfully reduce the harm to acceptable levels;
- Define the audit system necessary to ensure long-term success of the control measures.

In this chapter, we outline how monitoring of hazardous substances can be effectively integrated into the risk assessment process. A similar approach could be used for other harmful agents.

22.2 Identify all hazardous substances or agents

All 'substances' used in the workplace should be identified, noting the hazardous substances, including materials ranging from wood dust or mineral dusts through to cleaning and packaging materials. For all substances bought from external suppliers, a safety data sheet (SDS) should be obtained to enable the hazardous substances to be identified. The supplier has a legal duty to provide a SDS so this should be a straightforward step. In a work process, a number of substances may be reacted to form new substances. In these cases it will be necessary to identify the reaction products and by-products under planned operating conditions and any other products that could be generated under foreseeable failure situations. Useful information regarding the hazards associated with such substances can be obtained from information published by the HSE, trade associations, the technical literature – such as the ILO Encyclopaedia of Occupational Health and Safety, 'Hawley's Condensed Chemical Dictionary', 'Kirk-Othmer Encyclopaedia of Chemical Technology', Sax's 'Dangerous Properties of Industrial Materials', 'Patty's Industrial Hygiene and Toxicology'; or websites – such as MEDLINE.

Once you have an inventory of the hazardous substances associated with the task to be assessed you should identify those of concern, either because they are the predominant substances present or because they have relatively low occupational exposure limits (OELs) and are present in moderate amounts.

22.3 Identify the likely levels of exposure

It is necessary to assess the intensity and duration of exposure to the hazard and determine whether these exposures are likely to exceed the relevant OEL. Exposure assessments should include all foreseeable failure situations, all planned and emergency maintenance activities, all activities likely to be carried out by contractors working on the employer's premises and any potential releases into the environment.

Likely exposure levels can be assessed in several ways. For example, it is possible to use your judgement based on previous experience in similar situations or using simple common sense. If a worker is involved in handling a pharmaceutical agent in milligram quantities inside a fume cupboard then it is not unreasonable to assume that the level of inhalation exposure will be low. In contrast, in a process where the same agent is used in tonne quantities in a small plant with inadequate ventilation it might be reasonable to assume the level of exposure would be high.

For substances with good warning properties, e.g. substances whose odour detection thresholds or irritation thresholds do not exceed about 10% of the current British workplace exposure limits (WELs), subjective responses may give useful indications about exposure levels. Information on such warning properties can be obtained from publications such as Sax, Patty or Verschueren or websites such as MEDLINE.

It is also possible to use a variety of computer models to estimate exposure levels. We think the best is one known as Stoffenmanager, which was developed by a group of Dutch researchers to assists smaller organisations in managing risks of hazardous substances at work. The software tool provides support in performing a risk assessment, both for inhalation and dermal exposure. It also guides the user in selecting control measures that can form the basis for an action plan. Fortunately, Stoffenmanager is available in an English language version at www.stoffenmanager.nl (access is free once you register) and there is also a scientific paper describing the development of the tool (Tielemans et al., 2008).

Stoffenmanager assesses risks on the basis of hazards of substances or products combined with exposure estimates. There are two models incorporated into the software:

- One model that classifies hazards;
- A second model to estimate exposure.

There are some limitations to the application of Stoffenmanager, mainly because it relies on the R-phrase allocated to a product as part of a supplier's obligation under the regulations governing the supply of chemicals (you can find the R-phrase on the SDS, but note that the system of 'R-phrases' will change with the introduction of the Globally Harmonised System (GHS) for classifying and labelling chemicals). Therefore, it cannot be used with materials such as medicines, radioactive substances or waste products. The exposure model is also limited to supplied chemicals and cannot be used for chemicals that are formed during the process, such as diesel exhaust emissions or solder fumes. Also, the exposure assessments are limited to processes carried out at room temperature.

Stoffenmanager has the following modules:

- Basic information collection where you can enter your company data, departments and product data;
- Risk assessment where you can provide answers to a series of questions about the work situation to be evaluated;
- A control measures module to provide advice about measures to eliminate or control risk;
- An action plan module for progressing necessary steps for control.

There are other simple tools available for exposure or risk assessment for chemicals – often referred to as 'control banding' models. In Britain, the HSE developed 'COSHH Essentials', which is intended to fill a similar role to Stoffenmanager. Stoffenmanager has advantages over COSHH Essentials because the exposure model is more transparent in the former; i.e. it provides an estimate of exposure level not just advice about the appropriate controls that should be in place. COSHH Essentials is available at www.COSHH-Essentials.org.uk.

Clearly, relevant monitoring data can make a major contribution to deciding the level of exposure in a particular task or process. However, you should beware of making firm conclusions on the basis of a small number of measurements alone; remember that exposure may vary considerably from one worker to another and from one day to the next. It is far better to first make an assessment of the likely exposure by using your judgement or an exposure model. If you then make any measurements of the exposure level in the task they may confirm your original conclusion, in which case you have a much stronger basis for believing that the first conclusion about the exposure was correct. However, if the measurements contradict your prior view then you will need to make further enquiries or more measurements to come to a clear decision about the exposure associated with the task. There is a formal statistical process than can help with this type of decision making – it is Bayesian statistics and these techniques are increasingly being used by occupational hygienists.

One last point about exposure assessment, it is generally the case that we want to ensure that the exposure of almost everyone involved with a task will be acceptable and so for the exposure assessment we really want to estimate an upper percentile of the distribution of exposure, for example the 90th percentile such that nine out of ten workers involved with the task will have exposure below the value. Stoffenmanager attempts to estimate an upper percentile of the exposure distribution and you can estimate the 90th percentile of the exposure distribution from a set of measurements with simple statistics (see Chapter 7).

22.4 Identify all persons likely to be exposed

Identify all workers who are likely to be exposed to the substances of concern used in the task or process, how often they are exposed and for how long.

Ensure that the assessment identifies any maintenance and supervisory personnel who are likely to work on the process or work with equipment from the process.

It is also important to identify if any of the exposed persons are likely to be especially vulnerable, e.g. those sensitised to the substances, already exhibiting damage from substances or agents present used in the task – it would be imprudent to expose someone suffering with a respiratory disease to high dust levels.

22.5 Assess whether the exposures are likely to cause harm

Identify the likely consequences of exposure and whether such effects are minor or major, acute or chronic or can result from short-term or long-term exposures. This can be achieved by comparing the exposure data with the relevant exposure limit and examining any assigned R-phrases. It is also important to appreciate that the risk phrases are probably more correctly thought of as 'hazard phrases' and do not give any indication of the relative potential of the substances to cause harm.

If it is likely that substances may be rendered airborne, it is considered prudent to regard any substances assigned risk phrase R43 'May cause sensitisation by skin contact' as being potential asthmagens and treat them as having been assigned risk phrase R42 'May cause sensitisation by inhalation' and, if possible, to avoid the use of substances assigned risk phrase R40 'Limited evidence of a carcinogenic effect', as there is some suggestive evidence that the substance may cause cancer.

If you have estimated the level of exposure as the 90th percentile of the exposure distribution then comparing this value with the WEL will tell you whether most people involved with the task will have exposure below the limit. This should be sufficient to comply with the law.

However, given the high level of variability of personal monitoring results, the general long-term downward trend in OELs and the increasing numbers of substances identified to be carcinogens, mutagens or asthmagens over the years (e.g. the number of substances assigned R42 or R42/43 increased from 11 in Approved Supply List 1 of 1993 to 109 in Approved Supply List 7 of 2002), it may be prudent to minimise exposures to carcinogens, mutagens or asthmagens as far as possible, i.e. so that the highest measured exposures (or the 90th percentile) are not more than about 25% of the current WEL, and for all other substances are not more than the current WEL.

22.6 Consider elimination or substitution

If it is technically feasible to eliminate hazardous substances or agents, you should consider eliminating them. If they cannot be eliminated but can be obtained in a less hazardous form, e.g. if substances can be obtained as a solution rather than as a dry dust or can be obtained as a prepolymer rather than as a monomer, such less hazardous forms should be used, if practicable. If hazardous substances can be replaced by lower hazard or non-hazardous substances or their emissions reduced by adopting alternative processes, such changes should be made, so far as is technically feasible. However, it is important to ensure that replacement substances or processes do not introduce new hazards, e.g. ensure that the flash point of replacement substances are not significantly lower than those of the original substances (increasing the fire hazard) or that replacement of a welding process by an adhesive process does not introduce a respiratory or skin sensitisation risk.

22.7 Define additional control measures necessary to reduce the harm to acceptable levels

To identify the necessary control measures it is necessary to address the following:

- The methods of work;
- The circumstances and foreseeable deviations from normal procedure;
- The frequency of likely exposure;
- Whether exposures result from regular, planned or infrequent operations;
- The risks associated with maintenance activities.

Care should be taken to ensure that possible accidental exposures by inhalation or skin contact are considered. These include spillages, activities such as cleaning and maintenance that can disturb deposited material thereby making them airborne again or cause potential exposure to, or contact with, substances which are normally completely contained, entry into confined spaces that contain hazardous substances or which may be deficient in oxygen, and wearing contaminated clothing. Rules should be set that prohibit eating, drinking, smoking, applying cosmetics or similar, and discourage behaviour traits such as nail biting, to prevent substances hazardous to health entering the body by inadvertent ingestion.

The risk assessment should also include an examination of the current control measures.

Consider and define the preventative and/or control measures that will reduce risks to acceptable levels.

Once the current control measures have been assessed, any further measures that are deemed to be required must be listed. This may require a cost-analysis and the various jobs may have to be prioritised in terms of risk reduction. Control measures should be considered in terms of the advice provided in the chapter on control: i.e. in the order of total enclosure; partial enclosure with effective extract ventilation; effective extract ventilation; segregation of the worker from the process; general ventilation; good housekeeping; and the provision of personal protective equipment.

References and further reading

Tielemans E, Noy D, Schinkel J, Heussen H, Van Der Schaaf D, West J, Fransman W. (2008). Stoffenmanager exposure model: development of a quantitative algorithm. *Annals of Occupational Hygiene* 52(6): 443–454.

American Conference of Governmental Industrial Hygienists. *Documentation of the Threshold Limit Values and Biological Exposure Indices*. Cincinnati, OH: ACGIH. (Up to date documentation for relevant substances or agents can be purchased online from the ACGIH website – www.acgih.org.)

Encyclopedia of Occupational Health and Safety online in the ILO Safework website. www.ilo.org/safework_bookshelf/english/.

Handbook of Environmental Data on Organic Chemicals online. Available at www.knovel.com/web/portal/browse/display?_EXT_KNOVEL_DISPLAY_bookid=703.

Hawley's Condensed Chemical Dictionary online. Available at www.knovel.com/web/portal/basic_search/display?_EXT_KNOVEL_DISPLAY_bookid=704.

Kirk-Othmer (2004) *Encyclopedia of Chemical Technology* online. Available at www.mrw.interscience.wiley.com/emrw/0471238961/search.

Medline website: medlineplus.gov/.

Merck Index, 14th edition. Rahway, NJ: Merck Publishing Group.

National Institute of Occupational Safety and Health. *Pocket Guide to Chemical Hazards*. Pittsburgh, PA: NIOSH. Available free at www.cdc.gov/niosh/npg/.

Patty's Industrial Hygiene & Toxicology online. Available at mrw.interscience.wiley.com/emrw/9780471125471/home/.

Sax's Dangerous Properties of Industrial Materials online. Available at www3.interscience.wiley.com/cgi-bin/mrwhome/109802619/HOME.

23 Risk Communication

23.1 Introduction

In occupational hygiene we do not often make a quantitative assessment of risks in terms of the probability that someone in a group of workers will be affected by a disease. In most cases, we make assessments of exposure and then compare these data with some accepted limit value, for example the workplace exposure limit (WEL) in Britain. As we saw in the first section of this book, this approach is based on the simple premise that there is a close relationship between exposure and the eventual risk of any disease in an individual; and so controlling exposure below a specified level will actually control the risk below some important threshold.

The main part of the risk communication in occupational hygiene is about getting the message over about judgement of the quantitative level of risk on the basis of exposure measurements or a systematic risk assessment. However, it is important to realise that individual workers and managers may have very different perceptions of the risks and if these are not taken into account in the communication process then the real message may be lost. A person's perception of the risks from exposure to hazards at work may be as much determined by an 'emotional' response as factual information available to them.

23.2 Risk perception

There are four possible scenarios that we may encounter in risk communication, which are illustrated in Table 23.1. In this example, we consider the risks to be high if the exposures are above the limit value.

The reasons for the discrepancies between perception and reality, i.e. the 'calm down' and the 'watch out' scenarios, are dependent on many factors. For example, agents that are known to cause cancer or some other 'dreaded' consequence are generally perceived to have higher risks associated with them compared with other materials. Situations where there is no choice about whether an individual is exposed are generally seen as more risky than comparable situations that the person accepts voluntarily; for example working with a chemical versus using the same chemical in a hobby at home. Also, in workplaces where there is a pungent smell from a chemical the perception of risk may also be greater than in situations where there is no offensive odour from chemicals used.

Table 23.1 Risk and risk perception scenarios.*

'Business as usual'	**'Watch out'**
Risk is low and both the workers and managers agree that this is the case	Actual level of risk is high but the worker/manager perceives the risks to be low
'Calm down'	**'Crisis'**
Actual level of risk is low but the worker/manager perceives the risk to be high	The risk is high and both the workers and managers agree that the risk is high

*Adapted from 'Four Kinds of Risk Communication' by Peter M. Sandman. Available at http://www.psandman.com/col/4kind-1.htm.

Table 23.2 contains circumstances that can either increase or decrease the perception of risk.

23.3 Trust

Probably the most important factor in achieving effective risk communication is 'trust'. Trust is the foundation of the relationship between two people or between people and organisations. It has been shown that most workers in Britain have a fairly high level of trust in Health and Safety Executive inspectors because of the perceived altruistic role of their organisation. There is much less trust in other groups in society, for example in most surveys to assess trust, tabloid journalists and politicians generally score low.

It takes a great deal of effort to develop trust; there must be truth, openness, respect for and tolerance of the opinions of others, a commitment to improve the lot of others, keeping your word and avoiding harming others by either your actions or omissions. Trust is only gained through consistent efforts over a period of time, but one ill-thought action or word can destroy the relationship.

Table 23.2 Factors that either increase or decrease the acceptability of risks.

Risks are more acceptable if they are...	*Risks will be less acceptable if they are...*
Accepted voluntarily	Imposed by someone else such as an employer
Under the individual's control	Controlled by others
For the benefit of everyone	Of little or no benefit to anyone
Distributed fairly amongst the population	Unfairly affect some people and not others
Natural	Man made
Statistical, i.e. some unidentified people in the population are affected	Catastrophic for some identified people
Come from a trusted source	Come from some distrusted source
Familiar	Unusual or exotic
Affect only adults	Affect children

Some simple rules to help gain trust:

- Work with workers, managers and other stakeholders as a partner to provide reliable information, to dispel disinformation and to allay misplaced fears and concerns.
- Appreciate the concerns of your stakeholders and do not try to baffle them with science or statistics. Be sensitive to people's worries and treat people with respect.
- Be honest and open. Never mislead people or omit important information from your communications.
- Work with other credible information providers to give a consistent coherent message.

If you are in a situation where people need to 'calm down' then it is inevitable that there will be a certain amount of hostility. Do not take it personally and certainly do not ignore it because that is a recipe for further problems and erosion of trust. Here are some simple rules for dealing with hostility:

- Acknowledge the existence of the hostility;
- Listen to what is said and try to understand the perspective of the person concerned;
- Don't lose your temper and try not to get overanxious;
- Think about the types of questions you might get from a hostile group of workers and prepare your answers.

If you are in a 'watch out' situation then there is a need to increase awareness of the risks but not cause alarm or panic. This situation might best be addressed by some form of training or information provision from someone knowledgeable about the true level of risk present.

23.4 Communication

It is important to provide as much information as possible to help the individual come to a properly informed judgement about the real risks in a particular situation. For example, knowing that exposure to benzene can cause leukaemia can cause a panic-type reaction for people who have unknowingly been working with a mixture containing benzene, but being aware that the benzene is only present in trace quantities and the exposures are actually very low can be reassuring – particularly as it is known that benzene is not a particularly potent carcinogen.

It is important to choose your words carefully, no matter whether you are writing a note for the managing director or speaking to a group of workers. First, it is a good idea to try to avoid unnecessary jargon or if this is not possible to explain what it means when you first use it. There are some specific words that you should also consider carefully before uttering because the meaning may be different in common usage from the technical meaning. For example, in the chapter on risk assessment, we discussed whether or not

Table 23.3   Categorisation of risks.

Risk in any 1 year	Description	Example
>1 in 100	High	Death from any cause
1 in 100 to 1 in 1000	Moderate	
1 in 1000 to 1 in 10000	Low	Death from a road accident
1 in 10000 to 1 in 100,000	Very low	
1 in 100,000 to 1 in 1,000,000	Minimal	Death from murder
<1 in 1,000,000	Negligible	Death from a lightning strike

risks were 'acceptable', however saying to workers or residents near an industrial plant that some risk is 'acceptable' or 'insignificant' can give the impression that you do not really understand the importance of the situation; 'the risks may be acceptable to you but we have to work there every day'. Using the word 'significant' in a statistical sense may also be confusing for a non-technical audience. For example, a statistician may say the association between exposure to solvent vapours and the risk of headaches is 'not significant' and mean that the observation that higher solvent levels linked to higher incidence of headaches could have occurred by chance, but a lay person might just think that she/he is saying that the association is unimportant.

Some other potential misinterpretations include the following:

Saying, 'there is anecdotal evidence that exposure to chemical X causes birth defects' may be heard as, 'I have a lot of funny stories about people whose kids were made ill because they worked with this stuff'.

'It's safe to be exposed to 5 mg m^{-3} of cement dust; may be mistakenly understood as, 'cement dust is harmless'.

'We have used assumptions that give a conservative estimate of the risks' will almost certainly be understood as, 'they deliberately underestimated the risks we are experiencing'.

Remember it is sometimes difficult for people to grasp the concept of risk and very few people have a clear sense of the magnitude of risks in terms of the chance of something bad happening. Careful choice of words to describe risks can help. Table 23.3 shows six broad ranges of risk and corresponding descriptors and examples of situations within these categories.

For example, in any 1 year in a group of 100 people selected from the general population you might expect one to die from some cause. This is a 'high' risk. However, in the whole of Britain in the same year there will only be about five people who die from a lightning strike (about a 1 in 10,000,000 chance).

23.5   An example of quantitative risk assessment to aid risk communication

Of course in occupational hygiene we do not usually have information about the magnitude of the risk in terms of the probability of someone contracting a disease. However, it is possible to source this sort of information and it can help in discussing people's concerns about risk in specific circumstances. Here is an example that may help illustrate this. In the general population, about 15% of people die from lung cancer (lifetime risk 15 in 100), which is mostly due to cigarette smoking but there are a number of occupational carcinogens that are also known to cause lung cancer e.g. hexavalent chromium (Cr VI). For most occupational carcinogens, it is common to assume that there is no threshold for the exposure–response relationship, and so we expect that any exposure to Cr VI increases the risk. According to a World Health Organisation (WHO) analysis of the relevant epidemiological studies (WHO Air Quality Guidelines: http://www.euro.who.int/air/activities/20050223_4) the unit relative risk for lung cancer is about 4 in a 100 per $\mu g \ m^{-3}$ exposure to Cr VI over a whole lifetime (i.e. 24 h day^{-1}, 365 days year^{-1}, for 70 years). If this exposure was all received during work over 40 years this would correspond to about 8 $\mu g \ m^{-3}$ as an 8 h average in a workplace.

To convert the exposure for the lifetime unit risk to an exposure for the corresponding 'occupational' exposure for 40 years exposure we have used the following calculation, assuming 240 working days year^{-1}:

$$E_{work} = E_{lifetime} \times 24/8 \times 365/240 \times 70/40 = E_{lifetime} \times 8$$

In other words, a 40-year working lifetime is an eighth of the total time between being born and reaching your 70th birthday. If someone was exposed to 0.02 mg m^{-3} on average every day, 24 h day^{-1} then the equivalent exposure if all of that exposure was received at work would be 0.16 mg m^{-3}.

The unit risk for the workplace can then be calculated by dividing the lifetime unit risk (4 in 100) by eight, giving 5 in 1000.

Therefore, if we knew that a worker was being regularly exposed to about 10 $\mu g \ m^{-3}$ then they would have a working lifetime risk of (5 in 1000 multiplied by 10) 5 in 100 of dying from lung cancer, which we should describe as a 'high' risk. Someone exposed to about 1 $\mu g \ m^{-3}$ would have a risk of about 5 in 1000 (between 'moderate' and 'high'). So it is possible to use this information to explain the magnitude of their risk to a group of 100 workers regularly exposed to 1 $\mu g \ m^{-3}$ of Cr VI in their job. Assuming the group has a similar number of smokers to the national average then ultimately it is expected that about 15 of their number will die from lung cancer. For most the cause will be cigarette smoking but perhaps one person's cancer may be caused by the chromium exposure (the risk for exposure to 1 $\mu g \ m^{-3}$ is about 5 in 1000, which multiplied by the number of people at risk gives a predicted number of lung cancer cases of 0.5, i.e. a value fairly close to 1).

Information about unit risk for a range of chemical exposures can be found in the US Environmental Protection Agency IRIS website (www.epa.gov/iris/) and on the WHO Air Quality Guidelines website. One must be careful about using such information because it may have some limitations, particularly in relation to the range of exposures for which the unit risks are valid, but the limitations are discussed on the summary information provided by these resources.

The chromium exposure at 1 μg m^{-3} given in this example is much less than the current workplace exposure limit (50 μg m^{-3} in Britain), but there was still a moderate cancer risk at this level over 40 years. This underlines a very important point, that exposure below the workplace limits is not necessarily 'safe', and we should be careful about the terms that we use to describe results from monitoring. Exposure below a limit value is clearly in compliance with the law but may still have some associated risk. With this knowledge the workers can make more informed decisions about whether to request respiratory protection even if the exposure is below the limit or whether it might be best to quit smoking, which it can be explained will have a much bigger impact on the chance that the individual will die from lung cancer.

Armed with this information you are in a good position to help to discuss the risks with managers and workers. From your initial contact with the workplace it will be clear whether you are dealing with a 'watch out' or a 'crisis' type of situation, in our view it is probably more likely to be the former. In these circumstances you should carefully explain the cancer hazard from chromium exposure, the relatively low level of exposure present in the plant and that, if exposures continue at the current level, there is a chance that one of their numbers might eventually die from work-related lung cancer. The important thing to realize is that there is a considerable amount that can be done to reduce exposures and in most workplaces exposures decrease on average by about 5–10% each year, mostly as a consequence of improvements in process technology.

References and further reading

Bennett P, Calman K. (1999). *Risk Communication and Public Health.* Oxford, UK: Oxford University Press.

Calman KC. (2002). Communication of risk: choice, consent, and trust. *The Lancet* 360: 166–168. Available at http://www.thelancet.com/journals/lancet/article/PIIS0140-6736(02)09421-7/fulltext.

US Department of Health and Human Services (2002). *Communicating in a Crisis: Risk Communication Guidelines for Public Officials.* Rockville, MD: DHHS. Available at http://www.riskcommunication.samhsa.gov.

The Peter M. Sandman Risk Communication Website, containing a great deal of information about risk communication. http://www.psandman.com/.

Equipment Suppliers

3M United Kingdom PLC, 3M Centre, Cain Road, Bracknell, Berkshire RG12 8HT, United Kingdom, http://solutions.3m.com/wps/portal/3M/en_US/Oil-Gas/Home/Contact_Info/Global_Contact_Info/

ABLE Instruments & Controls Ltd, Cutbush Park, Danehill, Lower Earley, Reading, Berkshire RG6 4UT, United Kingdom, tel: +44(0)118 9311188, http://www.able.co.uk/

AIRFLOW Developments Ltd, Lancaster Road, Cressex Business Park, High Wycombe, Buckinghamshire HP12 3QP, United Kingdom, tel: +44(0)1494 525252, http://www.airflow.co.uk/

Berthold Technologies (U.K.) Ltd, Allied Business Centre, Coldharbour Lane, Harpenden, Herts AL5 4UT, United Kingdom, tel: +44(0)1582 761477, http://www.berthold.com/

BIRAL, PO Box 2, Portishead, Bristol BS20 7JB, United Kingdom, +44(0)1275 847787, http://www.biral.com/

Bruel & Kjaer UK Ltd, Bedford House, Rutherford Close, Stevenage, Hertfordshire SG1 2ND, United Kingdom, http://www.bksv.co.uk

Burkard Manufacturing Co. Limited, Woodcock Hill Industrial Estate, Rickmansworth, Hertfordshire WD3 1PJ, United Kingdom, tel: +44(0)1923 773134/5, http://www.burkard.co.uk/

Casella Measurement Ltd, Regent House, Wolseley Road, Kempston, Bedford MK42 7JY, United Kingdom, tel: +44(0)1234 844 100, http://www.casellacel.com/

Castle Group, Salter Road, Scarborough Business Park, Scarborough, North Yorkshire YO11 3UZ, United Kingdom, tel: +44(0)1723 584250, http://www.castlegroup.co.uk/

Cirrus Research Plc, Acoustic House, Bridlington Road, Hunmanby, North Yorkshire YO14 0PH, United Kingdom, tel: +44(0)1723 891655, http://www.cirrusresearch.co.uk/

Draeger Safety UK Ltd, Ullswater Close, Blyth Riverside Business Park, Blyth, Northumberland NE24 4RG, United Kingdom, tel: +44(0)1670 35 2891, http://www.draeger.co.uk/

ETS-Lindgren, Unit 4, Eastman Way, Pin Green Industrial Area, Stevenage, Hertfordshire SG1 4UH, United Kingdom, tel: +44(0)1438 730700, http://www.ets-lindgren.eu.com/

JS Holdings, Unit 6, Leyden Road, Stevenage, Hertfordshire SG1 2BW, United Kingdom, tel: +44(0)1438 316994, http://www.jsholdings.co.uk/

LOT-Oriel Ltd (for International Light), 1 Mole Business Park, Leatherhead, Surrey KT22 7BA, United Kingdom, tel: +44(0)1372 378822, http://www.lot-oriel.com/

Loxford Equipment Company Ltd, Wood Hall, Church Lane, Great Holland, Frinton-on-Sea, Essex CO13 0JS, United Kingdom, tel: +44(0)1255 851 555, http://www.loxford-equipment.co.uk/

Mirion Technologies, Inc, Bishop Ranch 8, 3000 Executive Parkway, Suite 220, San Ramon, CA 94583, USA, tel: +1(925)543 0806, http://www.mirion.com/index.php?p =locations#euro

Moldex-Metric AG & Co. KG, Unit 9, Glaisdale Point, Off Glaisdale Drive, Bilborough, GB-Nottingham NG8 4GP, United Kingdom, tel: +44(0)115 985 4288, http://www.moldex-europe.com/en/

Pulsar Instruments Plc, The Evron Centre, John Street, Filey, North Yorkshire YO14 9DW, United Kingdom, tel: +44(0)1723 518011, http://www.pulsarinstruments.com/

Quantitech Ltd, Unit 3, Old Wolverton Road, Milton Keynes MK12 5NP, United Kingdom, tel: +44(0)1908 227722, http://www.quantitech.co.uk/

RAE Systems UK, D5 Culham Innovation Centre, Culham Science Centre, Abingdon OX14 3DB, United Kingdom, tel: +44(0)1865 408368, http://www.raesystems.eu/

Shawcity Ltd, Unit 13, Pioneer Road, Faringdon, Oxfordshire SN7 7BU, United Kingdom, tel: +44(0)1367 246960, http://www.shawcity.co.uk

SKC Ltd, Unit 11, Sunrise Park, Higher Shaftesbury Road, Blandford Forum, Dorset DT11 8ST, United Kingdom, tel: +44(0)1258 480188, http://www.skcltd.com/

Thermo Fisher Scientific, Bath Road, Reading, Berkshire RG5 7PR, United Kingdom, tel: +44 7787 568038, http://www.thermo.com/

TSI Instruments Ltd, Stirling Road, Cressex Business Park, High Wycombe, Buckinghamshire HP12 3RT, United Kingdom, tel: +44(0)149 4 459200, http://www.tsiinc.co.uk

Chemical Analytical Services

Health & Safety Laboratory, Harpur Hill, Buxton, Derbyshire SK17 9JN, United Kingdom, tel: +44(0)1298 218099, http://www.hsl.gov.uk/

IOM Consulting, Research Avenue North, Riccarton, Edinburgh EH14 4AP, United Kingdom, tel: +44(0)870 850 5131, http://www.iom-world.org/

RPS Group Plc, Centurion Court, 85 Milton Park, Abingdon OX14 4RY, United Kingdom, tel: +44(0)1235 438 000, http://www.rpsgroup.com/

TES Bretby, Energy Services, PO Box 100, Bretby Business Park, Burton-upon-Trent DE15 0XD, United Kingdom, tel: +44(0)1283 554447, http://www.tes-bretby.co.uk/

Index

absorbed dose, 205–7
acceleration, 161–6, 169–70
accelerometer, 166–70
acetone vaporiser, 86
ACH, 27–8
acoustic pressure, 145
action values, noise, 147–8, 159–60
activated charcoal, 94–7, 102–4
activity emission potential, 26
acute
    exposure, 216–17
    health effects, 9, 63, 125, 221
adsorbent tubes, 42, 95–7, 102–4
Advanced REACH Tool, *see* ART
aerodynamic diameter – definition, 64–5
aerosol, 63–91, 111–22
aflatoxins, 114
air flow, 27, 189, 257–9
    measurement, 178–80, 237–41, 246–52
    natural air flow, 178, 183
air humidity, 175, 185–7
    sensitivity of measurements to, 80, 117,
        152
air pressure, 234, 242
    measurement, 235–7, 252–4
    static, 234, 239–40, 243–4
    velocity, 234, 239–41
air speed, *see also* air velocity, 234
air velocity, 234–59
    instrument calibration, 242
    instrumentation, 237–41
    low velocity measurement, 178–80
air-changes per hour, *see* ACH
ALARA, 206

ALI, 207
allergen, 115, 120–21, 137
alpha particles, 200, 202–3, 208
Anasorb adsorbent, 96
anemometer
    calibration of, *see* calibration –
        anemometer
    heated head, 238–9
    vane, 237–8, 246, 254–7
annual limits of intake of radionuclides, *see*
    ALI
APF, 262–4, 269–70
arc eye, *see* welders flash
arithmetic mean, 50, 250, 255–6
ART (Advanced REACH Tool), 55
asbestos fibres, 65–6, 74, 84–9
    control limits, 85, 88
    measurement of airborne concentration,
        84–8
assessment
    exposure, 18, 22–3, 129, 276–8
    risks to health, 8–12, 22–3, 31, 260, 275–81
    thermal risks, 185, 188–9
assigned protection factor (APF), *see* APF
atomic number, 199, 201–2

bacteria, 113–14, 118, 121
barometers, 242
barometric pressure, *see* air pressure
Bayesian statistics, 278
becquerels (Bq), 204
bellows pump, 106–7
beta particles, 203
bio-security, 112

bioaerosols, 262–4
biological hazards or biological agents, 14–17, 111–22
biological monitoring, 18–24, 36, 137
biological monitoring guidance values, *see* BMGV
biopersistence, 65
blanks – field or laboratory, 40, 58, 82, 103
BMGV (biological monitoring guidance values), 22
breakthrough, during vapour sampling, 97
breathing zone, 19–21, 68
bubblers, 95–6, 104–6

calibration
    anemometer, 242
    dust monitor, 75, 270
    light meter, 193
    rotameter, 40, 76–83
    sound level meter, 152–5, 157
    thermal equipment, 176
    vibration meter, 168–70
cancer, 285–7
    skin, 127, 216
candella (Cd), 191
carbon dioxide detection, *see* gas detection
carbon monoxide detection, *see* gas detection
centrifugal dust collector, 244
centrifugal sampler, 120
charcoal, *see* activated charcoal
Chartered Institute of Building Services Engineers (CIBSE) code, *see* CIBSE code
Chemical (Hazard, Information and Packaging for Supply) regulations – CHIP, 14, 127
chemical hazards or chemical agents, 4, 13–17, 61–110
Chromosorb adsorbent, 96
CIBSE code, 192, 196, 198
CIP-10 sampler, 72
clarity, 56
classified person – radiation, 209
clearance sampling, for asbestos, 85
clo, 186
coal dust, 72–3, 89
cold, 173–5, 186–90

colony forming units (CFU), 118
colorimetric detector tubes, 92–5, 99–100, 106–8
comfort – thermal, 174, 188
competent person, 12, 35, 245
conduction, 173–4
confined space, 28
containment, 115–16, 229, 241
contextual information, 51, 54, 132, 150
control, principles of good practice, 9, 227–8
control hierarchy, 228–31
control limit, *see* Control of Asbestos regulations
Control of Asbestos regulations (CA), 22, 85, 88
control of exposure, 9, 227–32
Control of Lead at Work regulations (CLW), 22, 57
Control of Noise at Work regulations (CNW), 23, 147, 153
Control of Substances Hazardous to Health regulations (COSHH), *see* COSHH
Control of Vibration at Work regulations (CVW), 23, 162, 165
convection, 173–4, 189
COSHH, 5, 14–15, 22–3
    bioaerosols, 111
    control advice, 233, 261, 275
COSHH Essentials, 11, 278
cowl sampler, 73–4, 84–8, 89
cyclone respirable sampler, 41, 69–72, 83–4

DAC, 207
data-logger, 75, 93, 101
DC shift, 169
decibel (dB) – definition, 143–4
deep-freeze stores, thermal environment, 175
derived air concentration of radionuclides, *see* DAC
derived limits, 207
dermal, 18–21, 125–40
dermal exposure, 22, 128
dermal uptake, 128, 135–6, 174
dermatitis, 125, 127–8
diffusive sampler, 94, 97–8, 108–9

direct reading instruments
   dust measurement, 11, 66–7, 75–7
   gas/vapour measurement, 93–4, 99,
      101–2
   radiation measurements, 214
   thermal measurements, 181, 182
   ventilation measurements, 237, 239
disabilities, 9
discomfort – PPE, 231, 262, 267
dispersion, 27–8
displacement, 163–4
dose
   noise, 157
   radiation, 199–201, 205–14
dosemeter
   film badge, 211–14
   personal noise, 148–52, 155–7
   thermoluminescent, 209, 211, 213
dosimeter, see dosemeter
Drager detector tubes, see colorimetric
      detector tubes
draughts, 187, 241
dry bulb thermometers, 178, 180,
      182–6
ducts, airflow measurement, 246–7
dust, 63–91
   airborne dust measuring techniques,
      66–89
   asbestos fibres, see asbestos fibres
   cloud behaviour, 67, 89–90
   direct reading instruments, see direct
      reading instruments for dust
      measurement
   filters for different types, 66–8, 89
dust lamp, see Tyndall beam

EH40, 14, 22, 127
electro magnetic fields (EMF), 216–17,
      221–2
electron, 199
elimination – of exposure, 228, 231, 279–80
emissions, 32, 134, 220
   process generated, 14–15, 26
endotoxin, 114, 120–21
exposure
   accidental, 7, 81, 280
   models, 18–21, 25–7, 277–8
exposure action values (EAV) – vibration,
      162

exposure limit value (ELV) – vibration, 162,
      165, 171
exposure-response, 4–5, 286

far-field, 27–9, 231
field-blank, see blanks
film badge – radiation, 209, 212–13
fit-testing, see RPE fit-testing
FIVES, 131–2
flicker, 191–2, 195, 197
flowmeter, 73–84, 105
Fourier-transform infrared (FTIR) gas
      analyzer, 101
frequency
   EMF, 216–17, 220,222
   noise, 144–7, 157–60
   vibration, 161–70
fugitive emissions, see passive emissions
fumes, 64, 229–30, 277

gamma rays, 200, 201
gas detection, 101–2
gases, 92–110
Geiger–Muller counter, 210
general ventilation, 27–9, 230–31
genotoxic, 5
geometric mean, 50
glare, 192, 197
gloves
   anti-vibration, 171
   chemical protective, 136–9, 264
grab sampling, see colourimetric detector
      tubes
gram-negative bacteria, 114, 121
gram-positive bacteria, 114
gray (Gy) – definition, 205

half-life, 22, 204
half-value layer, 209
hand-to-mouth – transmission, see
      ingestion
hazard
   definition, 4, 7
   identification, 8, 13–17, 276
hearing loss, see noise-induced hearing loss
hearing protection, 153, 158–60, 188
heat, 173–90
   strain, 175, 181–8
   stress, 173–6, 181–8

heavy metals, 89
HEPA filters, 116
hertz (Hz), 145, 216
humidity, *see* air humidity

illuminance, 191–7
impactors, 118–20
impingers, *see* bubblers
infrared radiation (IR), 200, 216–17, 220
ingestion, 18–22, 125–40
inhalable
    convention, 64–5
    dust measurement, 68–9, 72, 80–83, 89
injection exposure, 9, 18–21
intrinsically safe – electrical, 94, 238
IOM sampler, 69, 72, 80–84
Ionising Radiations Regulations, 199, 208
iPhone, 150
isotopes – definition, 199, 201–2

Kata thermometer, *see* thermometers, Kata

$L_{EP,d}$, 147–9, 155–7, 159
laboratory animal allergen (LAA), 115, 121
lasers, 220, 222–4
lead dust, 22, 69, 89, 137
Legionella, 113–14
LEV, *see* local ventilation
light meter, 193–5
lighting, 191–8
local exhaust ventilation, *see* local
    ventilation
local ventilation, 228–33, 257–9
log-normal distribution, 48, 51
lumen, 191
lux, 191, 193, 196

man-made mineral fibre (MMMF)
man-made vitreous fibres (MMVF)
manometer, 235–37, 249–50, 252–4
mass number, 199, 201–2
MDHS, 21
mean
    arithmetic, *see* arithmetic mean
    geometric, *see* geometric mean
mean radiant temperature – definition, 174,
    185
median, 50, 64
metabolic rate, 177, 185

metal fume fever, 65
mg m^{-3}, *see* also ppm, 6, 18, 82
micromanometers, 237
micrometre, 64, 65
microorganisms, 111–22
microwaves, 200, 216–17, 220–22
mm H$_2$O, 234–5
moulds, 114
MRE 113 sampler, 72–3
MSDS, *see* SDS
mycoplasma, 113
mycotoxin, 114

nanoparticle, 65, 132
natural frequency, 164
near-field, 27, 29
needle-stick injuries, 21, 113
neutrons, 199–203
noise, 143–60
noise-induced hearing loss, 143, 147, 265
non-stochastic health effects, 200, 206

occupational exposure limit, *see* OEL
occupational hygiene, 3–12, 18, 25
octave band analysis, 149, 157–60
OEL
    comparison with, 8, 21, 25, 31, 282
    definition, 5
    noise, 147–8
    radiation, 206–7, 218
    vibration, 165
oil mist, 89
organic vapour analyser, 101

para-aramid, 66
partial enclosure, 228–31, 280
pascal (Pa), 143–4, 234–5
passive emissions, 27
passive sampler, *see* diffusive sampler
pathogens, 112, 137
percutaneous uptake, *see* dermal uptake
personal noise dosemeters, *see* dosemeter
personal protective equipment (PPE), *see*
    PPE
pharmaceuticals, 89, 132, 137
photoionisation monitor, 101
physical agents, 4–9, 13–17, 141–223
piston-phone calibrator, 154, 157
pitot-static tube, 239–41, 246–52

planning a survey, 34–47
pore size, of filters, 68
Poropak adsorbent, 96
PPE, 11, 136, 227, 260–71
ppm, *see also* mg m^{-3}, 6, 56, 104
pregnancy, 9
primary standard, 40, 167, 193
probability, 50–51, 282, 285
pyrogens, 114

quality assurance, 39–40, 56, 117
quartz fibre electroscope, 211

radiant
  heat, 174–5, 183, 189
  power, 218
radiation
  background, 201, 207
  ionising, 199–215
  non-ionising, 216–24
  thermal, 249
Radiation Protection Advisor (RPA),
  199
radio waves, 200, 203, 216–17, 220–22
radon, 201, 204, 207, 214–15
REACH, 55
receptor, 25, 29, 134, 137
record keeping, 53–9
rectal temperature, 182, 185–6
reporting, 53–9
Reporting of Injuries, Diseases and
  Dangerous Occurrences Regulations
  (RIDDOR), 161
resonant frequency, 164, 217
respirable, 64–5
respirable dust – convention, 68–73,
  83–9
respirator – fit-testing, *see* RPE fit-testing
respiratory protective equipment, *see* RPE
risk, 3–12, 275–6
  acceptability of, 260–61, 285
risk assessment, *see* assessment of risks
risk communication, 282–7
risk perception, 13, 261, 282–3
root-mean-squared (RMS), 161–4, 221
rotameter, 76–81, 95, 105
RPE, 138–9, 260–71
  fit-testing, 265, 269–70
  heat stress, 174, 184

safety data sheets, *see* SDS
samples
  long-term, 32, 50, 100
  personal, 36, 38, 69, 85, 117
  short-term, 32, 50, 100, 106–8
  static, 38–9, 85
sampling bag for gas collection, 100–101
sampling methods, 21, 37
sampling strategies, 37–9, 132
sampling train, 76, 105
SCOEL, 5
SDS, 14–15, 127, 276–7
SEG, 37
segregation, 28, 228–9
Separation, 28
sievert (Sv) – definition, 205
silica dust, 89
silica gel as absorbent material, 94, 96
similarly exposed group, *see* SEG
SIMPEDS cyclone, *see* cyclone respirable
  sampler
skin, *see* dermal
skin notation, 18, 127
SLM, 11, 40, 147–55
smoke tube kit, 241–2, 256–7
snow blindness, 216
soap bubble calibrator, 76–80
sound dosimeters, *see* noise dosemeters
sound level meter, *see* SLM
sound pressure level, 143–4
source-receptor, 25, 134,137
sources
  hazards, 19–21, 25–7, 229–31, 241
  heat, 174–5, 183
  light, 191
  noise, 144–8, 155, 159
  radiation, 200, 208–10, 217
  vibration, 168–70
speed of light, 216
static pressure, definition, 234
statistics, 50–52
stochastic health effects, 200, 206
Stoffenmanager, 277–8
stratum corneum, 135, 220
substance emission potential, 26
substitution, 228, 231, 279–80
suction inlet, performance of, 257–9
sun protection factor (SPF), 219
surveys, 34–47

sweating, 136, 173, 184
swing hygrometer, 43, 176, 182–3
synthetic mineral fibres, 66, 88

tachometer, 245
temperature, air, 173–90
Tenax adsorbent, 96
thermal environment, measurement of,
    176–85
thermoluminescent dosemeter, *see*
    dosemeter, thermoluminescent
thermometers
    convention, 64–5
    globe, 174–6, 180–85
    kata, 178–9
    wet-bulb, 175–6, 178, 182–5
Threshold Limit Value (TLV), 175
time-weighted average, *see* TWA
total enclosure, 228–31, 243, 280
trust, 283–4
turbulent – air-flow, 241, 247, 257
TWA, 6, 262
Tyndall beam, 89–90, 242

ultraviolet radiation (UV), 16, 218–19, 223
unit risk, 286
unsealed sources, 206, 210, 214
uptake, 127, 135–8

vane anemometer, *see* anemometer, vane
vapour pressure, 26, 185
vapours, 92–110
velocity pressure
    definition, 234
    measurement, 239–41

vibration, 23, 161–72
    hand-arm, 161–2, 164–7, 171
    whole-body, 161, 164, 171
video recording camera, 36
viruses, 4, 112–13
VITAE, 131–2
VOC (volatile organic chemicals), 101
volatile organic chemicals, *see* VOC

walk-through survey, 15
Walton–Beckett eyepiece graticule, 85–6
warehouses, thermal environment of, 175
wavelength, 145–6, 199–203, 216, 218
WBGT (wet bulb globe temperature),
    175–8, 181–6
weighting – noise, 146–7
WEL – definition, 5, 22
welder's flash, 216
welding fume, 73, 89, 229–30
wet bulb globe temperature, *see* WBGT
wet-work, 126–9
whirling hygrometer, *see* swing hygrometer
wind chill factor, 189–90
wind tunnels, 242
work-rest scheduling, 185
Workplace (Health, Safety and Welfare)
    Regulations, 175, 192
workplace exposure limit, *see* WEL
worst case sampling, 37–9, 54

X-rays, 200–206, 209, 212
XAD adsorbent, 96

yaw, 238
yeasts, 114–15